Comments & Feedback

"Some of my patients are very excited about your program – because it works! Some of them are reducing their medication and others are coming off their medication." Dr. W. Bayer, NY

"McCulley's book is phenomenal! -- he's done something that the experts said was impossible, and he's still not taking any medication! His book is a must-read for all doctors and diabetics. There's something about those engineers being able to solve complex problems ..." Dr. D. Courtney, PA

"This book is empowering. I plan to keep this book handy in my office." Journal of the National Medical Association (JNMA)

"After reviewing my blood work, my doctor told me that all signs of my diabetes were gone! And, the pain in my foot from the neuropathy is gone (so I don't need the cane anymore!)." D. Carter (diabetic who used the book's super meal program for 4 months to beat his diabetes)

"I couldn't get my blood sugar below 300 with medication. After 3 weeks on your super meal program, it was back to the normal range! My doctor was shocked." E. Gallagher (diabetic from NYC)

"I like that you included a spiritual aspect instead of just talking about the body (physical). Our people underestimate the power of the inner spirit." Rev. J. Cherry, Rochester, NY

"I like your flow charts – diabetics finally have a roadmap that shows them where they are and where they're going." [A diabetes educator]

"Thank you, DeWayne – you've given me and other people hope by sharing your story." A. Peters (diabetic support group member)

"You explain diabetes in a way that makes it easier for people to understand the disease. And, you give us simple steps to follow in order to get better!" [An audience member after a diabetes lecture to a group of wellness consultants and diabetics]

Acknowledgements

I am truly indebted to many people for their encouragement and support:

- My mother, my sister Marguerite, and my daughter Cynthia who helped me through my recovery from near-Death (diabetic coma); my mother and my brother Gregory who went to the churches to ask them to pray for me while I was in the coma; my other brothers and sisters; Cynthia's mother Carole, and her grandfather and grandmother (Mrs. & Mrs. M. Austin).

- My doctor, the ambulance team, and the hospital nurses and doctors who never gave up despite my being so close to death.

- People from my hometown church who helped us while we were growing up: Uncle Claude, Aunt Vonnie, Ms. Bloodsaw, Ms. Wiley, Ms. Dunnavant, Ms. Ragster, Ms. Malloy, Ms. James, Ms. Saunders, Ms. Brodie, Deacon Daniels, Deacon Ragster, Deacon Wilkins, Deacon Wiley, Pastor Collins . . .

- My high school teachers and college professors: Ms. Batten, Ms. Davis, Ms. Jankovich, Mr. Husnick, Mr. Bohach, Mr. Phillips, Mr. John Houlihan . . .

- Various friends/associates and people from work who provided their insights and continued to encourage me: Ed B., Larry P., John P., Ray, Marcella, Thomas, Jim, Pam, Daryl, Doug, Art, Joyce, Rick, Linda, Barb, Dave, Javier, John H., Russ, Terrie; Joe N., Bert, Helen, Keith, two of my Xerox managers Ted and Pat, Dr. R. Williams, Dr. Dawn, Ron, Barb F.

- People involved with the heart/diabetes associations and the diabetic support groups that I facilitated: Alfreda, Beverly, Duncan, Tamiko, Michael, Helen, Marion, Pat, Christina, Margaret, Alvin, Mary, Rena, Audrey, Eric, Valerie, Ruby, May, Dorothy, Annie, Loretta, Dana.

- People from churches, colleges, companies, wellness groups, community organizations, who provided contacts, references, encourage-ment, support, and the opportunity to speak publicly: Sally, Dr. Shirley, Sue S., Dr. Lynn, Sue, Cy, P.J., Juanita, Debbie, Rev. Mackey, Audrey, Bob, Rose; George, Professor Dan, Linda, Nelson, Carol, Elaine, James, Joe, Sarah, Bernard, Dianne, Dorothy, Phantom Chef, Dr. Rita, Dr. Raj, Dr. Samikkannu, Dr. DiPrima, Dr. Bayer, Dr. Kalidas, Nalita, Dr. Moore, Rev. J. Cherry.

- People who have helped after the book/DVD were released: Sylvia & Joe Provenza, John & Barbara Smith, Dr. Courtney, Sue & Cy F., PJ E., Tasso S., Charlie Fox, Bill Norwood, Neil & Barb B., Rich S., Mike H.

About the Author

In March 2002, DeWayne went into a diabetic coma with a blood glucose level of 1337 – more than twelve hundred points above normal. Despite a set of complications that included hyperglycemia, dehydration, two blood clots, pneumonia and four insulin shots a day, DeWayne was able to use his engineering and biochemistry background to methodically and completely wean himself off the insulin and other drugs to lower his average glucose level to 92.5 mg/dl and his hemoglobin A1C to 4.4%, reversing his Type 2 diabetes – all in less than 4 months. He credits his recovery to God, the doctors and nurses, his mother, his daughter Cynthia, his engineering background, and a set of serendipitous events that helped him through his recovery.

DeWayne believes he was very fortunate to have obtained a full college scholarship, an invaluable college education (B.S., E.E., Pennsylvania State University), and a good job as an engineer, first with Hughes Aircraft Co., then, with Xerox Corp. Because he believes it is important to give back to the community, DeWayne volunteered as a math tutor for the Urban League and one of the local high schools in the 1980s and 1990s. Today, DeWayne is working with Parwel (www.parwel.com), a health services company, to provide diabetes education and integrative health services to corporations, organizations and individuals – to help people struggling with diabetes, high blood pressure, obesity, fatigue, and heart disease.

As an engineer, DeWayne was trained to research, analyze, test, draw logical conclusions, and write technical reports based on complex engineering and machine data. Ironically, DeWayne was able to use that same training to research, analyze, test and draw logical conclusions from the hundreds of clinical studies to help him design a diabetes wellness program and write this book. In addition, the encouragement that DeWayne received from his mother, his daughter, and various people (from work, the local churches, the wellness industry, and the American Diabetes Association support group he was facilitating), also helped him to write this book. DeWayne's hope is that this book (and his new diabetes education program) will inspire you and others the way he was inspired – by people he would never have met if it weren't for his experience with diabetes.

Notice to Readers

This book is written with the express purpose of sharing the author's experience of his recovery from a near-death diabetic coma and all the invaluable information of hundreds of clinical studies and medical references from doctors, healthcare professionals, scientists, nutritionists and other experienced healthcare advocates. Consequently, the information in this book is provided for informational purposes only and is by no means meant to be a substitute for the advice provided by your own doctor and other healthcare professionals. It is imperative that you always consult with your doctor to discuss your health state and determine your specific course of action. The author shall have no liability or responsibility to any person or entity with respect to any loss, damage or injury, caused or alleged to be caused directly or indirectly by the information contained in this book.

The information in this book is not intended to prescribe any form of treatment for any illness or medical condition. This book should only be used as a guide in interacting with your doctor, dietitian, diabetes health coach and other healthcare professionals, and should not be considered a substitute for expert medical advice. In fact, you should utilize the guidelines for doctor appointments in Chapter 11 to help improve the relationships with your doctor and other healthcare professionals.

The U. S. Food & Drug Administration has not verified any therapeutic claims expressed or implied in this book. You (the reader) are responsible for making any decisions regarding the suitability and validity of the information provided in this book. Always consult with your doctor before you implement any changes to your diet, supplement usage, exercise regimen, or lifestyle.

Table of Contents

Diagrams & Tables

Can't Wait? – Want to Get Started Now?

Start with these "super" meals and contact the author to register for a free teleseminar.

Super Breakfast

This type of vegetable-based breakfast provides a more sustained level of energy and key nutrients that diabetics (and non-diabetics) are missing when they consume the more traditional grain-based breakfast, which leads to that mid-morning "crash" or craving.

- 1 ½ cups steamed spinach (or 1 cup steamed broccoli)
- 2 oz. baked wild salmon (or sardines, or an organic egg)
- ½ yellow pepper, mushrooms, spices to season the vegetable/meat
- 1 tbsp. extra virgin olive oil (add after steaming vegetables)
- 16 oz. filtered water
- 1 slice of toasted sprouted grain bread (optional addition)

Super Dinner

This type of dinner sets the stage to help the body cleanse/detoxify and repair itself while you sleep.

- 1 cup steamed Brussel sprouts and 1 cup steamed broccoli
- 5 oz. baked skinless chicken/turkey breast (or 5 oz. wild salmon)
- ½ red pepper, mushrooms, spices to season the vegetable/meat
- 1½ tbsp. extra virgin olive oil (add after steaming vegetables)
- 1 slice of sprouted grain bread
- 16 oz. filtered water (or 16 oz. white tea)
- Optional meal: a raw salad that contains the aforementioned foods with Romaine lettuce and organic salad dressing

Super Snack

The following nutritious snacks require very little time to prepare.

- 1 apple, a handful of walnuts/almonds, a glass of water
- 1 cup of grapes, a handful of trail mix/pulse food (nuts/seeds), water
- 8 oz. organic/raw juice, mix in 2 tbsp. of freshly ground flaxseed
- 1 cup of yogurt, add in ground flaxseed, blueberries; glass of water
- 4-5 whole grain crackers, 2 oz. canned salmon/tuna, water

Note: For alternatives of your favorite foods, use the table (page 354).

Chapter 1. Introduction

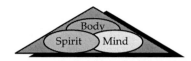

Background, Facts & Figures

I discovered firsthand that your perspective on life truly changes once you face Death and survive a life-threatening coma and a disease such as diabetes. Because I consider this is a true blessing to have fully recovered from a near-death experience and from a disease that has no documented medical cure, I feel a responsibility to share that experience. Ironically, what I learned over the years as an engineer in terms of design, planning, testing, data analysis, and writing prepared me to successfully fight this disease and write this book. Of course, I realize that my recovery from diabetes may be an anomaly due to my engineering background and a series of "accidents" that helped me through my recovery. But, since I am not completely certain that this was an anomaly, I hope that by sharing this information, others with similar health problems will be inspired to improve their health or the health of a loved one. If this information helps someone, then, I will know that this was all worth it.

There are many good books written about diabetes, but I was unable to find a book that provided a systematic and organized approach with specific wellness protocols for fighting the root causes of this insidious disease. As a result, I was frustrated and confused concerning what to do when I couldn't get clear answers as to the right foods to eat/not eat and why my blood glucose level was so high. And, when the dietitian couldn't explain how the foods in her diet plan would help my diabetes, I became very concerned. Then, after my unexpected recovery, I was surprised by the number of people who had questions about how I recovered.

That's when my mother, my daughter and a few other people at work suggested that I write a book. But, I thought they were just being kind. Besides, I didn't really want to invest the kind of time it would require to write a book. After I gave several presentations to churches, wellness consultant forums and community groups, some of the audience participants asked if I had a book or was planning to write a book. With a strong push from my daughter, my mother and several other people, I finally relented to at least analyze the market need for a new book about diabetes.

The following is a summary of the key points from my market needs analysis that, in some cases, surprised me, and finally convinced me to write this book.

- There are more than 21 million people in the United States and 170 million people worldwide with diabetes (95% Type 2).
- Every hour more than 2,000 people are diagnosed as a diabetic in the United States.
- The number of people worldwide with diabetes is expected to rise to 366 million by 2030 – more than doubling in just 25 years. What is more disturbing is that the increase is based on obesity rates remaining stable. Unfortunately, obesity rates continue to rise.
- There are more than 41 million Americans with Metabolic Syndrome X, a strong pre-cursor to becoming diabetic. Metabolic Syndrome X is characterized by a combination of indicators including obesity, high insulin levels, internal inflammation, high blood pressure, high cholesterol, and fatigue.
- There are millions of non-diabetic people who struggle with similar health issues that diabetics struggle with, including high blood pressure, high cholesterol, fatigue, obesity, kidney problems, and cardiovascular problems. Consequently, non-diabetics have some of the same needs for health-related and nutrition-related information.
- Many of the diabetics I met had tried to change their eating and exercise habits, but with little success due to misinformation about nutrition, exercise and blood glucose testing.
- The majority of the diabetics I met had resigned themselves to taking some type of drug to control their diabetes.

- There were some diabetics who believed that they were doing well by taking drugs to control their blood sugar. They were either unaware or didn't care about the long term effects of the drugs.
- There were some diabetics who were comfortable living *with* the disease instead of determining how to live *without* the disease – because they were unaware of better options to fight the disease.
- I found that most diabetics were doing something wrong in at least 6 of the 8 areas associated with diabetes management and blood glucose control, namely: nutrition, exercise, blood glucose testing, drug therapy, education, doctor visits, spiritual health, and record-keeping. And, in many cases, the diabetic or the healthcare person didn't know they were doing anything wrong in those areas!
- I was not able to find a book that addressed how to control and reverse diabetes in measurable terms that the average person could track on their own. There was no book that could answer my basic questions about the disease and its root causes. During my recovery I referred to several books and websites, many of which were out-of-date, had vague information or conflicted with each other.
- My daughter felt that people would learn a lot more if what I presented were written down – so that people would not have to take so many notes.
- After several presentations, people kept inquiring if I had written a book. They felt that I had a powerful message that needed to be shared on a larger platform.
- My mother kept meeting people who would ask her how she lost weight, lowered her cholesterol and remained so active at her age.
- The blood glucose levels of most diabetics returned to normal when they implemented some of my nutritional principles. Non-diabetics also experienced positive results.
- Although people are living longer, they are not necessarily living healthier. More people are relying on drugs, ending up in hospitals; living in pain; and, dying of diseases due to the lack of knowledge and poor lifestyle choices.
- Many people do not have a personal computer and access to the health-related information on the Internet. They need a hardcopy book that provides that information.

Facts & Figures

The following are additional facts and figures that further convinced me to write this book.

- Diabetes continues to grow at epidemic levels as it affects more children and kills more people each year than AIDS and breast cancer combined. The average life span of a diabetic is shortened by 13.5 years and costs more than $250,000 per family over 20 years.
- Average annual medical costs for a diabetic is $13.243 versus $2,560 for a non-diabetic, a difference of more than $10,000 a year.
- More than 50 million Americans with high blood pressure and 150 million being overweight/obese provide a strong feeder base for cardiovascular disease, cancer, diabetes, and arthritis.
- "Diabetes is the fifth-deadliest disease in the United States, and it has no cure. The total annual economic cost of diabetes in 2002 was estimated to be $132 billion, or one out of every 10 health care dollars spent in the United States." American Diabetes Association
- At least 13% of African-Americans have diabetes and African-Americans are twice as likely to develop the disease. This is due to African-Americans being more likely to have one or more of the following risk factors: high blood pressure, overweight/obesity, high cholesterol, poor nutrition, a sedentary lifestyle, and economic/environmental impacts due to societal biases.
- "Diabetes is the leading cause of new cases of blindness in people ages 20-74. Each year, from 12,000 to 24,000 people lose their sight because of diabetes." American Diabetes Association
- More than 4 out of every 5 diabetics will develop one or more of the following complications: kidney disease (nephropathy), eye disease (retinopathy), nerve disease (neuropathy), or heart disease (cardio-vascular disease).
- Two out of every 3 diabetics will die of a heart attack or stroke.
- According to a study by the Yale University School of Medicine, more than one fifth of the patients with Type 2 diabetes have decreased blood flow to the heart, but no symptoms to suggest there is a problem. Known as myocardial ischemia, this condition occurs when the heart does not receive enough blood to meet its metabolic needs, usually due to plaque build-up in the coronary arteries.

- "Heart disease strikes people with diabetes, twice as often as people without diabetes." American Heart Association
- "Heart disease, *not* breast cancer, is the number killer of women in the United States." American Heart Association
- Diabetes treatment costs more than any other disease (over $132 billion annually), but diabetes treatment also generates the most revenue for the healthcare industry (over $210 billion annually!). Is this a conflict of interest for an industry that is more focused on a "sick" care strategy that creates drug-dependent patients – instead of a "health" care strategy that cures the actual ailment or disease?
- "Doctors must shift their focus from treating disease alone to tailoring treatments to individual patient needs." American Journal of Medicine Feb 2004

The Controversy

According to medical science there is no cure for Type 2 diabetes. Since the medical treatment protocol primarily focuses on suppressing the symptoms of the disease, medical science is right – there is no cure for Type 2 diabetes. And, there will be no cure as long as the public is satisfied with medical science using drugs and surgery as their answers to this disease. According to medical science I should be dead or on insulin. So how do you explain me beating diabetes? Luck? God? Coincidence?

When several diabetics told me they had lowered their sugar level, increased their energy, lost weight, and (some) had reduced their medication, I was surprised to say the least. And, when my mother told me she was able to reduce her cholesterol and blood pressure by making some nutritional changes, I began to wonder that maybe it was not luck. So, I conducted research into nutritional science, biochemistry, and findings from clinical and epidemiological studies. In the meantime, my daughter and several people at work asked me to document what I had done so that they could share the information with family members and friends. Then, when other people including my doctor asked me what I had done to wean myself off insulin, lose weight and lower my blood glucose, I began to think that maybe I should share this with other people, especially diabetics. And, so, the journey began . . .

Purpose of this Book

The primary purpose of this book is to provide wellness information so that diabetics and other people are aware of other options to fight diabetes and prevent the unnecessary suffering, drugs and surgeries. As God said: **"My people perish for lack of knowledge." Hosea 4:6**.

This book provides the knowledge (procedures and protocols) that will prevent people from perishing due to the lack of knowledge about diabetes. Based upon the etiology of Type 2 diabetes and the analysis of its pathogenesis, this book identifies the root causes of Type 2 diabetes and provides medical-endorsed measurements/tests that track the progress of a diabetic's recovery. However, this book is *not* a medical book and is not meant to replace the personal advice and support you receive from your physician and other healthcare professionals. In fact, the book is designed specifically to be used as a reference guide while working with your doctor, dietitian, diabetes health coach and other healthcare professionals to improve your health.

This book defines a diabetes wellness program, which is an integrated Body-Mind-Spirit approach to the healing process for people who are fighting a systemic, degenerative disease such as Type 2 diabetes. This wellness program enables you to become a *victor* of wellness, instead of a *victim* of drugs and disease, based upon the following five principles.

1. The Body, Mind and Spirit must work in harmony and balance for the entire being to be healthy.
2. Proper nutrition, (no drugs), exercise, education and spiritual health are the key planks to successfully fight the primary root causes of most systemic, degenerative diseases (including diabetes).
3. There are 5 "live" nutrient-rich foods (from God) that align with the body's blueprint and internal healing mechanisms.
4. There are 5 "dead" nutrient-poor foods (made by man) that trigger many of today's diseases and prevent the body from using its internal healing mechanisms.
5. Because a disease (such as diabetes) is a condition that is "acquired" primarily due to the *absence* of proper nutrition, then a disease (such as diabetes) can be "unacquired" with the *presence* of proper nutrition.

This wellness program aligns with the body's need and ability to heal itself and prevent the diabetes from causing further damage – when that body is fed the proper food and spiritual nutrients. This program works because it addresses the *real root causes* of Type 2 diabetes – insulin resistance, inflammation, nutritional deficiency, oxidation, and toxicity; and, is based upon personal experience and hundreds of clinical studies. As a result, the body relearns how to properly metabolize food and increase glucose uptake, providing a higher level of energy within a matter of weeks. This diabetes wellness program is designed to help you:

- Increase glucose uptake, reduce blood glucose levels, and increase the utilization of insulin in the body by consuming specific foods, juices, nutrients, herbs, and food-based supplements.
- Prevent, control or reverse the long-term complications of nerve, kidney, eye, and heart diseases; and other complications including obesity, high blood pressure, cholesterol, and homocysteine – based on specific wellness protocols.
- Learn how to reduce belly fat, reduce body fat and lose weight properly and permanently.
- Customize the wellness protocols to fit your specific health needs, based on your blood glucose testing and other medical tests.
- Design meals with the 5 "live" nutritious foods that heal the body; while avoiding the 5 "dead" processed foods that harm the body.
- Avoid the 7 most common mistakes that many diabetics make.
- Progress from no blood glucose control to complete control and reversal of diabetes by using a well-structured six-stage process.
- Learn how to properly handle stress and conquer your inner demons.

Author Sidebar: I do not consider my diabetes wellness program to be an official "cure" for Type 2 diabetes, despite all of the evidence. As an engineer, I do not believe in anecdotal data – I believe in the data from independent, qualified test labs and similar resources. A series of double-blind, placebo-controlled clinical studies need to be performed to properly validate (or discredit) my diabetes wellness program. Hopefully, there is a company that would be interested in pursuing this endeavor for the betterment of our country and the world.

Chapter 2. My Coma & Recovery

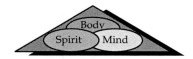

My Coma

Surprisingly, I became ill in a very short period of time and almost died without any warning. This is very important to grasp because death can come upon us very quickly when we continue to ignore the signs, such as weight gain, fatigue, or an increase in blood pressure. Interestingly, this is the false trap that we all fall into – what I call the "False Illusion of Health". How many times have you heard about someone having a stroke or heart attack and you just talked with that person just a few days ago and he/she looked completely healthy? And, despite this type of health crisis occurring on a regular basis, we never translate that health crisis happening to us. And, for those of us who are ill with a health problem such as diabetes, obesity, or high blood pressure, we ignore our doctors and live with this false hope that "It'll go away" – what I call "The State of Denial". That is what happened to me.

It was March 2002, work at Xerox was busy as usual, especially with the recent reorganization and restructuring within the company. As our engineering teams had become smaller and lost key talent, we had to become more efficient in getting work done. I had stopped playing basketball and tennis, and was eating more processed foods, gaining weight, increasing my cholesterol level and ignoring the warning from my doctor to change my eating habits. As a result, I had gradually put on 45 pounds within several years. I had started to drink more and urinate more frequently, but I thought that it had something to do with my prostate. So, I scheduled a doctor's appointment for April.

I awoke the morning of March 19, 2002 in a semi-paralyzed state – my arms and legs felt rubbery, similar to how your arm or leg feels when you sleep on it. Because I didn't feel right, I had decided to go back to sleep to get some extra rest and go to work later that morning. But, for some strange reason I decided to call 911 and was rushed to the hospital by the local ambulance. I found out later that if I had gone back to sleep, I would have died in my bed that morning.

According to the doctors, I went into a non-ketotic hyperglycemic hyperosmolar (NKHH) coma, with a blood glucose level of 1337, and almost died. In fact, the doctors had called my mother (who lives in Pennsylvania) to tell her that by the time she arrived in New York, I would probably not be alive. But, for the grace of God, and the expertise of the doctors and nurses, I somehow survived the coma, the blood clots, and death.

My Daughter's Arrival

At the time I went into the hospital, there was a terrible snowstorm that made it almost impossible to travel. My daughter, Cynthia, had called the airline to get a plane as soon as possible. When the operator told her it was going to be expensive, Cynthia said: "I don't care what it cost! I need to get to my father, he's in the hospital!" The operator told her that she could get a discount for bereavement if she obtained a notification from the hospital, which she did. I must have been in pretty bad shape, because when Cynthia arrived at the hospital she didn't recognize me when she entered my room. In fact, she turned around and asked the nurse "Where's my father? This must be the wrong room." When the nurse told her "Well, that's Mr. McCulley." Cynthia was devastated – she had never seen her father so sick, overweight and close to death.

Every night Cynthia called my mother, who would provide Cynthia with encouragement that "God will get your father through this coma." Cynthia also relied on her mother, who was also concerned with my condition. Cynthia and her mother talked several times a day just to maintain some sense of hope and to support each other. Consequently, this allowed Cynthia to calm down and focus on what needed to get done while I was in the hospital.

When I came out of the coma and was fully cognizant of my surroundings, Cynthia told my mother that night, "Grandma, Dad's out of the coma, but he still looks pretty bad." My mother told Cynthia, "Tell your father to pray." Cynthia said "But I've never seen my Dad pray before." My mother said, "Cynthia, all my children know how to pray – they were all raised in the church." So the next day Cynthia told me "Grandma said that you should pray." I said "Okay." and, that night, and the following morning, I prayed like I had never prayed in my life. I found out later that the nurse talked to my mother every morning and had seen me praying. She told my mother "I have some good news for you. I saw your son praying this morning." My mother smiled and said, "That's good to hear."

My mother also provided Cynthia with guidance concerning what foods to buy since my kitchen was stocked with a lot of snacks and junk food, e.g. cookies, pies, cakes, soda, bottled juice, frozen dinners, etc. With my mother's help, Cynthia pulled herself together and was very instrumental in keeping my spirits up, even though things didn't look very promising those first few days. Hopefully, Cynthia will utilize that same strength to help fulfill her own destiny the way she obviously redirected mine.

Hospital Events

I was in the intensive care ward for the first seven days of my hospital stay. There were several times that I could have died, but there were several interesting events, some of which I believe redirected my fate:

- There was a lot of disagreement concerning why my blood glucose level was so high. Some of the hospital doctors were convinced that I was an alcoholic, until my doctor showed up to set the record straight. Otherwise, without my doctor's help, I'm not sure if I would have received the proper treatment at that critical time when my life was still in the balance.
- I remember the head nurse – her energy, her drive, and her commitment to keep me alive. I believe she didn't go home that first night and was very responsible for keeping me alive during that critical time. (I sent a letter to the hospital personnel department a

couple months later thanking her and the other medical staff for not giving up on me).

- For some reason, one night, I couldn't go to sleep no matter how hard I tried. Then, a nurse came in to give me some medication. But, something told me to ask her: "Why are you giving me this medication? What is it for? I haven't been given any medication at night before now." Then, the nurse realized that she was in the wrong room! She apologized profusely and left immediately.
- As my health started to improve, one of the people from my engineering team stopped by to visit. At work, we call him "Elton John". I believe it's because of his hairstyle and the fact that he plays the piano. Later that day, when one of the nurses asked me how I was doing, I said, "Pretty good, Elton John just stopped by to say Hi." Because the doctors and nurses thought that I might be developing dementia, they provided almost hourly encouragement and advice during the rest of my hospital stay to improve my health.

Out of the Hospital

My daughter drove me home after thirteen days in the hospital. Finally, I thought that I would get some much-needed rest. But, we needed food so we drove to the grocery store and spent more than two hours going up and down the aisles trying to find the foods that my mother had told Cynthia to buy for me. This was torture because my legs were rubbery and I didn't have much energy. After about an hour, I felt shaky and a little dizzy. I realized that my blood sugar was low and that I was in danger of going into another coma. Cynthia had bought me some candy bars for emergencies, but she was in another part of the store, and, I didn't have time to find her. I went to the candy bar aisle and found one of my favorite candy bars, Almond Joy. I opened one of the bags and quickly ate two of the candy bars and the shakes subsided. I thought: "Wow, is this what I have to look forward to for the rest of my life?"

Although I was out of the hospital, I was placed on short-term disability and could not return to work. Because of the severity of my diabetes, I was required to take 4 insulin shots a day to control my blood glucose and prevent a future coma episode. In addition, because of bouts with dehydration, blood clots (deep vein thrombosis), oxygen deprivation, pneumonia, and high cholesterol, I had to take other drugs including Coumadin (to thin my blood) and Lipitor (to lower my cholesterol). Although the drugs were keeping me alive, my overall health was not improving and I was not getting any stronger. I was extremely fatigued, overweight (by 60 pounds), and felt faint/dizzy because my body was unable to effectively convert the food to energy. Because of my fear of needles, it was extremely difficult psyching myself up every several hours to inject myself with the insulin. In fact, I briefly considered having a home nurse give me my insulin injections, but at $100 a visit, four times a day, it didn't take long to figure out that I'd better get over my fear of needles. A home nurse did visit during the first week to ensure that I was injecting myself properly with the two different insulins and to answer any questions.

My Mother and Sister's Arrival

Three weeks had now passed, and Cynthia needed to return to work. But, she was very concerned about leaving me alone. My mother told Cynthia that she didn't need to worry because she was going to fly here to pick up where Cynthia had left off. Cynthia was very surprised especially since my mother had never flown before in her life! In addition, despite the financial costs of a plane ticket and missing work, my sister Marguerite decided to accompany my mother.

When my mother and sister arrived, they didn't waste any time in getting the house in order. They inspected each room and quickly identified a set of activities that needed to get done. In addition, because of the information they had received from Cynthia, they concluded that it was imperative to collect all my unopened snacks and junk food and return them to the grocery store. They made me pack up my cakes, pies, potato chips, sodas, TV dinners, cookies, bottled juices, etc. and return them to the Wegman's grocery store. This was quite embarrassing, but what choice did I have? Face my mother? It was easier to face the store clerk. When the store clerk saw the three carts of food that I was returning, she asked me why. I meekly whispered and pointed to my mother who was standing behind me with a stern look on her face. I think the clerk felt sorry for me, so she accepted the returned food and gave me a store credit of almost $250! During the next month, I didn't have to pay for any food that I bought from the store. Thanks to my mother and the Wegman's grocery store, it was financially beneficial for me to eat healthy.

My mother felt it was necessary that I learn how to cook properly so she wrote several recipes for some of her dishes. My mother and my sister both showed me how easy it was to prepare a healthy breakfast, lunch, snack and dinner in very little time. They also dragged me to other stores to purchase other items such as the Foreman Grill, a blender, a nonstick frying pan, and a steamer.

People ask me all the time how I was able to turn around my bad eating habits so quickly. I point out that it wasn't really me – it was my daughter, mother and sister who drove all of the changes. Hmm-mm . . . three women – I didn't have a fighting chance now that I think about it. They didn't feel sorry for me when we went grocery shopping. They would go up and down each aisle at least 3 times while I held onto the grocery cart because my legs were so weak. There were many times when I just wanted to rest, but they would always have something that needed to get done: go to the store, clean out the garage, clean the bedrooms, do the laundry . . . I believe they were killing me and enjoying it at the same time. Ironically, my doctor believes this push from them and not feeling sorry for me may have accelerated my healing.

After about two weeks, my mother and sister felt that they had accomplished what needed to get done, so they returned home.

The Accidents

During my recovery, there were several serendipitous accidents that my mother refers to as "blessings that were meant to happen."

The 1st accident (or blessing) occurred when the head nurse didn't go home when her shift ended the day I entered the intensive care ward of the hospital. She was instrumental in keeping me alive during those initial critical hours when it appeared I was not going to make it.

The 2nd accident occurred when my daughter bought the diabetes book, titled *The Insulin Control Diet* by Dr. Calvin Ezrin and Robert Kowalski. At the time, I didn't realize how important this one book was going to be in my understanding the science of diabetes. As it turned out, this was the only book that I came across during my recovery that explained diabetes from a scientific perspective including how insulin really worked as a fat storage hormone and an instigator in critical vitamin/mineral losses and deficiencies. It also explained the importance of glucagon and why diabetics have so much trouble managing and controlling blood glucose highs and lows. When I asked my daughter how she selected this book, she had no logical answer since she herself knew very little about diabetes. She wasn't certain how her hand was guided to select that one book from so many others.

The 3rd accident occurred just before I was discharged from the hospital. One of the nurses, who was a diabetes educator, gave me a ticket to a diabetes health conference being held locally at the Hyatt Regency Hotel. I was fortunate to be invited to this conference where I met hundreds of diabetics, health care professionals, doctors, nurses, pharmacists, and medical sales people. I saw many people who were without limbs, in wheelchairs, wearing coke-bottled glasses, limping, and severely overweight. Everyone that I talked with was helpful in sharing their knowledge about diabetes. What I learned about diabetes during this conference would have taken me at least a month to learn on my own. Ironically, I learned a lot about what *not* to do if I wanted to defeat my diabetes. And, the knowledge, spirit and unselfishness of everyone provided me the focus that I needed to fight this disease. In addition, fear was a key motivator and became my catalyst for change because I didn't want to lose a limb, my eyesight or end up in a wheelchair.

Because of my poor health, I had difficulty exercising. I tried to exercise to lose some weight, but I didn't have the energy. And, even when I had some energy, the exercising just made me hungrier, leading me to eat more and eventually put on more weight! Also, it was frustrating and scary to exercise and see my blood glucose level go even higher when I thought that exercise would help me to lose weight and lower my blood glucose. I found out later that the intense exercise triggered my liver to release stored glycogen, which caused my blood glucose to rise.

With so much time on my hands I didn't know what to do to slow down the progression of the disease to prevent amputation and possible blindness. Then, came the 4th accident that changed everything! One evening, while I was sitting at the kitchen table crying and feeling sorry for myself, my elbow accidentally hit one of the biblical pamphlets that my mother had left for me to read. The pamphlet fell on the floor and opened to a page displaying the scripture **Leviticus 17:11: "The life of the flesh is in the blood."** I didn't really know what that meant, so I mistakenly interpreted it to mean that "since my flesh was dying, the answer to my problem was in my blood"; and, that I needed to increase the number of times that I was testing my blood each day to find the answer to my deteriorating health. By testing my blood up to 8 times a day including 1 hour and 2 hours after meals, I was able to collect a tremendous amount of data in a short period of time. As a result, I was able to quickly eliminate the foods that were causing my blood glucose to spike, e.g. cereal, pancakes, wheat bread, bananas, bagels, orange juice, apple juice, rice, low-fat salad dressing, toast, French fries.

Right after my mother, sister and daughter had returned home, the 5th accident occurred one morning when I was preparing my breakfast and noticed that I had run out of my favorite cereal. Because my blood glucose that morning had been a little on the low side (65 mg/dl), I started to get weak and a little dizzy. I didn't want to eat a candy bar, so I went to the refrigerator to see what my mother had prepared for me. I found some Brussel sprouts in a plastic container. I hated Brussel sprouts. However, because I was getting weaker, I didn't have much choice, so I quickly heated the Brussel sprouts with some olive oil and a leftover piece of salmon. Surprisingly, when I measured my glucose level 2 hours later, I noticed that it had not spiked as it had in the past! I was very excited, but, then, I thought maybe it was a fluke because my glucose level had started at such a low level. Anyhow, I felt that I had nothing to lose so I decided to eat Brussel sprouts again for lunch, my mid-afternoon snack and dinner. Each time, my glucose leveled off 2 hours after the meal! A few days later when I went back to my favorite cereal, my glucose level returned to a higher level after breakfast. So, I decided to change my concept of breakfast and eat a green vegetable as my carbohydrate in place of the traditional cereal or other grain. With each passing day, my glucose levels were steadily coming down. (I found out later during some research that the juice from Brussel sprouts and the juice from stringbeans are very nourishing for the insulin cell receptors and the body's glucose management system).

It didn't take me long to modify the hospital's diet plan and develop a healthy nutritional plan while slowly and methodically reducing my insulin injections, one to two units at a time. This, in turn, lowered my body's resistance to insulin and reduced my average blood glucose level from 300^+ to 200^+ to 120^+, and, finally to 88.5 mg/dl (with less than a 10 mg/dl deviation) within four months. Also, my hemoglobin A1C was reduced to 4.4% (normal range is 4.2 to 5.5%).

Interestingly, I discovered that many of the so-called "healthy" foods recommended by the dietitian were "killer" foods for diabetics! For example, cereal, rice, pancakes, bananas, toast, wheat bread, mashed potatoes, orange juice, and apple juice all caused my blood glucose to rise and remain high. Once I eliminated these foods, my cravings for refined carbohydrates diminished greatly and my blood glucose level stabilized.

During those 4 months I was able to reduce my insulin dosage from 60 units to 0 units and, within another month, I was totally drug-free – no more Coumadin or Lipitor. Also, my energy level continued to grow while my need for food decreased. Because my body was doing a better job utilizing the nutrients from the food I was eating, my body did not require as much food (fuel) to produce the necessary amount of energy that I required on a daily basis.

Doctor Visits

The doctor visits to the ophthalmologist went very well. Fortunately, there was no major damage to my eyes as the swelling of my lenses eventually subsided and my vision returned to normal within three months. The visits to my primary care physician also went very well. In fact, my primary care physician was always supportive and encouraging;

and, wanted to know what I was doing to be recovering so quickly. He was very interested in how I figured out how to safely wean myself off the insulin, and asked for a copy of my charts.

Unfortunately, the visit to the endocrinologist did not go as well. When I showed him my blood glucose charts and how I had started to wean myself off the insulin, he was very concerned. He felt that I was taking too aggressive of an approach to this serious disease. He prescribed several shots for pneumonia, flu, and other ailments because a diabetic's immune system is weakened, making his body more susceptible to infections and other diseases. When I suggested that I wanted to strengthen my immune system with nutrition instead of weakening it with the shots, the endocrinologist vehemently disagreed with this strategy. When I left the office, the nurse warned me that I was going through a "honeymoon period" and that, because of the seriousness of my diabetes, it would just be a matter of time (2 to 3 months) before I would need to return to taking more insulin. When I left the doctor's office, I ran into two patients in the lobby who overheard that I was weaning myself off insulin. They were surprised and interested in how I was weaning off insulin, but I didn't really know what to say at that point. I had assumed that everyone knew how to wean off insulin, and, that I was just learning what everyone else already knew.

When I returned to my car, I broke into a cold sweat because I wasn't certain what to do. This was very unsettling to me because my doctor, who has been treating diabetics for 26 years, did not review my blood glucose charts or support my using the charts to gradually wean myself off the insulin. I believe that he was trying to protect me from having another diabetic coma incident, but I was concerned about my body becoming dependent on the insulin injections. I sat in the car and prayed for the strength and the guidance to do the right thing. My inner voice told me to continue with what I was doing; and, so I continued to wean myself off the insulin, first the Humalog, then, the Lantus – until I eventually reached zero units.

Back to Work

Now that my blood glucose levels were stabile, my doctor gave me the authorization to return to work. But, he did have some reservations because he felt the stress of the job might trigger another diabetic attack.

At work, people were very kind and, some would stop by my office to ensure that I was okay and had not gone into another coma. I wanted to get back to my life as an engineer, but at least one or two people would stop by each day with questions about diabetes. I was surprised to discover that some of the people I knew or worked with were either diabetic or had a relative who was diabetic. They had heard about how I had wrestled with this disease and was no longer on insulin. And, they wanted to know how I did it. When I tried to explain, I usually forgot something important, so I started writing down some of the key points on a notepad. The notepad gradually turned into a 10-page document.

Several people including my daughter suggested that I expand the document into a book, but I didn't think I had enough information for a book; plus, I didn't really want to invest that kind of time into writing a book. After a year of excuses for rationalizing why I didn't want to write a book, I finally relented and, after completing the market-needs analysis, I started writing a book in mid-2003.

As my health continued to improve, I was able to transition from half-days at work to full days within a month. My company's engineering management and the personnel department supported me by not putting pressure on me while my team picked up some of my responsibilities. Consequently, I did not feel any stress during that critical time of my recovery; and, I was able to gradually increase my responsibilities at my own pace until I was operating at full capacity once again. And, just when I thought things were finally returning to normal, I would accidentally run into someone who was either diabetic or had a family member who was diabetic. Then, I would spend the next several minutes sharing information with them that seemed to lift their spirits – but they still had more questions.

Support Group & Church Meetings

Then, another one of those accidents occurred when a member of a local diabetic support group, Alfreda, asked me to come to their meeting and share my story about diabetes. Coincidentally, Alfreda had catered a picnic for the organization I worked for a couple years ago and she had heard what happened to me from a secretary who used to work for one of my previous managers. After I shared my story with the diabetic support group, I was surprised by their energy and enthusiasm for someone they had never met. Then, I was asked by the local director of the American Diabetes Association (ADA) to facilitate the diabetic support group meetings. It just happened that the person who had been facilitating the support group meetings had left for a better job opportunity a few weeks earlier. I also found out later that some of the people in the support group had gone to the ADA director to ask me to facilitate their meetings.

This was a key event because I met some wonderful people like Alfreda, Marion, Mary, Alvin, Rena, Pat, Christina, and Margaret who shared their stories about diabetes, including their personal concerns and frustrations with fighting this disease. They helped me to build my confidence with other people in the support group that I didn't know. I was able to use this forum to share the knowledge that I had acquired during my recovery. But, because we only met once a month, it was difficult to build any momentum. Also, the information wasn't getting to enough (new) people, and the ADA director and I didn't know how to address this.

Another accident occurred when one of the local churches asked the ADA director to give a presentation on diabetes as part of their Men's Day Program. But, at the last minute, the ADA director couldn't make it. So, she called and convinced me that I could do the presentation even though I had never done anything like this in a public forum. Since I was not comfortable with speaking in public (especially about something that I was just learning about), I reluctantly accepted to give the talk – as long as I was allowed to read the information from my notes.

When I arrived at the church, I was very nervous for three reasons: one, I didn't like speaking publicly especially in front of people I didn't know; two, I hadn't had enough time to practice reading my notes; and, three, I didn't know how I would take a full thirty minutes to talk about diabetes. After I was introduced, I slowly walked to the podium, trying to collect my thoughts. I started out thanking the church for inviting me and talking about my upbringing in a small town and church in Pennsylvania. I wasn't certain how to segue into the diabetes talk, so I said something like: "God blessed me with the perfect disease for an engineer – diabetes." Of course there were a lot of dumbfounded looks in the audience, which made me more nervous. So, I repeated part of my statement to try to collect my thoughts: "God blessed me with the perfect disease, a disease that medical science says has no cure." I heard a few "amens" from the audience congregation, so I repeated the statement: "God blessed me with a disease that medical science says has no cure. I had a blood sugar level of 1337 and took 4 insulin shots a day. Today, I no longer take any medication, my average glucose level is 92.5 and my hemoglobin A1C is 4.4%." I heard more "amens" from the congregation, which relaxed me and the next thing I knew I was talking about diabetes and how to proactively control the disease with the right foods and more frequent testing. The 30 minutes flew by very quickly.

When I tried to wrap up my talk, the congregation wouldn't let me because they had a lot of questions. I said that I was not prepared to answer any questions because this was not my field ("I'm an engineer not a doctor."). But, I agreed to write down the questions I couldn't answer and would have someone get back to them. Well . . . 20 minutes later, I had somehow answered all of their questions. During the next program intermission, several people approached me with more questions. This eventually led the church to setting up a diabetes support group that I facilitated with some wonderful people like May, Eric, Valerie, Dorothy, Ruby and Annie.

Then, another church that heard about the presentation asked me to give a similar talk to their congregation about my experience with diabetes; and, another church asked me to come to their Saturday Morning Breakfast. Then, a wellness group asked me to give a presentation; and, a correctional facility asked me to provide a presentation on obesity and diabetes; and, a senior citizens retirement facility invited me to discuss how to eat healthy on a fixed income; and, on and on it went.

Then, the scope of what I was doing was expanded when one of the directors of the American Heart Association asked me to work with several of the local churches tied to their Healthy Heart Program. As a result, I conducted several well-received diabetes seminars with a number of churches, including Baptist, Pentecostal, Methodist, Seventh Day Adventist, and Christian. And, then, I was accidentally invited to a health fair held by the local Hindu temple, where I met some wonderful doctors and other healthcare professionals. I have truly been blessed to have met so many wonderful people that I would never had met if I had not been a diabetic.

But, because this was beginning to take up too much of my time, I created a document of all my notes and information and had copies printed for the churches and other local groups. This allowed me to return to my normal life as an engineer. But, the document led to more questions that caused me to add more pages to the document. Then, the document became too expensive to continue to have copies printed. So I finally relented to write a book that would provide all the detail that wasn't in the document and would answer all the questions that I normally discussed during my presentations. Now that the book is completed, everyone will have the necessary information that's been missing and my life will finally return to normal.

Update by the Author

I am developing new products (e.g. cookbook, audio CD book, wellness journal) and partnering with a health services company (Parwel) to provide diabetes education/coaching services to corporations, organizations and individuals. Go to www.deathtodiabetes.com for a list of new products and services.

Chapter 3. Diabetes Overview

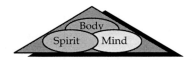

Diabetes History

Diabetes was identified as a medical problem centuries ago, but it didn't become a major health issue until people increased their consumption of processed foods while reducing their physical activity during the past 15 years. This has lead to a steady increase in the number of overweight and obese people, with an increasing percentage of them developing insulin resistance and eventually becoming diabetic.

Consequently, diabetes, specifically Type 2 diabetes, has rapidly become one of the most chronic diseases in the United States and worldwide, with more than 7% of the adult population affected. Type 2 diabetes is more common in the elderly and minority populations that are influenced by economic/societal biases, specifically Native Americans, African Americans, Hispanic Americans, and Asian and Pacific Island Americans. In these populations, Type 2 diabetes may be present in 10% to 50% of the adult population. However, this is only the tip of the iceberg of an epidemic of impaired glucose intolerance, insulin resistance, and an increased risk of cardiovascular disease.

Diabetes has been linked to the Western lifestyle, as it is uncommon in cultures consuming a more primitive diet. As cultures switched from their native diets to more commercial processed foods, their rate of diabetes increased, eventually reaching the same proportions seen in Western societies. A great deal of research has been conducted into the possible root causes of diabetes, with most of the prevalent ideas falling into the following categories: dietary indiscretion, obesity, endocrine imbalance, heredity, unknown virus, psychic stress, and environmental. This disease literally affects every cell in the body and the essential biochemical and metabolic processes involved with those cells.

As a result, diabetes is much more than a "blood sugar" disease – high blood sugar is just one of the *symptoms* of the disease. Unfortunately, the drug therapy is primarily directed at these *symptoms* (to lower the blood sugar level) and *not* at the underlying biochemical and metabolic *root causes* (to get *rid* of the disease), especially **excess insulin production**.

Obesity appears to be a significant factor, particularly considering the fact that more than 90% of Type 2 diabetics are overweight or obese. And, because diabetes appears to run in families, genetic factors may be important in determining susceptibility to diabetes. These genetic factors represent the "loaded gun" that presents a danger to your health. The poor eating habits and sedentary lifestyle represent "pulling the trigger" of the loaded gun. In effect, if you do not "pull the trigger", then, the "loaded gun" cannot damage your health. Unfortunately, since many siblings "inherit" the cooking and eating behaviors from their parents and relatives, it is the *environmental, dietary* and *lifestyle behavioral* factors that "pull the trigger" and fuel this disease. To support this contention, there are many clinical studies with significant evidence that diet and exercise can effectively control this disease and slow down many of its complications. The controversy and confusion is associated with the attributes of that diet, leaving many diabetics confused and frustrated with fighting this disease. Hopefully, this book will clarify those attributes and eliminate the confusion by focusing on the underlying biochemical, metabolic, and hormonal root causes of this disease, e.g. hyper-insulinemia, insulin resistance, inflammation, nutritional deficiencies, toxic overload, oxidation, and acidity. Interestingly, in my research, I found that even non-diabetics were affected by these same root causes, leading to obesity, high blood pressure, and high cholesterol.

What has become apparent through years of medical research is that diabetes is not simply a matter of one or two things having gone wrong. It is a complex condition with a multitude of biochemical, metabolic and hormonal imbalances. Consequently, although the conventional medical approach of using insulin or oral drugs to treat the symptoms of diabetes may be effective in the short term, it is not effective in the long term. An effective approach would be one that reduces the high level of insulin resistance and improves the health of the trillions of sick cells.

Types of Diabetes

There are primarily three (3) types of diabetes, Type 1 Diabetes, Type 2 Diabetes, and Gestational Diabetes.

Type 1 Diabetes (insulin-dependent diabetes mellitus, IDDM) is associated with the inability of the pancreatic beta cells to produce insulin. This disease is classified as an autoimmune disease that attacks and kills the insulin-producing beta cells. The pancreas continues to form beta cells, but they are rapidly killed off by the malfunctioning immune system. Type 1 diabetes used to be called childhood-onset diabetes, because it primarily afflicted children whose immune systems had not fully matured. But today adults in their 20s and 30s are now developing this disease.

Type 2 Diabetes (non-insulin-dependent diabetes mellitus, NIDDM) is associated with **excess insulin production** and the body's inability to effectively utilize the insulin produced by the pancreas, leading to more insulin production. This is known as insulin resistance. Type 2 diabetes used to be called adult-onset diabetes, because it primarily affected older adults. But today with more children being overweight and sedentary, they are now developing this disease.

Gestational Diabetes is also associated with excess insulin production and the body's inability to effectively utilize the insulin produced by the pancreas. But, Gestational Diabetes only occurs during pregnancy and usually disappears after the delivery of the baby.

Please Note: Despite the similarities, Type 2 Diabetes is a much different disease than Type 1 Diabetes. Type 2 Diabetes is a *lifestyle* disease with trillions of metabolically defective cells. Type 1 Diabetes is an *autoimmune* disease with dead or dormant pancreatic beta cells that are not producing insulin. The focus of this book is the lifestyle-driven Type 2 Diabetes. However, many of the wellness principles can be applied to Type 1 Diabetes and Gestational Diabetes with the proper medical, lifestyle and nutritional guidance.

Author's Note: This chapter is important because the more I understood about this disease, the easier it became to defeat the disease.

Blood Glucose Management (Normal Operation)

The human body contains more than 70 trillion cells, many of which help to regulate the body's blood glucose (blood sugar) level by pulling in the glucose out of the blood. The blood glucose level is regulated within a narrow range from 80 mg/dl to 120 mg/dl using two hormones secreted from the pancreas: insulin and glucagon.

Insulin is normally secreted by the beta islet cells of the pancreas when the blood glucose level starts to rise, usually due to the consumption of food. Although there is always a low level of insulin secreted by the pancreas, the amount secreted into the blood increases as the blood glucose rises. Similarly, as the blood glucose level falls, the amount of insulin secreted by the pancreatic islets goes down. Insulin has an effect on a number of cells, including the muscle cells, red blood cells, and fat cells which absorb glucose out of the blood, having the net effect of lowering the high blood glucose level returning it to the normal range.

On the other hand, glucagon is secreted by the alpha islet cells of the pancreas when the blood glucose level starts to sink and goes too low, usually between meals and during exercise, to bring the glucose level back up. As the blood glucose level goes down, more glucagon is secreted. Like insulin, glucagon has an effect on many cells of the body, but most notably the liver. The effect of glucagon is to make the liver release the glucose it has stored in its cells into the blood stream, with the net effect of increasing blood glucose. Glucagon also induces the liver (and some other cells such as the muscle cells) to make glucose out of building blocks obtained from other nutrients found in the body.

If the blood glucose level rises above 120 mg/dl this can be normal if the person has eaten within 2 to 3 hours, but even after eating, the glucose level should be below 180 mg/dl. Above 180 is termed "hyperglycemia" which translates to mean "too much glucose in the blood". If the blood glucose level is below 70, this is termed "hypoglycemia".

In addition to insulin and glucagon, another hormone called leptin may play a vital role, especially if the diabetic is significantly overweight. Leptin is a recently discovered hormone that is produced by the fat cells.

Leptin tells the body and brain how much energy it has, whether it needs more energy (a sign of hunger), and whether it should get rid of some energy (and stop being hungry). In other words, leptin tells the brain (hypothalamus) when to eat, how much to eat, and, most importantly, when to stop eating. Based on a recent study, it appears that leptin may affect blood glucose levels through two different brain-body pathways: one that controls appetite and fat storage, and another that tells the liver what to do with its glucose reserves. Further studies are underway to better understand leptin's role in obesity and its link to diabetes.

Are You Diabetic?

During a physical exam your doctor may discover that you have a high fasting blood glucose reading above 126 mg/dl. Your doctor will follow up with one or more of the following tests to determine if you are diabetic:
- Fasting Blood Glucose Test
- Oral Glucose Tolerance Test

Fasting Blood Glucose Test
For this test you will be required to fast (not eat) for at least eight hours on two separate days. Your doctor will draw your blood and measure your glucose level each time. If your blood glucose level is 126 mg/dl or greater both times, then, you are diabetic. If your doctor is not fully certain that you are diabetic, then, he/she will perform the Oral Glucose Tolerance Test.

Oral Glucose Tolerance Test
For this test you will be required to fast for at least eight hours. Your doctor will give you a sugar solution to drink and measure your blood at one-hour intervals during the next three hours. If your blood glucose level is 200 mg/dl or greater each time, then, you are diabetic.

Marginal Cases (Pre-diabetes) & Risk Factors

For marginal situations where the fasting blood glucose is above 100 mg/dl in combination with two of the following risk factors, a patient may have impaired glucose tolerance (IGT), an indication that he/she is becoming insulin resistant or pre-diabetic. The risk factors for Type 2 diabetes include the following:

- Abdominal (belly) fat: a waistline greater than 40 inches (for a man), or 35 inches for a woman
- Overweight/obesity: Body Mass Index (BMI) greater than 25
- Poor nutrition: too much processed white rice, potatoes, bread, pasta, and other refined flour products; too many cookies, cakes, pies, bottled juices, soda, ice cream, and other sweets; and, not enough fiber, water, plant oils, and nutrients from vegetables and fruits
- Sedentary lifestyle: very little physical activity or exercise
- Age: 45 years or older
- High blood pressure (130/80 or higher)
- High triglycerides (over 150), Low HDL cholesterol (under 40 for men, 50 for women)
- High C-reactive protein, high homocysteine and/or small, dense LDL particles, indicators of high levels of internal inflammation
- Non-Caucasian ethnicity: Hispanic American, African American, Native American, Asian American (partially due to societal "isms")
- A family history of Type 2 diabetes or cardiovascular disease
- Acanthosis nigricans: patches of thick, brownish, velvety skin on the neck, underarms, or groin; also, just below the breasts in women
- Poor mental health, e.g. depression
- A history of gestational diabetes during pregnancy
- Tobacco/alcohol consumption

If your doctor believes that you have impaired glucose tolerance, he/she may suggest a change in eating habits and exercise to lose several pounds and reduce the insulin resistance, preventing the onset of diabetes. This is a major opportunity to *prevent* Type 2 diabetes, but, unfortunately, most of us do not listen to our doctor because we do not want to make changes to our lifestyle.

Then, when we get the bad news, we are either in denial, surprised or angry that we have been diagnosed as a diabetic. As our health gets worse, we expect our doctor to perform a miracle and fix us with some "magic pill". This is not fair to our doctor, who's earlier warning was ignored; and it's not fair to our family, who depends on us.

If your doctor has warned you about your weight, blood glucose level, blood pressure, or one of the aforementioned risk factors, then, you should take heed because he/she is trying to save your life. If you have not been to your doctor in a while, you should set up an appointment as soon as possible. It is a lot easier to *prevent* diabetes than it is to control and reverse it.

If you exhibit more than three of the aforementioned risk factors, you may have what is being called Metabolic Syndrome X, a condition driven by years of high insulin levels and inflammation in the body. And, the more of these risk factors you have, the greater the chance that you will develop insulin resistance and become pre-diabetic; and, eventually diabetic. Excessively high insulin levels over a period of years will develop into hyperinsulinemia and the accumulation of excess fat particularly in the abdomen area – all due to insulin resistance. The excess fat releases chemicals called cytokines that block the insulin receptors which triggers the pancreas to release two to three times more insulin. This can inhibit the breakdown of homocysteine, which can eventually lead to internal inflammation and damage to various body parts such as the arteries and kidneys.

If you have more than three of these risk factors, talk to other family members to understand your family history. Because of the embarrassment of the disease and because some cultures/families just didn't talk about this or other diseases, there may be an (unspoken) family history that is usually passed down via poor eating habits, negative attitudes and negative behaviors – some of which may be compounded by environmental and societal biases. As a result, a silent disease like diabetes is allowed to progress from one generation to the next, with each new generation acquiring the disease sooner than the previous generation.

Acceptance of the Diagnosis

Once you have been diagnosed with diabetes, you will go through several stages of emotions: surprise, denial, anger, suspicion, acceptance and resolve. This is normal. Unfortunately, many people, once diagnosed with a disease, remain in a state of denial and/or anger and miss a major opportunity to prevent the disease from taking hold and their health deteriorating to a serious level. Discuss your problem with a family member or close friend, and acquire more knowledge about the disease. Sometimes, just talking about your health problem or becoming better informed helps to alleviate some of the fear and anger.

Author's Note: It may appear to be somewhat overwhelming when you try to figure out what you should do. I was fortunate because my daughter initiated many of the early activities by working with the doctors and nurses to obtain my insulin, the needles, the blood glucose meter, the test strips and the lancets. Also, the hospital had one of their home nurses visit me to ensure that I knew how to properly test my blood glucose and inject myself with the insulin. The nurses seemed to sense the fear and anxiety I had and were able to diffuse it with their patience and insight – they seemed to know what questions I was going to ask and helped to put me at ease with their quiet confidence and caring demeanor. There is no doubt in my mind that all of this help enabled me to get going in the right direction almost immediately. My mother and my sister were also a tremendous help at the beginning by showing me how easy it was to prepare nutritious meals. Their help made it easier for me to accept the diagnosis, absorb a tremendous amount of information, and allow me to move forward instead of languishing in self-pity.

Once diagnosed, some people do make some minor changes to their diet and/or exercise hoping that these changes will deter the disease. Some people even experience some initial success (e.g. weight loss), but, unfortunately, they underestimate the devastation that the disease can cause and are unaware that the disease is still lingering and silently progressing throughout their body. As a result, the disease takes a foothold while they relax and eventually the disease "returns" stronger and more formidable, requiring additional changes to diet, exercise, and, possibly, the need for diabetic drugs.

Treatment Guidelines

Your doctor will recommend a treatment protocol based on your blood glucose readings from the aforementioned blood glucose tests. In general, your doctor will recommend the following, but keep in mind that these are only guidelines that may be modified for your specific situation.

Glucose Reading (mg/dl)	Diagnosis	Treatment
100 to 125	Impaired glucose tolerance (Pre-diabetes)	Nutrition, exercise
126 to 140	Diabetes	Nutrition, exercise
141 to 200	Diabetes	Nutrition, exercise, oral drugs
201 and higher	Diabetes	Nutrition, exercise, oral drugs/ insulin

Figure 1. Diagnosis & Treatment Guidelines

Author's Personal Note: In my case, the doctors had to put me on insulin (Humalog and Lantus) immediately because my blood glucose level was so high that it was life-threatening and they knew that the oral drugs would not be effective in getting my blood glucose under control.

Impact of Diabetes

There are more than 190 million people worldwide and more than 21 million people in the United States with diabetes, with more than 95% having Type 2 diabetes. In the United States alone, there is at least an additional 41 million people who are unaware that they are diabetic, pre-diabetic, or have Metabolic Syndrome X. Every hour over 2,000 people are diagnosed as a diabetic. Type 2 diabetes in adults has increased from less than 10% in 1982 to more than 30%, with more than 85% of the adults diagnosed with Type 2 diabetes being obese. Type 2 diabetes in children has increased from less than 4% in 1982 to more than 20%, with more than 85% of the children diagnosed with Type 2 diabetes being obese. More than 80% of all diabetics will develop some form of cardiovascular, kidney, eye, or nerve disease.

I could go on and on with more statistics explaining how diabetes impacts our health. But, most people don't really care that much about statistics. So, I created the following diagram that provides a better overall picture of the health impact and seriousness of diabetes on an annual basis in the United States.

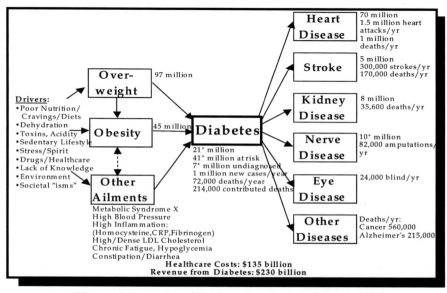

Figure 2. Impact of Diabetes (Annually) in the U.S.

As you can see from the diagram, diabetes is primarily being driven by a large population of overweight/obese people who have a profile of poor nutrition, a sedentary lifestyle, and a high dependency on drugs. Diabetes, in turn, appears to be a key driver of heart disease, stroke, kidney failure, and other circulatory-related diseases. Diabetes has reached epidemic levels and will continue to grow as the top chronic disease in terms of affected population, healthcare cost, and revenue -- as the combination of an overweight population, a sedentary lifestyle, the inability to handle stress, and the dependency on processed foods and drugs will continue to fuel these numbers -- with no apparent end in sight.

Although healthcare costs and out-of-pocket expenses will continue to rise, the revenue (from blood glucose testing tools, surgeries (amputation, eye, heart), doctor appointments, medical tests, hospital stays, dialysis, and drugs) far exceeds the expenses, making diabetes a lucrative business for the healthcare industry.

Type 2 Diabetes

Type 2 diabetes is a complex, insidious disease that slowly and silently destroys your body one day at a time. This silent killer destroys your organs one by one, by attacking and damaging the small capillaries and blood vessels that feed your heart, brain, feet, kidneys, and eyes – this is called microvascular disease. Diabetes accelerates the biological aging of the organs and tissues, but most of this aging is not painful or visible to the unsuspecting diabetic. As the disease progresses, the majority of diabetics develop two or more of the following complications:

- Additional weight (fat) gain, leading to low energy and fatigue, obesity, high blood pressure, dehydration, high cholesterol, arthritis, toxicity and other acidic, inflammatory ailments.
- Kidney disease (nephropathy), leading to kidney failure and dialysis.
- Eye disease (retinopathy), leading to blindness.
- Nerve damage (neuropathy), leading to amputation of a lower limb; and other nerve-related conditions.
- Gum (periodontal) disease, leading to the loss of teeth and other infections.
- Heart disease (due to high blood pressure, high homocysteine, thick blood), leading to a heart attack or stroke.
- A higher susceptibility to other infections and diseases due to an underlying mechanism of internal inflammation and a weakened immune system.

Like Oprah said during one of her TV shows about diabetes: "There's no such thing as a little sugar problem . . . this is a very serious problem in our country."

Because most diabetics do not feel any pain or discomfort for at least several years, they choose to ignore the disease.

Then, when they begin to have kidney problems or feel pain or discomfort, usually in the feet, they visit their doctor. Unfortunately, that usually leads to some type of drug therapy, but the disease continues to progress, leading to more drug therapy. And, most diabetics believe the drugs are working because their blood glucose level is lowered and they are not experiencing any pain. But, the disease continues to progress as the body builds up its resistance to insulin requiring even more drugs, leading to one or more of the aforementioned complications.

Insulin Resistance & Inflammation

Type 2 diabetes is *more* than a "blood sugar" disease! It is a combination of **insulin resistance** and **inflammation**. Insulin resistance and inflammation prevent your body's cells from effectively using the insulin produced by the pancreas. That is, the insulin receptors on the surface of each cell are damaged (inflamed), ignoring the presence of insulin in your blood and refusing to allow glucose from your blood to enter your cells. The cells in your body require the glucose (as fuel) in order to produce energy. Without this fuel, your cells cannot produce energy and you will feel tired. This is one of the primary reasons why many diabetics lack the energy to exercise or feel the need to take a nap in the middle of the day.

Under normal circumstances, when you eat food, it is broken down and converted to glucose, and the glucose level in your blood begins to rise. This signals the pancreas to secrete insulin into your bloodstream. The cells in your body, such as the fat cells and muscle cells, contain these "doors" (insulin receptors) that sense the presence of insulin. Insulin acts like a "key" and causes these "doors" in the cell membranes to open. When these "doors" open, the glucose in your blood is transported into your cells and processed to provide you with energy. Any extra glucose is stored as glycogen in your liver and muscle cells for future use (e.g. exercise). At this point, the glucose level in your blood lowers and returns to normal, usually within 2 hours after eating.

But, that isn't what happens when you are a diabetic. Everything is the same up to the point when these "doors" (insulin receptors) sense the presence of insulin. At that point, the damaged cell "doors" do not respond to the "key" insulin and do not open and let in the glucose. Although some of the glucose is stored as glycogen by the liver and muscle cells, the majority of the glucose begins to "back up" in the blood causing the blood glucose level to continue to rise. The pancreas senses that the blood glucose level is still rising, so the pancreas ramps up and secretes more and more insulin to try to "push" the glucose into the cells and bring the glucose level down.

As the glucose level continues to rise, the liver and muscle cells, due to a limited storage capacity, are unable to store any more glucose and become resistant to insulin. Consequently, the extra glucose is converted to fat by the liver and stored throughout the body in places that do not have limited storage capacities: the abdomen, hips, waist, and the blood (as triglycerides). In the meantime, the kidneys try to help by removing glucose from the blood. This leads to frequent urination, which leads to a strong thirst and constant drinking, which leads to more urination and a depletion of vitamins and minerals. The high levels of insulin in the body trigger the increase in fat storage -- especially in the abdomen area, which includes the omentum layer of fat surrounding the bowel. The high levels of insulin also inhibit the metabolism (breakdown) of fat as the amount of fat and the number of fat cells in the body continues to increase. The excess fat cells release chemicals called cytokines that block the insulin receptors, leading the pancreas to churn out two to three times more insulin. After years of high insulin levels force-feeding the glucose into the resistant cells, some of the insulin-producing beta cells in the pancreas may burn out. This, in turn, causes insulin levels to fall, leading to a further rise in the glucose level. And, as the glucose level rises even more, this can eventually lead to further cell membrane damage, cell starvation, severe dehydration, and organ shutdown triggering a coma state.

As depicted in the following diagram, the lack of communicative response from the damaged (inflamed) cell receptors ("doors") to open up and let in the glucose leads to low energy, fatigue and an increased resistance to insulin. This ongoing insulin resistance and inflammation leads to an increase of oxidation (free radical damage), inflammation (cell membrane/tissue damage), and toxicity (poisoning and acidity).

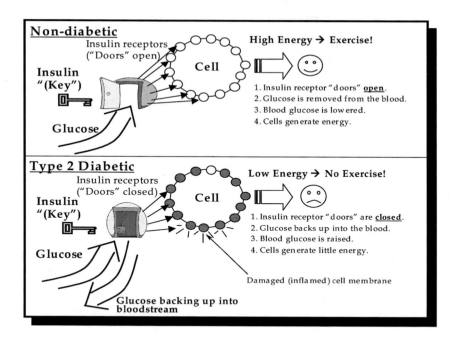

Non-diabetic

Insulin receptors
("Doors" open)

**Insulin
"(Key")**

Cell

Glucose

High Energy → Exercise!

1. Insulin receptor "doors" **open**.
2. Glucose is removed from the blood.
3. Blood glucose is lowered.
4. Cells generate energy.

Type 2 Diabetic

Insulin receptors
("Doors" closed)

**Insulin
"(Key")**

Cell

Glucose

Low Energy → No Exercise!

1. Insulin receptor "doors" are **closed**.
2. Glucose backs up into the blood.
3. Blood glucose is raised.
4. Cells generate little energy.

Damaged (inflamed) cell membrane

**Glucose backing up into
bloodstream**

Figure 3. Type 2 Diabetes at the Cellular Level

In addition, ongoing diabetes leads to the following problems:

- A depletion of vitamins (B-complex, Vitamin C, Vitamin E) and minerals (calcium, potassium, magnesium, chromium), many of which are excreted in the urine due to the kidneys trying to get rid of the excess glucose. The loss of these nutrients prevents proper carbohydrate/protein/fat metabolism, electrolyte balance, nerve protection, insulin regulation, muscle relaxation, and antioxidant protection from free radicals.
- An increase in the production of cholesterol by the liver due to the insulin activating the HMG-CoA reductase enzyme.
- A conversion of the extra glucose to fat, increasing the triglycerides, LDL cholesterol, and blood viscosity (thickness).
- A prevention of the breakdown of homocysteine, causing an increase of cell inflammation leading to a buildup of plaque in the artery walls, which become rigid, thicker and more narrow.

- An increase of inflammation markers such as homocysteine, C-reactive protein (CRP), fibrinogen, and lipoprotein(a), leading to thick, sticky and slow moving blood.
- An increase in advanced glycated end products (AGEs), which are formed when glucose damages the protein in the cells, preventing the normal function of those cells and accelerating the aging of the cells.
- An increase in blood pressure due to the hyperinsulinemia, thicker blood and narrowed, more rigid arteries.
- An increase in blood pressure due to the retention of salt and water and poor filtering of the blood by the kidneys, which may stimulate the liver to produce more cholesterol.
- A gradual development of pancreatic beta cell dysfunction.
- Development of blood clots due to the thicker, sticky blood, eventually leading to strokes and heart attacks.

Also, the extra insulin drives the glucose level down too low triggering hormonal hunger – this is why diabetics feel tired (low glucose level) and hungry (hormonal hunger). If the pancreas does not secrete enough glucagon to counter-balance the extra insulin, the glucose level is driven down too low, and may trigger an attack of low blood sugar.

When the blood glucose level rises too high and remains too high, the glucose molecule attaches itself to cells permanently and is eventually converted to a poison called sorbitol that destroys the cells. This process gradually leads to blurred vision, burning foot syndrome, tingling, and the loss of feeling in the extremities.

Why Diabetics Remain in a Diabetic State

When many people are initially diagnosed with diabetes, they fail to heed the warnings of their doctors and they fail to take any action. Why? Because they do not feel any pain or have any major symptoms that impact their daily lives. Other diabetics, who do heed the warning, lose weight or begin taking a diabetic drug to control their blood glucose. Unfortunately, both of these groups are doomed because they do not understand what is really going on inside their bodies. They fail to realize that the disease is primarily due to excess insulin and trillions of defective cells not operating properly; and, that these cells need to be repaired and that the environment the cells are living in (the body's internal terrain) needs to be cleaned up.

The following flow diagram is a high level depiction of what goes on in a diabetic's body. Insulin resistance is the result of a vicious metabolic cycle ("doom loop") of eating an excess of refined, processed carbohydrates that cause rising blood glucose levels, triglycerides, inflammation and insulin surges. This leads to blood glucose "crashes" and fat storage, causing fatigue, increased appetite, hunger and strong cravings for more refined carbohydrates. And, the additional fat increases the body's need for more insulin. If the diabetic is also eating a lot of fatty animal meat, this increases the production of homocysteine and fat, which leads to more insulin resistance within the fat cells. And while the fat cells normally release a protein hormone called leptin to signal that plenty of fat is stored and to reduce the appetite level, this does not appear to occur in some diabetics and obese people. If the diabetic does not use proper nutrition and exercise to break this vicious cycle, he/she will gain more weight as the disease and its complications continue to progress.

Even with drug therapy to lower the blood glucose level, these vicious "cycles of doom" will cause the disease to continue to progress because **the drugs don't address the excess insulin production**. For example, insulin injections help to lower the blood glucose level in the short term. But, over a period of time, the extra insulin stimulates the production of more fat cells, which triggers the body's need for more insulin and more calories (more food). In addition, the insulin inhibits the body from metabolizing and breaking down the fat; increases the internal inflammation mechanism due to high homo-cysteine; and, depletes the body of the key vitamins and minerals that help to metabolize carbohydrates and proteins in addition to the fats. As a result, the body has trillions of defective cells that are in a continual cycle of not using the glucose in the blood and requiring more insulin, which increases the production of more fat and inhibits the metabolism and breakdown of fat as a fuel. As depicted in the following diagram, **this is how many people become fat and more than 90% of Type 2 diabetics remain fat while developing other complications.**

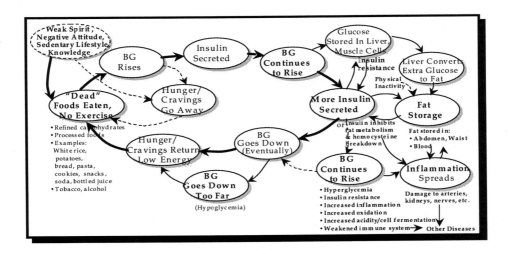

Figure 4. Metabolic Doom Cycle

The high insulin levels (and high glucose levels) lead to a reduction in the production of serotonin (a feel-good hormone) and the eventual increase of cortisol (the stress hormone). This depletion of serotonin leads to negative feelings of depression, anxiety, or despair, which increases the stress level, triggering a rise in cortisol. Stress creates the "fight or flight" response, which causes the release of cortisol. This, in turn, triggers the release of other hormones such as epinephrine, and stored glycogen (to prep the cells) causing a rise in the blood glucose and insulin levels. But, because the glucose can't get into the cells (due to the insulin resistance), the body lacks the energy to properly handle the stress and becomes frayed. This is why some diabetics become fatigued when under severe stress. **This is one of the major reasons why some Type 2 diabetics develop emotional issues – too much stress, compounded by too much cortisol and too little serotonin.**

However, I believe that some diabetics do try their best to modify their nutrition and exercise habits. But, because of misinformation about the proper foods to eat/not eat, they unknowingly fuel the disease. As a result, they become frustrated and disappointed. Unfortunately, they blame themselves when, in fact, it is really not their fault. And, this form of self-blaming can further fuel the disease emotionally.

The following is a summary of the major reasons why diabetics remain in a diabetic state due to emotions, behaviors, and misinformation.

- Some diabetics are indifferent and stubborn, refusing to make the behavioral changes to their nutrition, exercise, and lifestyle. Some do not want to take on the responsibility for their own health – it's easier to deny, ignore, pretend, complain or blame someone else.
- Some diabetics believe the drugs are working because their glucose level is lower. They are unaware that the disease is more than just controlling their blood glucose level.
- Some diabetics love their food more than their health! They are chemically, hormonally and emotionally addicted to their favorite foods -- making it very difficult to break the poor eating habits.
- Some diabetics try to get by with minimal changes to their eating habits and exercise, hoping that it will be sufficient. Some even experience some success with weight loss and a lower glucose level, but it's short-lived because their bodies still produce excess insulin.
- Many diabetics are unaware that it actually cost more to eat the "dead" food because of the extra expenses for over-the-counter drugs, prescription drugs, doctor appointments, surgeries, hospital visits, health insurance premiums, etc.
- Some people, including diabetics, believe that eating healthy is boring, expensive, and time consuming. They feel due to their busy schedules and family commitments that they don't have the time to eat properly. Also, they believe that healthy foods are more expensive and just don't taste as good as convenience and fast foods.
- After several years of fighting the disease, some diabetics become drained emotionally and spiritually. As a result, they "give up" and "give in" to the fact that the best they can do is to live with the disease and the drugs.
- Many diabetics don't believe that eating properly can make that much of a difference; and, if it did, it takes too long to reap the benefits. It's easier to just take a drug.
- Societal prejudices and "isms" that negatively affect education, employment, families, and other institutions, lead to misinformation, financial strain, anger, denial, inadequate insurance, and poor healthcare.

- There is a defense mechanism that "protects" people when, after years of being told "there's no cure for diabetes" that the opposite might be true. Some diabetics will spend energy trying to convince themselves and others that "It can't be true – that's impossible. I've been living with this disease a long time, I should know."
- Many diabetics associate with family members and friends who enable or support their bad eating habits. They do not associate with people who will tell them that they are getting fat or eating unhealthy.

Refer to Chapter 13 for countermeasures to overcome these issues.

Short Term Complications

There are four major diabetes-related short-term complications that you need to be aware of:
- Hyperglycemia (high blood sugar)
- Hypoglycemia (low blood sugar)
- Ketoacidosis
- Hyperosmolar syndrome

Hyperglycemia (High Blood Sugar)

If your blood glucose level goes too high, you may experience one or more of the following symptoms: frequent thirst (polydipsia); frequent urination (polyuria); fatigue; frequent hunger (polyphagia); blurry vision; dry mouth; dry or itchy skin; recurrent infections.

This is known as hyperglycemia. But, it is important to remember that many people with Type 2 diabetes may not have any of these symptoms. The classic symptom of being hungry frequently stems from the fact that the diabetic cannot utilize glucose well as an energy source within their cells. The glucose is circulating in the blood, but the cells cannot absorb it to use it as a fuel. The excess glucose also "spills" into the urine, leading the diabetic to urinate frequently (the second classic symptom of diabetes). This leads to the third classic symptom of frequent thirst because the body can sense that excess water is being lost because of the frequent urination.

IMPORTANT! If your blood glucose level goes too high, you may go into a coma if you do not take corrective action immediately. If you ignore the symptoms and it progresses, you may go into a non-ketotic hyperglycemic hyperosmolar coma. **Call 911** if necessary.

How high and how fast your glucose level rises and how much glucose is converted to fat when you eat is dependent on several nutrition-related factors that will be discussed in Chapters 6 and 7.

Hypoglycemia (Low Blood Sugar)

Hypoglycemia is an abnormally low level of glucose or sugar in the blood. The most common form is called functional hypoglycemia (FH) and is caused by an inadequate diet that is too high in refined carbohydrates. An over-consumption of refined carbohydrates causes the blood glucose level to rise rapidly, stimulating the pancreas to secrete an excess of insulin. This excess insulin removes too much glucose from the blood, resulting in an abnormally low blood glucose level. If the pancreas does not secrete enough glucagon to counter-balance the extra insulin, the glucose level is driven down too low, and may trigger an attack of hypoglycemia.

If your blood glucose level goes too low, you may experience one or more of the following symptoms: dizziness, disorientation, anxiety, sweaty palms, hunger.

WARNING! If your blood glucose level goes too low, you may go into a coma if you do not take corrective action immediately. So, be aware of the symptoms and take action immediately. **Call 911** if necessary.

This is known as hypoglycemia. To (temporarily) correct the problem, eat/drink something immediately, e.g. a glass of orange juice, a candy bar, some glucose tablets. Afterwards, prepare a small balanced snack, e.g. an apple or a handful of grapes, a soft-boiled egg or a handful of nuts/seeds, and a glass of raw vegetable juice.

If you are experiencing very low blood glucose levels, it may be due to one or more of the following:
- Skipping a meal, not eating enough during a meal
- Not eating enough quality carbohydrates such as vegetables
- Eating too much refined flour and sugar products during a meal
- Eating too much animal protein that does not get digested properly
- Exercising too strenuously or exercising on an empty stomach
- Too strong of a diabetic drug dosage
- A combination of other drugs
- Drinking too much alcohol
- A highly stressful situation

Make the necessary corrections to prevent another low blood glucose episode, e.g. stop eating refined carbohydrates and other processed foods; eat more quality protein such as fish, nuts and seeds. Vitamin and mineral supplementation may be necessary to supply tissues that are markedly depleted. Also, digestive enzymes may be needed to ensure proper absorption of food for the digestion of proteins, carbohydrates, and fats. Discuss this with your doctor if your low glucose levels do not subside after you've made the corrections to your eating habits.

Note: If you are experiencing low blood sugar in the middle of the night, test at 2 a.m. for a few nights. If your readings are low at that time, discuss with your doctor to lower your evening drug dosage.

Author's Personal Note: Low blood sugar happened to me, usually due to my missing a snack or over-exercising. As I became healthier, the low readings subsided. In fact, after I recovered, I noticed that even when my readings went low, I no longer felt weak or light-headed. I suspect that my pancreas had begun to work more effectively releasing glucagon to trigger the release of stored glycogen and allowing my brain to make better use of the available glucose in my blood.

Ketoacidosis

Ketoacidosis and hyperosmolar syndrome are two other short-term complications, but they are a lot more serious and require medical intervention, and therefore, should be treated as *medical emergencies*. You should not try to handle these complications on your own. Instead call your doctor and have someone drive you to the hospital, if possible.

Ketoacidosis is a condition that usually occurs in Type 1 diabetics when there is no insulin with very high glucose levels (usually above 400 mg/dl) and no energy production. In order to get energy, the body burns fat, which produces acidic ketones as a byproduct. These ketones poison the blood, which turns from alkaline to acidic leading to one or more of the following early symptoms: very tired and sleepy; weakness; great thirst; frequent urination; dry skin and tongue; leg cramps; fruity odor to the breath; upset stomach, nausea.

If the condition goes untreated, it progresses to the following symptoms: vomiting; shortness of breath; sunken eyeballs; very high blood sugars; rapid pulse; rapid breathing; low blood pressure; unresponsiveness, coma. **At this time, medical intervention is necessary to prevent death.**

Hyperosmolar Syndrome

Hyperosmolar syndrome is a condition that usually occurs in Type 2 diabetics when there are very high glucose levels (usually above 700 mg/dl) leading to severe dehydration and loss of electrolytes (e.g. sodium, potassium). Hyperosmolar syndrome is similar to ketoacidosis in that ketones are produced (but they don't make the blood as acidic) and there is a high glucose level (but it is usually much higher). While ketoacidosis happens very quickly, hyperosmolar syndrome usually develops over a period of days or even weeks with the following symptoms: frequent urination; great thirst; weakness; dry skin and tongue; leg cramps; sunken eyeballs; rapid pulse; decreased mental awareness; paralysis of the arms and legs ("rubbery" arms and legs); unresponsiveness, coma. Symptoms for hyperglycemic hyperosmolar syndrome are linked to dehydration rather than acidosis, so a fruity odor to the breath and an upset stomach are less likely.

WARNING! Diabetics and family members need to know how to recognize these conditions and realize that treatment with a piece of fruit will not work. The diabetic needs medical treatment immediately. **Call 911.**

Preventive Measures

Measurement of ketones in the urine is very important for diabetics with infections or on insulin pump therapy due to the fact it gives more information than glucose tests alone. Since ketones travel from the blood into the urine, they can be detected in the urine with ketone test strips that are available at any pharmacy.

Check the urine for ketones whenever a blood glucose reading is 300 mg/dl or higher – if a fruity odor is detected in the breath, abdominal pain is present, nausea or vomiting is occurring, or you are breathing rapidly and short of breath. If a large amount of ketones are detected on the test strip, ketoacidosis is present and immediate treatment is required.

Long Term Diseases & Complications

Diabetes gradually deteriorates the body over a period of years as the glucose clogs and damages the small capillaries that feed the kidneys, eyes, feet, and heart. As a result, at least 4 out of every 5 diabetics develop one or more of the following long term diseases and complications:

Kidney disease (Nephropathy): Kidneys normally filter out waste products from the blood, but when the kidneys become damaged, the waste products remain in the blood and protein leaks into the urine, leading to kidney failure and dialysis.

Eye disease (Retinopathy): The signs of damage to the eyes include blurry vision, spots, and loss of vision, which can lead to blindness if the macula is damaged and there is a loss of blood supply to the retina. Other eye diseases that diabetics may acquire include cataracts and glaucoma.

Nerve disease (Neuropathy): The signs of nerve damage include the loss of feeling (touch) in the feet, tingling and burning, which can lead to foot ulcers, gangrene and amputation. If motor or autonomic nerves are damaged, this can lead to the loss of muscle control, causing problems such as gastroparesis, a disorder in which the stomach takes too long to empty causing erratic blood glucose levels. Other problems affect breathing, sexual function, bladder control, and bowel control.

Cardiovascular disease (CVD): The signs of cardiovascular disease include high homocysteine, high C-reactive protein (CRP), and high blood pressure -- which can lead to a heart attack or stroke. Cold feet/hands and sexual dysfunction may be signs of circulatory (or nerve-related) problems.

Other complications: They include excessive weight gain, high blood pressure, high cholesterol, high triglycerides, high inflammation, and fatigue. There may also be a higher susceptibility to other illnesses and infections, including periodontal (gum) disease.

The 7 Most Common Mistakes

Based on my research and my personal experience working with many diabetics, I discovered that most diabetics make the same mistakes! The following is a list of the seven most common mistakes, primarily due to misinformation and the lack of knowledge.

1. **Weight loss focus:** Some diabetics focus on trying to lose weight instead of trying to get healthy. Focusing on losing weight may work in the short term but because this may drive bad eating habits, it is a temporary fix that eventually leads to more weight gain.
   Counter-measure: Focus on getting healthy by eating properly to control your blood glucose level and improve the health of your cells. Once you improve the health of your cells and get your blood glucose level under control, the weight loss will occur naturally and permanently, as the body is able to burn fat as fuel.

2. **Poor Nutrition:**
   Breakfast/Other Meals: Many diabetics either don't eat breakfast or they eat a grain-based breakfast, e.g. cereal, grits, toast, bagel. Most diabetics eat a refined carbohydrate-loaded, fiber-deficient dinner.
   Counter-measure: Eat a green, leafy vegetable-based breakfast, e.g. 1-2 cups of steamed spinach (or broccoli) topped with 1 tbsp. of extra virgin olive oil, 2 ounces of baked wild salmon, 1 slice sprouted grain bread, and 16 ounces of filtered water. Optional: For additional sustenance, include a glass of raw vegetable juice, mixed with a tbsp. of freshly ground flaxseed. If you have multiple illnesses, stay away from most processed grains, especially wheat, during the initial stages of recovery. Also, eat a similar meal for dinner with an extra vegetable or legume (1-2 cups), additional monounsaturated/Omega-3 fats (1 tbsp.), and additional lean protein (3-4 ounces).
   Over-focus on avoiding carbohydrates: Many diabetics try to avoid eating carbohydrates to "force" their blood sugar level lower. Diabetics mistakenly believe that all carbohydrates are bad.
   Counter-measure: Ensure every meal has a *wholefood* carbohydrate such as a green, leafy vegetable, and avoid the *refined* carbohydrates.

3. **Blood glucose testing:** Most diabetics test too infrequently, they don't record the test results, and/or they don't take the proper corrective actions based on the test results.
   Counter-measure: Increase your blood glucose testing and record the readings to evaluate so that you can make corrective actions to what you're eating and how you're exercising. Of course, if you do not make any corrective actions based on the readings, then, you are wasting your time with the extra testing.

4. **Denial & stubbornness:** Some diabetics live in denial and do not believe that they will end up with kidney failure, amputation, blindness, heart attack or stroke -- despite the overwhelming statistics that show that more than 4 out of every 5 diabetics develop one or more of these health complications. Other diabetics are too stubborn to change their eating habits or lifestyle because they love to eat.
   Counter-measure: Talk to a family member or a friend, or join a support group. Discuss your fears and concerns with your doctor or other healthcare professional. Educate yourself about the disease.

5. **Lack of exercise:** Most diabetics either do not exercise or they exercise improperly.

   Counter-measure: Implement a consistent aerobic/weight-resistance exercise program that you will enjoy and fit into your daily schedule and lifestyle. But, you must provide your body with the proper fuel (by eating right) in order to generate the energy to exercise.

6. **Food & Lifestyle Addictions:**

   Food addiction: Many diabetics are unknowingly addicted to the chemicals in their favorite foods. This makes it difficult to stop eating these foods even though the diabetic knows these foods are harmful to their health and contain very little, if any, nutritional value.

   Counter-measure: Begin eating more of the nutrient-rich foods, such as green, leafy vegetables, to change your body chemistry and reduce the chemical addiction. The changing of your body's chemistry is a critical step towards breaking your food addiction. Start with a nutritious breakfast, and eventually add a nutritious dinner to help change that chemistry. These nutritious meals will help the body reduce the insulin resistance and inflammation of the cell receptors – allowing the cells the opportunity to gradually repair themselves.

   Lifestyle addiction: Most diabetics enjoy and are used to their current lifestyle and do not want to lose their freedom. Ironically their "lifestyle" is in reality their "deathstyle".

   Counter-measure: Make small changes. If you educate yourself about this disease you will discover that you will eventually lose that precious freedom if you allow the disease to take hold in your body. We all love our freedom, but you don't have to sacrifice your life for that freedom.

7. **Reliance and belief in drugs:** Most diabetics rely on the drugs to control their blood glucose instead of making the nutrition and lifestyle changes to help the body heal itself.

   Counter-measure: Begin eating the nutritious foods to reduce the need for the drugs, which beget more drugs and toxic side effects that further deteriorate the body's health. Once you start taking drugs to compensate for poor eating habits and a sedentary lifestyle, you start down a very slippery slope that gradually leads to more drugs and poorer health.

Myths

Here are several myths and misunderstandings about diabetes, nutrition and other related topics.

Myth: Diabetes is just a little sugar problem – it's not that serious.
Truth: Diabetes is a disease that affects trillions of cells in the body and, gradually, leads to complications such as heart attack, stroke, amputation, kidney failure, and blindness. So, diabetes is serious . . . very serious.

Myth: Eating sweets and your genetics cause diabetes.
Truth: Eating sweets does not cause diabetes – they make you fat, which can lead to diabetes. Although your genetics can play a partial role in diabetes, the eating and cooking habits that are passed down from one generation to the next are more significant contributors, when combined with a sedentary lifestyle. Look at your genetics as being the "loaded gun" and your eating habits/lifestyle as "pulling the trigger". As long as you don't pull the trigger, the loaded gun can't harm you! Your body may have a genetic predisposition to acquire diabetes, but, if you make better decisions than your ancestors about food, exercise, and lifestyle, then it is not a forgone conclusion that you will become diabetic.

Myth: There is no cure for diabetes – once a diabetic, always a diabetic.
Truth: The treatment protocol for Type 2 diabetes is drug therapy, which is designed to suppress the symptoms of the disease and not address the root causes of the disease. And, therefore, the disease cannot be cured. However, there is sufficient clinical evidence that shows lifestyle changes (such as nutrition, exercise, testing, and spiritual health) can prevent and control Type 2 diabetes. And, once the diabetes is under control, further lifestyle changes may reverse the effects of the disease – if the treatment focuses on repairing the trillions of defective cells.

Myth: Diabetes is not as serious if you are taking pills instead of insulin.
Truth: Diabetes should be taken as seriously regardless of whether you are taking pills or injections. Unfortunately, because we live in a drug-tolerant society that sees pills as "normal", we don't really believe our health is in any danger if we are taking pills. Either way, the diabetes will still progress and lead to other health complications. In fact, pills lull

diabetics into a comfort zone and a false sense of wellness that eventually fails them.

Author's Note: A co-worker thought that he was safe taking a pill, but today is on insulin because the disease continued to progress.

Myth: You can control your diabetes by avoiding the carbs.
Truth: You may be able to temporarily lower your blood glucose level, but you can't avoid a major macronutrient such as carbohydrates and expect to get healthy. Besides, not *all* carbohydrates are bad – it's the *refined* carbohydrates such as white bread, pasta, and cereals that are the problem. However, good carbohydrates, such as broccoli and Brussel sprouts, actually provide some of the missing saccharides, which help to repair the cells and reduce the insulin resistance.

Note: Recent research indicates that cells have a thin carbohydrate ("sugar") coating (glycocalyx) of glycoproteins and glycolipids that support cellular communications and the immune and endocrine systems.

Myth: It costs more to eat healthy foods.
Truth: It *does* cost more to eat healthy foods – in the short term. Fresh vegetables and fruits cost more than a box of macaroni and cheese. Sprouted-grain bread cost more than wheat bread. Organic brown rice cost more than white rice. However, as your health improves, you will **save money** with over-the-counter drugs, prescription drugs, doctor visits, physical exams, hospital stays, and the quantity of groceries.

Myth: Most people (including diabetics) do not like taking drugs.
Truth: Surprisingly, most people prefer to take drugs – in lieu of making changes to their lifestyle, nutrition, or exercise regimen. Most people will deny that they like taking drugs, but the facts show that more than 65% of the people in the United States take prescription and/or over-the-counter drugs; and, more than 60% take multiple drugs. This is due to our intolerance to personal pain and suffering – why suffer if there's a drug that will eliminate the pain? Also, there is the belief that the drugs are "working" because they do what they are advertised to do, e.g. reduce pain, lower blood pressure, lower blood glucose, lower cholesterol. It will require a major paradigm shift in our thinking to move away from drugs as the solution to our health problems.

Chapter 4. The Diabetes Control & Reversal Model

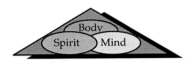

The Diabetes Wellness Program

This diabetes wellness program is an integrated body, mind and spirit strategy that enables the diabetic to turn on the body's internal healing mechanism by *avoiding* the processed foods such as white rice, potatoes, bread, pasta, cereals, snack foods, and sweets while eating more of the nutritious foods such as vegetables, fruits, fish, plant oils, beans, and nuts. These nutritious foods help to initiate a cleansing, detoxification and repair of trillions of defective cells to reduce the insulin resistance and inflammation. Vegetables, wheat/barley grass and raw vegetable juicing can accelerate the reduction of insulin resistance and inflammation; increase absorption of nutrients into the cells; strengthen the immune system; and, rebalance the body biochemically and hormonally. This eventually provides the diabetic with much needed energy to initiate and expand his/her exercise regimen, which also helps to cleanse and detoxify the body. The consistent consumption of nutritious foods with proper nutritional supplementation allows the entire body to begin a rejuvenation process to repair and rebuild itself. These nutritious foods enable the body to function in a harmonious manner; and, the body in turn operates in harmony with the mind, preventing depression and drug/medication overuse, two major problems with diabetics or anyone with a major disease.

A person who has been a Type 2 diabetic for several years eventually becomes a "walking pharmacy" because of the dependence and belief in drugs. First it's the diabetes, which brings its own set of drugs and side effects; then it's problems with the kidneys that bring another set of drugs and side effects. Then, it's problems with the eyes, the nerves, and the heart, each bringing its own set of drugs and side effects. This makes it very difficult for the body to fight back and try to heal itself because of all the drugs and their side effects. Consequently, the disease continues to spread the damage to other body organs, while the drugs suppress and "hide" the symptoms and give the diabetic a false belief that everything is getting better – but, the body continues to deteriorate ever so slowly and silently.

This diabetes wellness program guides you through six stages of recovery and repair. As you continue through each of the six stages, your body will rebalance itself biochemically, hormonally, emotionally and spiritually. How long will it take? The responses of individuals will obviously vary, but, as long as you wean your body off as many drugs as possible, the approximate timeline will be anywhere from 4 months to 18 months for most people. In extreme cases it may take longer, especially if you have been diabetic for several years and you have trillions of damaged cell membranes. Your degree of success will depend upon your level of knowledge and your commitment. But, in general, the timeline can be accelerated by leveraging one or more of the key "living" elements, e.g. nutrition, exercise, testing. Similarly, the timeline can be longer if you do not leverage these key elements, and, especially if your body is still handling different drugs that add to the body's inflammation and toxic load, inhibiting the healing process. Once you see how your body responds positively to the changes to nutrition, exercise, and testing, the easier it will be to estimate your personal timeline as you progress from one stage to the next.

This wellness program will require a personal accountability, instead of placing the blame for your health problems on your doctor, your family, or God. Consequently, the program empowers you to develop and maintain a positive attitude with life as well as an open mind to new ideas about health and nutrition. You become a *victor* of wellness instead of *victim* of disease and drugs.

Note: References to the term "diabetes" throughout this book are primarily associated with **Type 2 diabetes**.

The 8 "Living" Elements

There are eight major "living" elements, or activities, which must be managed to properly control (and possibly reverse) Type 2 diabetes. Most diabetics are aware of two of them – nutrition and exercise. The following is a complete list of the eight "living" elements:

- Nutrition
- Exercise
- Blood Glucose Testing
- Recordkeeping/Analysis
- Drugs/Medications
- Mind & Spirit
- Education
- Doctor Visits/Physical Exams

The following chapters will elaborate on the best practices and principles of these eight elements so that you can better manage and control your diabetes.

The Diabetes Control & Reversal Model

The foundation of this diabetes wellness program is a six-stage model that guides the diabetic through diabetes management, control and reversal.

Stage 1 No BG Control: is the stage where the majority of diabetics usually find themselves in the beginning, with an average fasting blood glucose (BG) level that is greater than 126 mg/dl or an oral glucose test measurement greater than 200 mg/dl.

Stage 2 BG Control with Drugs: is the stage where most diabetics transition to when they underestimate the disease and are unable to improve their cell health and control their blood glucose level with nutrition and exercise. During this stage the diabetic and his/her doctor are trying to use drugs to help lower the diabetic's blood glucose level and eventually bring it within the normal range.

Stage 3 BG Control with Reduced Drugs: is probably the most difficult stage for a diabetic to reach once he/she and the doctor have chosen to use drug therapy to lower the diabetic's blood glucose level and, hopefully, improve the health of the cells. It becomes a more difficult battle because the cells have to deal with the disease *and* the drugs, which bring along their own side effects and impedance to the body's healing process.

Stage 4 BG Control without Drugs: is the stage that some diabetics reach when they are able to control their blood glucose with nutrition and exercise (and no drugs). They are able to reduce the amount of insulin resistance and inflammation in their cells, enabling the cells to repair themselves. Unfortunately, many diabetics relax during this stage because they are not aware that there is still work to be done to actually reverse and eradicate the disease. As a result, they regress back to Stage 1 when their average glucose level eventually rises above 126 mg/dl and remains there.

Stage 5 BG & HbA1C Control: indicates that the average blood glucose level and hemoglobin A1C are both consistently within the normal range without the need for any drugs.

Stage 6 BG & HbA1C Tighter Control: indicates that the cells are healthy as the average blood glucose level and hemoglobin A1C are consistently within a tighter range without the need for any drugs; and, the disease is totally reversed – no insulin resistance and no inflammation. In addition, other critical health parameters are within their normal ranges, e.g. blood pressure, body mass index, minerals, enzymes, homocysteine, cholesterol.

Based upon the etiology of Type 2 diabetes, the analysis of its pathogenesis, and the sciences of disease, including pathophysiology, pathological anatomy, biochemistry, and psychopathology, the following diagram provides a high level overview of the six stages and the eight "living" elements of Type 2 diabetes control and reversal. This model is very flexible and can be customized to suit your health needs and lifestyle.

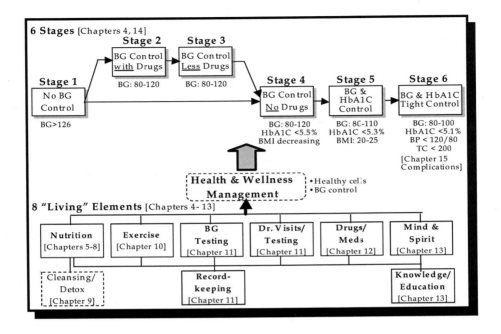

Figure 5. The Diabetes Control & Reversal Model

The next several chapters (Chapter 5 to Chapter 13) will provide more details about the eight "living" elements and how they can affect the health of your cells, your blood glucose control, and your appetite. Chapter 14 will provide details about each of the six stages and what you should be doing with each of these eight elements to progress from one stage to the next stage. These details will help you to better track your progress and determine what you need to do to get to the next stage. Chapter 15 will provide wellness protocols that address the long-term complications associated with diabetes, including kidney disease, eye disease, nerve disease, and heart disease. Chapter 15 will also address other complications, including high blood pressure, high cholesterol, and high homocysteine. For your convenience, in the above diagram, the chapter reference for each component of this model is shown in brackets.

Chapter 5. The Major Macronutrients

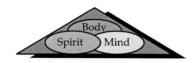

The 4 Macronutrients

Sometimes it is confusing trying to figure out how carbohydrates, proteins, fats, vitamins, minerals, fiber, calories and all of the other nutritional components fit into an overall eating plan or diet. The following sections will help to clear up some of that confusion.

There are four major macronutrients that the cells of your body require every time you eat — to maintain its balance biochemically and hormonally, to generate energy, to communicate with other cells, and to keep the body and mind healthy from disease. Coincidentally, there are four macronutrients that reside in every cell in the human body:

Carbohydrates, which come primarily from plants, e.g. land vegetables, fruits, grains, sea vegetables, other plant foods; and, from man-made processed foods, e.g. bread (flour), pasta, cereal.

Proteins, which come primarily from animals and plants, e.g. fish, nuts, seeds, beans, eggs, chicken, beef, turkey, vegetables.

Fats, which come primarily from animals and plants, e.g. olive oil, flaxseed, nuts, fish, meat, dairy; and, from man-made processed foods, e.g. margarine, potato chips, French fries, store-bought baked goods.

Liquids, which come primarily from plants and the earth, e.g. water, tea, raw juice; and, from man-made beverages, e.g., soda, coffee, bottled juice.

The following section provides an overview of each of these macronutrients, including some examples of each.

Carbohydrates

The primary purposes of carbohydrates are to provide energy, enhance immune function, and support cellular communications. Carbohydrates are converted into energy so that cells can function and do their jobs effectively. Carbohydrates also help cells to communicate with each other, and help to modulate the immune system (for protection) and the endocrine system (for hormonal balance).

There are two major types of carbohydrates:
Complex carbohydrates (oligosaccharides, polysaccharides): are found in large chains of saccharide molecules in plant foods, e.g. land/sea vegetables, fruits, whole grains. They take more time to metabolize, providing a steady release of glucose into the bloodstream and a sustained level of energy throughout the day (from meal to meal).

Simple carbohydrates (monosaccharides, disaccharides): include glucose, mannose, galactose, fucose, xylose; and maltose, lactose, sucrose. They support immediate energy production by metabolizing very quickly in the bloodstream.

Note: Recent research has identified eight *essential* monosaccharides (glyconutrients) that are the building blocks for chains of saccharide molecules, or glycans. They combine with proteins and fats to create glycoforms, the structures on cell surfaces that cells use to communicate with each other. These saccharides, which support the immune and endocrine systems, include: mannose, glucose, galactose, xylose, fucose, N-acetylglucosamine, N-acetylgalactosamine, and N-acetylneuraminic acid. The primary sources of these saccharides (glyconutrients) are mushrooms, fungi, seaweed, aloe vera, saps, gums, herbs, and seeds; the secondary sources are vegetables, fruits, legumes, and grains.

Calorie Size of a Carbohydrate:

Every gram of a carbohydrate provides 4 calories of energy. For example, an apple contains about 25 grams of carbohydrates, which is equal to about 100 calories. But, don't forget that an apple does have about 1 gram of plant protein, so the total calories of an apple are 104 (100 + 4).

Proteins

The primary purposes of proteins are to provide the building blocks to produce new tissue, and to repair damaged skin, bones and muscles. Proteins create the antibodies that help fight off disease and the hormones that regulate various functions in the body. Proteins also help to control the release of glucagon, which stimulates the release of glycogen when the blood glucose level falls too low. Proteins help to maintain the body's acid-alkaline (pH) balance and regulate the amount of fluid in the cells by balancing the potassium and sodium levels.

Proteins are made of building blocks called amino acids. Amino acids are involved in muscle and bone growth, tissue repair, energy production, and the formation of the brain's neurotransmitters. There are 25 amino acids in the body, 8 *essential* and 17 non-essential. The 8 essential amino acids must be obtained from food: isoleucine, leucine, lysine, methionine, phenylalanine, threonine, tryptophan and valine. Meat, poultry, fish, milk, eggs and cheese are considered complete sources of protein because they contain these eight essential amino acids. The other 17 are called nonessential because the body can make them: alanine, arginine, aspartic acid, carnitine, cysteine, gamma-aminobutyric acid, glutamine, glutathione, glycine, histidine, homocysteine, hydroxyproline, ornithine, proline, serine, taurine, and tyrosine.

The human body builds over 50,000 known proteins and over 15,000 enzymes from the amino acids, including digestive and metabolic enzymes. All enzymes are made from the amino acids, sometimes with vitamins acting as coenzymes and sometimes with mineral activators. Amino acids play a key role in normalizing moods, attention, concentration, aggression, sex drive, and sleep. When a person eats protein, the body must break it down into the individual amino acids before it can use them in specific metabolic pathways. A lack of amino acids can be followed by an inability to produce the digestive enzymes that are necessary to break down protein into it's component amino acids. This can lead to a cycle of poor nutrition because the body needs amino acids in order to get amino acids from the food that is eaten.

There are four major types of protein:
Plant/Non-animal: nuts, seeds, beans, lentils, whole soy foods (tofu, tempeh, miso), blue-green algae (e.g. spirulina, chlorella); sea vegetables, land vegetables; and grains (amaranth, quinoa).

Sea animals: fish (e.g. wild salmon, tuna, sardines, mackerel, trout) and seafood (e.g. shrimp, lobster, crab).

Land animals (Meat): beef, chicken, turkey, pork, lamb, and wild game (deer, bear).

Land animals (Dairy): yogurt; cow's milk, cow's cheese, raw milk; eggs, organic eggs from free-range chickens; and goat's milk, goat's cheese.

Note: The above food sources (except for the soy products and some of the plant products) provide complete proteins. The egg is considered the perfect protein food because it contains all the amino acids and is very easy to digest.

Calorie Size of a Protein:
Every gram of a protein provides the same number of calories as a carbohydrate - 4 calories of energy. For example, one egg contains about 6 grams of protein, which is equal to about 24 calories. But, don't forget that the egg has about 0.5 grams of carbohydrates and about 5 grams of fat, so the total calories of an egg are 71 (24 + 2 + 45).

Fats

The primary purposes of fats are to form cell membranes, keep cell walls supple, cushion your organs and protect you from temperature extremes. Fats help to slow down the absorption of carbohydrates, trigger the feeling of "fullness" when you eat, and keep your skin and hair healthy.

There are four major types of fats:
Monounsaturated fats: are mainly found in foods that come from plants and are liquid at room temperature. They include olive oil, hazelnuts, almonds, Brazil nuts, avocado, cashews, sesame seeds, pumpkin seeds, and walnuts.

Polyunsaturated fats: come mainly from plants and are liquid at room temperature, and contain Omega-3 and Omega-6 *essential* fatty acids (EFAs). Omega-3 EFAs include alpha linolenic acid (ALA), eicosa-pentaenoic acid (EPA) and docosahexaenoic acid (DHA). Plant oils such as flaxseed contain ALA. Marine oil (from crustaceans) and fish oil from wild salmon contain EPA and DHA. Polyunsaturates that are rich in Omega-3 EFAs include flax oil, hemp oil, pumpkin seeds, walnuts and oily fish, such as wild salmon, sardines, mackerel, trout and herring. Omega-6 EFAs include linoleic acid (LNA), gamma linolenic acid (GLA), and arachidonic acid (AA). Polyunsaturates that are rich in Omega-6 EFAs include evening primrose oil (EPO), borage oil and black current seed oil.

Saturated fats: are a major part of the phospholipid component of cell membranes. They are also a major component of healthy cells, the preferred fuel for the heart and muscles, and serve as cancer-fighting genetic "regulators" in the body. Unfortunately, when animals are fed corn, growth hormones and antibiotics, this compromises the saturated fats. However, saturated fats from animals that are wild or grass-fed and are not given growth hormones or antibiotics are much healthier. Saturated fats are found mostly in animal products and are solid at room temperature. They include meat and dairy (milk, cheese). Saturated fat is also found in tropical oils such as coconut and palm oils.

Trans fats: are man-made and reside in various processed foods including margarine, French fries, potato chips, pretzels, fried foods, and store-bought cookies, pies and cakes. Trans fats, or "partially hydrogenated oils", were originally created to prolong the shelf life of packaged foods.

Calorie Size of Fats:
Fats are the most concentrated source of energy for your body, providing 9 calories per gram versus 4 calories per gram for carbohydrates and protein. For example, a tablespoon of olive oil contains about 14 grams of fat, which is equal to about 126 calories.

Liquids

Liquids are important because they help to hydrate the cells and digest the solid foods that we consume. Most liquids such as canned juice, lemonade, tea and raw juice are actually carbohydrates but they all contain the most critical nutrient that we sometimes overlook – water. Water is the one macronutrient that your body requires more than any other macronutrient, especially since the human body is more than 72% water and the blood is 90% water.

Because the body loses about 3 quarts of water each day, the body must be in a continuous state of proper hydration. To accomplish this, the water must be of a high enough quality such that it can help remove the toxins and pollutants that accumulate in the body. In addition, since water is involved in every function in the body, it must act as a conductor of electrochemical activity, such as neurotransmission, by moving water from one nerve cell to another smoothly and effectively. This movement is created by magnetic forces in the body, which keep the movement in balance. As water flows, changes in pressure create movement across the cell membranes. Any changes in pressure will allow proteins, minerals and other nutrients being carried by the blood to escape into spaces between vessels and deprive the cells of these vital nutrients to sustain life. When water in the blood is contaminated with chemicals from the food and environment, it enters the cells and changes their structure, which in turn could lead to changes in DNA and the start of the disease process.

There is a direct connection between the quality and content of the water in the body and how the body responds to disease, especially since many people are dehydrated. The percentage of water in the body decreases with age from a high of 70% to as low as 50%. This is due to an increase in fat, a decrease in muscle tissue, and a decrease in the body's ability to regulate the balance of sodium and water caused by a decrease in kidney function. Consequently, it is even more important to consume quality water and foods that contain quality water on a daily basis.

There are several types of liquids:

Filtered water: helps to optimize the hydration of your cells, and acts as the transport medium for nutrients and waste.

Bottled water: is a form of filtered water, but some of the bottled water contains contaminants due to poor filtering and the breakdown of the plastic container, leaking PCBs into the water.

Tap water: contains heavy metals, chemicals, bacteria, waste and other contaminants that may be detrimental to your health in the long term.

Raw juice: can be extracted from fresh raw vegetables, wheat/barley grasses and fruits to provide vital nutrients including filtered water.

Blended juice: can be obtained by mixing fresh or frozen vegetables/ fruits in a blender to provide vital nutrients including fiber.

Tea: includes green tea, white tea, hibiscus tea and other herbal teas that contain antioxidants and other phytonutrients.

Processed juices: include bottled and canned juices, which contain a lot of sugar and high fructose corn syrup, and are stripped of their vital nutrients.

Other beverages: include soda, diet soda, and coffee, etc.

Note: Since most of these liquids (beverages) are classified as simple carbohydrates, their caloric value must be accounted for as part of the meal's total calorie count.

Calorie Size of Liquids:

Water provides zero (0) calories, but other liquids, which are primarily carbohydrates, provide 4 calories per gram. For example, a cup of apple juice contains about 29 grams of carbohydrates, 0.2 grams of protein, and 0.3 grams of fat, which is equal to about 120 calories (116 + 0.8 + 2.7). This is a major oversight by some diabetics who fail to count the carbohydrate calories from their beverages and other drinks.

Chapter 6. The 5 "Live" & 5 "Dead" Foods

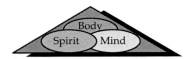

The 7 Nutrient Factors

Now that you know there are four macronutrients (carbohydrates, proteins, fats, liquids), how do you determine which macronutrients are the healthier ones? Based on numerous nutrition-based studies, there are seven (7) critical nutrient factors that promote optimum health and help to determine whether a specific macronutrient will be beneficial to your health. The seven critical nutrient factors are: vitamins, minerals, antioxidants, fiber, enzymes, oils, and water.

- **Vitamins:** provide specific micronutrients to protect, cleanse and nourish the cells, tissues and organs, and to help metabolize foods. Examples of vitamins: Vitamin A, Vitamin B-complex, Vitamin D.
- **Minerals:** provide specific micronutrients to support various biological functions including the growth of bones and teeth, muscle contraction, blood pressure, nerve transmission, blood formation, energy production, fluid regulation, macronutrient metabolism, acid-alkaline balance (pH), and various other enzymatic reactions. Examples: calcium, potassium, magnesium, chromium, vanadium.
- **Antioxidants:** provide protection from cancer cells, free radicals and oxidation. Examples: Vitamin C, Vitamin E, selenium, beta-carotene, CoQ10, indole-3-carbinol.
- **Enzymes:** help to digest, assimilate and metabolize foods to provide fuel and energy. Metabolic enzymes are made by the body to cause chemical reactions that keep the body operating and performing necessary functions. Digestive enzymes are provided by the body to help digest, absorb and utilize the nutrients from food. Food enzymes (within raw food) help to digest carbohydrates (amylase), protein (protease), fat (lipase), and fiber (cellulase).

- **Fiber:** helps to cleanse and detoxify the body by removing waste, cholesterol and toxins. Examples: pectin, psyllium, bran, plant sterols.
- **Oils:** help to lubricate the tissues, arteries, joints, skin and other organs. Examples: olive oil, flax oil, fish oil.
- **Water:** provides hydration to cells and acts as a transport to carry other nutrients to the cells, tissues, and organs.

Healthy/Unhealthy Macronutrients

Given the importance of these seven nutrient factors, it would follow that a healthy carbohydrate, protein or fat will contain most or all of these seven nutrient factors. Similarly, an unhealthy carbohydrate, protein or fat will not contain most of these seven nutrient factors. For those of you who are knowledgeable in nutritional science, there shouldn't be any surprises with the following definitions of healthy and unhealthy macronutrients. All I've done is "quantify" whether a macronutrient is healthy or unhealthy based upon the number of nutrient factors contained within that macronutrient.

Healthy/Unhealthy Carbohydrates

Specifically, colorful vegetables, fruits, and other plant foods (e.g. spinach, blueberries, mushrooms) qualify as healthy carbohydrates because they contain most or all of the seven nutrient factors. Some whole grains (e.g. oat, amaranth) qualify as healthy carbohydrates because they contain most of the seven nutrient factors: vitamins, minerals, fiber, antioxidants, and enzymes. These healthy carbohydrates satisfy the major objectives of nutritious food, namely to nourish, protect, and cleanse the body. These carbs also help the cells to communicate with each other.

Processed foods and junk food qualify as unhealthy carbohydrates because they lack most of the seven nutrient factors and they cause your blood glucose level to rise leading to insulin spikes, a depletion of vitamins/minerals, inflammation, and a weakened immune system. In addition, these foods do not satisfy the three major objectives of nutritious food. Processed foods and junk food include bottled juice, potato chips, cookies, crackers, donuts, soda, jellies, ketchup, snacks, white rice, potatoes, bread, pasta, and other flour-based products.

Healthy/Unhealthy Proteins

Nuts, seeds, beans, fish, organic eggs, and some whole soy products qualify as healthy proteins because they contain at least four of the nutrient factors; and, do not contain an excess amount of saturated fat. Organic dairy, grass-fed, lean animal meat, and wild animal meat qualify as healthy proteins because they contain at least four of the nutrient factors and do not contain the growth hormones, antibiotics and excess saturated fat that conventional meat and dairy products contain.

Corn-fed animal meat and eggs from animals raised with antibiotics and growth hormones/steroids and processed soy qualify as unhealthy proteins because they lack most of the seven nutrient factors. These foods can cause an increase in the production of homocysteine, cholesterol, and stress hormones in the body, leading to inflammation, clogged arteries, increased fat production, a strain on the kidneys, cancerous tissues, lack of cell energy, and a weakened immune system.

Healthy/Unhealthy Fats

Monounsaturated fat found in extra virgin olive oil and almonds qualifies as a healthy fat because it helps to lubricate the artery walls and the various joints in the body and prevent inflammation. Monounsaturated fat is high in Vitamin E and helps to lower inflammation, oxidation and cholesterol and offer protection against certain cancers.

Some polyunsaturated fats found in fish oil, flax oil and walnuts qualify as healthy fats because they contain one or more of the three major Omega-3 essential fatty acids (EFAs): alpha linolenic acid (ALA), eicosapentaenoic acid (EPA), and docosahexaenoic acid (DHA). These Omega-3 EFAs help regulate the body's blood sugar level, prevent the increase and spread of internal inflammation, raise the body's metabolic rate, and thin the blood to reduce the danger of blood clotting, high blood pressure, strokes and heart attacks.

Trans fats, some of the saturated fats from animals, and some of the polyunsaturated fats that contain Omega-6 EFAs qualify as unhealthy fats. The trans fats reside in various processed foods including margarine, French fries, potato chips, cookies, and fried foods. The unhealthy saturated fats are found mostly in animals that are corn-fed and given growth hormones and antibiotics; and, include processed meats such as hot dogs, bologna, and lunch meats. Other unhealthy saturated fats are found in processed tropical oils such as refined coconut and palm oils, which are found mostly in store-bought cookies, cakes, and snack foods. The Omega-6 polyunsaturated fats are found in vegetables oils such as soy, corn, sunflower, safflower, and cottonseed; and, some are found in processed meats. These foods can cause an increase in the production of homocysteine, cholesterol, and stress hormones in the body, leading to inefficient insulin utilization, inflammation, clogged arteries, increased fat production, cancerous tissues, lack of cell energy, and a weakened immune system.

Using these definitions of "healthy" and "unhealthy" macronutrients based on the number of nutrient factors as a guideline, all foods can be grouped into two major categories:
- "Dead" food
- "Live" food

These terms may sound a little melodramatic, but I believe that they get the point across without having to explain the rationale of each term in detail. In addition, I found these terms to be very effective in making specific points during my presentations. Also, these terms tie nicely into the book's title and the photograph on the front cover.

"Dead" food inhibits the body from healing and leads to disease and early *death*. "Dead" food is man-made, processed food that lacks most of the seven nutrient factors. Coincidentally, these foods, along with a sedentary lifestyle, are connected with the development of many of the major systemic diseases such as heart disease, diabetes and cancer.

"Live" (pronounced līv e) **food** helps the body to heal, fight disease and stay *alive*. "Live" foods are primarily raw, unprocessed, lightly-cooked or partially processed foods that contain most of the seven nutrient factors. The term "live" does not necessarily mean that the *food* is alive, but it does contain the nutrients that keep the body *alive*. Coincidentally, these foods are connected with the prevention and reversal of many of the major systemic diseases and ailments.

The 5 "Dead" Foods

There are five major "dead" foods. When consumed in excess with a sedentary lifestyle, these processed foods turn the body acidic, cause inflammation, and slowly damage or kill the body's cells and create neurochemical imbalances that trigger unhealthy food cravings. These chemical imbalances, in turn, devastate your health physically, biochemically, hormonally, emotionally and spiritually. Over a period of years, this leads to systemic ailments/diseases such as high blood pressure, diabetes, heart disease, and cancer. The five "dead" foods include most food products that contain refined sugar, high fructose corn syrup, refined flour, trans fats, saturated fat, alcohol, caffeine, nicotine, and other harmful chemicals.

1: Refined white sugar includes all foods made with high fructose corn syrup, corn syrup, refined sugar, sucrose, maltose, dextrose, molasses, brown sugar, artificial sweeteners, and processed honey as well as foods/beverages such as soda, diet soda, bottled juice, soft drinks, candy, jams, jellies, cookies, cakes, pies, some cereals, and some condiments.

Health impact: These refined carbohydrates are high glycemic foods that cause your blood glucose level to rise, triggering food cravings and insulin surges that lead to fat production, inflammation, depletion of vitamins/minerals, low energy and a weakening of your immune system. Many of these processed foods contain high fructose corn syrup (HFCS), which is more dangerous than refined sugar because HFCS increases hunger cravings and fat production. This can lead to systemic diseases such as diabetes, heart disease, cancer, arthritis, Alzheimer's and osteoporosis. Although artificial sweeteners and sugar-free foods do not contain the refined sugar and calories, their chemical makeup can increase the tendency to overeat and damage the nervous system.

2: Refined white flour includes all foods made with refined flour or starch such as white bread, enriched bread, white pasta, white rice, macaroni, cereals, crackers, donuts, pancakes, pastries, biscuits, spaghetti, cakes, pies, and other processed foods; and, starchy vegetables such as white potatoes and corn.

Health impact: These refined carbohydrates are also high glycemic foods that cause your blood glucose level to rise, triggering food cravings and insulin surges that lead to fat production, inflammation, depletion of vitamins/minerals, and low energy. And, the increased production of serotonin (and tryptophan) provides a false sense of well being and security. Bleaching agents produce a chemical called alloxan, which makes white flour look "clean", but alloxan may damage the pancreatic beta cells in some people, reducing their production of insulin. You can minimize the negative effects to your health by eating the organic whole grain, high fiber version of these foods. Many of these processed foods contain a lot of nutrient-poor chemicals, which are linked to other systemic diseases such as heart disease, cancer, arthritis, Alzheimer's and osteoporosis. However, if you have multiple health issues, it may be necessary to temporarily stop eating all flour, starchy vegetables, grains and grain-based foods (especially wheat). This is due to the embedded chemicals and toxins in these foods that may be compromising your immune system and desensitizing the insulin receptors of your cells. However, once your body has cleansed and detoxified itself and begun to heal, you can gradually re-introduce healthier versions of these foods during the latter stages of your recovery.

3: Trans fats include all processed foods made with hydrogenated oil, such as stick margarines, French fries, potato chips, pretzels, cookies, fried foods, donuts, crackers, store-bought baked goods, and packaged foods. The process of creating hydrogenated oil destroys the essential fatty acids in the oil and replaces them with deformed trans fatty acids.

Health impact: Trans fats are shaped differently from their original form, creating deficiencies and imbalances throughout the metabolism, including fatty deposits in the arteries. It is believed that trans fats in the nerve cell membranes don't fit as well as the normal Omega-3 fats, so they cause the nerve cells to communicate less efficiently and the brain cannot function optimally. Trans fats in processed foods also promote heart disease, cancer, and other degenerative diseases. These processed foods lead to fat production, inflammation, clogging of the arteries, and damaged cells (DNA structure). These foods also prevent your body from burning fat and effectively utilizing insulin as this synthetic fat clogs your insulin receptors. Many of these processed foods are linked to other systemic diseases such as arthritis, Alzheimer's and osteoporosis. Stick margarines contain more trans fats than the soft versions that come in a tub; and, some of the soft margarines now contain no trans fats. But, be wary of some margarines and processed foods that claim that they contain "no trans fat" – check the list of ingredients to be certain there is no partially hydrogenated oil.

Foods such as French fries are a "triple-killer" because (1) they contain starchy potatoes, which behave just like refined sugar and raise your insulin level; (2) they contain trans fats; and (3) they contain acrylamide, a proven carcinogen (cancer-causing agent). Acrylamide is formed when refined carbohydrates such as potatoes and cereals are cooked beyond 250 degrees Fahrenheit. Acrylamide levels are highest in potato and cereal-based products subjected to heat processing such as frying, grilling, or baking.

4: Saturated fats, which are solid at room temperature, are found in animal meat, organ meats, processed meats, lunch meats, fried foods and some dairy products (cow's pasteurized, homogenized milk, cheese, butter, ice cream). These fats contain arachidonic acid, which is found in the fat and muscle tissues of animals. Arachidonic acid is essential for your health, but it can be destructive at high levels, leading to inflammation and heart disease. Saturated fats are also found in coconut oil, palm oil and other tropical oils. Some of the Omega-6 poly-unsaturated fats in vegetable oils such as soybean, corn, sunflower and safflower can also be destructive to your health.

Health impact: Excess consumption of saturated fats can lead to inflammation, excess fat production, increased leptin production (loss of appetite control), clogging of the arteries, cancerous tissues, and reduced insulin utilization. Conventional animal meat is obtained from animals such as cows that are fed corn, and chickens that are fed soybeans and grain. These animals are given growth hormones, antibiotics and other chemicals, which collect in their muscle and fatty tissues and produce antibiotic-resistant bacteria – all of which are passed onto us when we consume these meats on a regular basis. Virtually all packaged meat products including bologna, hot dogs, pepperoni, salami, ham, spam, lunchmeat, bacon, sausages and most breakfast meats contain mostly saturated fat and the preservative sodium nitrate, which is known to cause seizures and cancer.

Milk in its natural form is very nutritious, but many of the nutrients are destroyed by homogenization and pasteurization. As we get older, our body produces less of the lactase enzyme (to break down the milk sugar, lactose), making milk difficult to digest. This can make milk problematic, because it can prevent the proper absorption of nutrients into the blood and restrict the elimination of the toxic waste from the blood, leading to the formation of mucous, congestion, colds, and allergies. Milk contains a white, tasteless, odorless protein called casein, which is the principal protein of cow's milk and is the curd that forms when milk is left to sour. It is the basis of cheese and is used to make strong wood glue, plastics, adhesives, paints, and certain processed foods. You can minimize, but not completely avoid, the negative effects to your health by drinking raw milk or goat's milk; or, by eating low fat cheeses, leaner meats or organic meats from cows and chickens that are fed grass on a free range. These saturated fats are a major component of healthy cell membranes and fuel for the heart and muscles.

Polyunsaturated vegetable oils such as corn oil and sunflower oil should be avoided and definitely should not be heated because they break down easily, becoming rancid, producing carcinogens, and causing excess inflammation. These oils do not raise your total cholesterol, but they may lower the good cholesterol lipid, known as high-density lipoprotein (HDL) and cause inflammation that can lead to heart disease.

However, **extra virgin coconut oil** is actually a *healthy* saturated fat because it contains the healthy form of saturated fat that is very stable, the medium chain fatty acids. Therefore, virgin coconut oil is the best oil for sautéing, cooking and frying. The healthy medium chain fatty acids in coconut oil do not circulate in the bloodstream like other fats, but are sent directly to the liver where they are immediately converted into energy, just like carbohydrates. Therefore, the body uses the fat in coconut oil to produce energy, rather than be stored as body fat.

5: Drugs include alcohol, tobacco, caffeine, over-the-counter (OTC) drugs, prescription drugs, and recreational drugs.

Health impact: Alcohol and tobacco devastate the liver, lungs and cardiovascular system causing cancer, heart disease and other diseases. Caffeine is a stimulant that may trigger insulin surges. Excess caffeine may cause the body to produce an oxidative chemical called alloxan that may damage the pancreatic beta cells in some people, reducing their production of insulin. Many OTC and prescription drugs cause serious side effects that can lead to liver, kidney or heart failure. Long term use of most diabetic drugs overworks the pancreas, which usually leads to insulin injections and reduced production of insulin by the pancreas, leading to a **lifetime dependence on insulin injections**! Also, these drugs "fool" the body by altering the biochemical and hormonal functions within the body, leading to **chemical dependencies** and the suppression of symptoms that later manifest themselves as a disease.

Many "dead" processed foods are easy to recognize because they contain one or more of the following harmful chemicals: high fructose corn syrup (HFCS), hydrogenated oil, MSG, sodium nitrate, or inorganic sodium. These food chemicals cause the body to expend a lot of energy to "break down" the food, producing excess waste and toxins. Also, these chemicals cause inflammation and prevent the proper utilization of insulin and the uptake of glucose into the cells.

- HFCS, a by-product of corn processing, was discovered to cause diabetes in animals, but it is a common ingredient in many processed foods, including unsuspecting foods such as ketchup, relish, yogurt, jelly, some cereals, fruit juices, and applesauce.
- Hydrogenated oil is a synthetic fat that is not easily metabolized and tends to clog the insulin receptors of the cells, leading to a decrease in insulin sensitivity.
- Monosodium glutamate (MSG) is an excitotoxin that overexcites your cells to the point of damage, acting as a poison. MSG can be hidden in food labels, e.g. hydrolyzed vegetable protein, gelatin, yeast extract, malted barley, broth, casein, rice syrup
- Sodium nitrate is used to preserve processed meats, and inorganic sodium is used to preserve processed foods in cans and packages.

Note: The food manufacturers manipulate the sugar, fat, and salt in their foods to ensure that the consumer will still like the taste of their foods.

The 5 "Live" Foods

There are five major "live" super foods. When consumed on a regular basis, these foods create a biochemical/hormonal balance that reduces insulin production, controls appetite, nourishes the cells, strengthens the immune system, prevents inflammation, and helps to heal the body physically, biochemically, hormonally, emotionally and spiritually. The five "live" super foods include vegetables/fruits, filtered water, lean protein, monounsaturated/Omega-3 fats, and organic whole grains. For those familiar with proper nutrition, there should be no surprises here.

1: Vegetables/Fruits, Other Plants include bright-colored, tasty foods that are full of critical nutrients. *Vegetables* include green/leafy vegetables such as spinach, broccoli, Brussel sprouts, bok choi, kale, romaine lettuce; asparagus, cabbage, cauliflower, celery, cucumbers, okra, peppers, stringbeans, other greens (collard, turnip); sea vegetables such as chlorella and sea plankton; and, grasses such as wheat, barley, alfalfa; and, fermented foods such as sauerkraut. Vegetables of other bright colors (green, red, yellow, purple, orange) include artichokes, avocado, bean sprouts, beets, carrots, chickpeas, mushrooms, parsley, peppers, sweet potatoes, tomatoes, and zucchini. *Fruits* include dark, bright colored fruits such as açai berries, blackberries, blueberries, cherries, cranberries, elderberries, strawberries, apples, grapes, and goji berries; plus, apricots, avocado, figs, grapefruits, kiwi, lemons, limes, mangosteens, melons, papaya, peaches, pears, plums, pomegranates, prunes, and raspberries.

Health impact: Green, leafy vegetables such as spinach, asparagus, broccoli, Brussel sprouts, cabbage, string beans, and celery contain fiber which slows down their absorption helping to delay the emptying of the stomach and thereby smoothing out the absorption of sugars into the blood. Avocado is an excellent fruit for diabetics because it contains monounsaturated fat, magnesium, potassium, folate, antioxidants such as Vitamin E, and fiber, which helps to remove cholesterol from the blood and improve bowel regularity and the health of the colon. Fruits such as apples, berries, cherries, grapefruit, and pears also contain fiber to help slow down the absorption of the sugar.

In addition to the high levels of *fiber*, these vegetables and fruits contain *water, antioxidants, protein, enzymes, vitamins, minerals* and specific *saccharides* that help nourish, protect and cleanse the body; and, support cell-to-cell communications. Specifically, vegetables and fruits contain pigment-related phytonutrients called *polyphenols, flavonoids* and *carotenoids* that promote cardiovascular health. Polyphenols are in the deeper-colored plant foods such as blueberries, strawberries, grapes, and green tea. Flavonoids can be found in blueberries, cranberries, currants, teas and olives. Carotenoids can be found in orange and yellow foods such as cantaloupe, mangos, carrots and sweet potatoes.

Some of these specific phytonutrients include the *neoxanthin* carotenoid and *chlorophyll* (in green, leafy vegetables such as spinach, arugula, Swiss chard, collards and kale); *lycopene* carotenoid (in red foods such as tomatoes and watermelon); *anthocyanins* (in blue and purple foods such as blueberries, grapes, plums, beets and cherries); *allicin* (in white foods such as garlic, mushrooms, onions, bananas, and white fleshed, peaches and nectarines); *capsanthin* carotenoid (in red foods such as paprika, red bell peppers, and red chili peppers); *alpha/beta carotene* (in orange foods such as pumpkin, carrots, sweet potatoes, apricots and mangoes); *beta-cryptoxanthin* carotenoid (in orange-yellow foods such as oranges and tangerines); *hesperetin* flavonoid (in citrus fruits such as grapefruit, lemons and oranges); *indole glucosinolate* (in cruciferous vegetables such as cabbage, broccoli and Brussel sprouts); *lutein* carotenoid (in yellow-green foods such as kale, spinach, parsley, avocados, peas, carrots and squash); *quercetin* flavonoid (in onions, blueberries, elderberries and raisins); and, the polyphenols *ellagic acid* and *tannins* in pomegranates, cranberries, blueberries and green tea.

It is well known that the *chlorophyll* in wheat grass and vegetables detoxifies carcinogens found in cooked muscle meats or barbecued foods. Chlorophyll has also been recognized for its anti-inflammatory, anti-mutagenic, and antioxidant properties. Chlorophyll has been cited as strengthening the immune response; therapeutic for inflammation of the ear and the mucous membrane of the nose and sinuses; supportive of normal kidney function; accelerating wound and ulcer healing; and reducing fecal, urinary and body odor in geriatric patients. This makes chlorophyll very beneficial to diabetics.

Vegetables and fruits also contain *Vitamin C, potassium, magnesium, folic acid*, and *enzymes* that are beneficial to diabetics. These nutrients help to prevent inflammation and fight diseases such as cancer and heart disease by preventing/killing cancer cells, breaking down homocysteine to prevent plaque buildup, and relaxing the artery walls to prevent high blood pressure. Vegetables and fruits contain soluble fiber, which has a lowering effect on blood glucose and cholesterol levels.

Vegetables such as broccoli, Brussel sprouts, cauliflower, cabbage, and kale of the cruciferous (cabbage) family contain *Indole-3-carbinol (I3C)* and *Diindolylmethane (DIM)*, phytonutrients that have been found to provide protection from certain cancers. Indole-3-carbinol is a member of the class of sulfur-containing chemicals called glucosinolates that is formed from parent compounds whenever cruciferous vegetables are crushed or cooked. Indole-3-carbinol and other glucosinolates (e.g. sulforaphane) are antioxidants and potent stimulators of natural detoxifying enzymes in the body. Indole-3-carbinol and other glucosinolates are believed to be responsible for the lowered risk of cancer by increasing the conversion of the bad estrogen (estradiol) to a weaker estrogen (estrone), protecting against breast and prostate cancers. Diindolylmethane (DIM) improves the breakdown and synthesis of substances in the body by improving the balance of testosterone and estrogen (estradiol). One of the many glucosinolates, *sulforaphane*, found in broccoli, protects the body against colon cancer. Interestingly, the bioavailability of indoles is increased by light cooking (e.g. steaming).

Vegetables such as garlic, onion, leek, asparagus, shallots, chive and scallions are members of the allium family that contain *thiosulfonates*, which are known to promote a more favorable HDL-LDL ratio, less inflammation, lower blood pressure and increase immunity. But they have also been found to provide protection from certain cancers. Like their cruciferous cousins, when thiosulfonates are cut or smashed, the sulfur compounds release biotransformation products, including *allicin, ajoene, allylic sulfides, vinyl dithin* and *D-allyl mercaptocysteine*. Some of these are considered anti-atherosclerotic, antioxidant, or anti-cancer agents, while others are antibacterial, antiviral, antifungal, and an inhibitor of platelet aggregation. As a result, all of these foods are very beneficial to diabetics.

Vegetables such as spinach and rhubarb and fruits such as apricots and apples contain organic acids that act primarily as antioxidants, cancer preventives, liver protectors and inflammatory mediators. The acids include oxalic in spinach, rhubarb, tea and coffee; tartaric in apricots and apples; cinnamic in aloe and cinnamon; caffeic in burdock and hawthorn; ferulic in oats and rice; gallic in tea, coumaric in turmeric; salicylic in spearmint; and tannic in nettles, tea and berries.

Fruits such as lemons, limes, and grapefruit are very beneficial to diabetics because they alkalize the body and reduce the acidity from the excess sugar, and they contain a lot less sugar than other fruits. These tart fruits contain *Vitamin C, bioflavonoids, water,* and *other phytonutrients* that help to maintain the body's defenses, and provide cholesterol-lowering and anti-cancer benefits. For example, lemons contain high levels of *Vitamin C* and *limonoid/limonene phytonutrients* that help to lower cholesterol levels and provide anti-cancer benefits. Lemon is also very effective for strengthening the gums and teeth, and preventing and curing acute inflammations of the gum margins, pyorrhea, and other oral diseases. Since these phytonutrients are found in the whole lemon, pith and peel included, it is best to make use of the whole lemon. Though the lemon juice is sour in taste, its reaction in the body is alkaline and as such it is valuable in the treatment of gout, rheumatism, sciatica, lumbago, and the pain in hip joints, which result from too much acid in the body. A sufficient intake of lemon juice prevents the deposit of uric acid in the tissues and thus reduces the possibility of an attack of gout. Grapefruit contains the *flavonoid narigenin,* which is believed to reduce the risk of some cancers. Grapefruit can improve blood circulation and lower blood cholesterol levels. Research has shown that grapefruit seed extract (rich in citrus bioflavonoids) is effective against some intestinal pathogens such as Candida albicans and other candida species (fungi), some E. coli (bacteria) species and Staphylococcus aureus (bacteria). It is effective as part of the natural treatment of constipation, flatulence and abdominal discomfort, as well as for bladder infections, thrush and vaginal candida infection. *However,* grapefruit juice increases the availability of some drugs in the body, causing potentially dangerous side effects. These included heart rhythm disturbances, impaired kidney function, blood pressure changes and anemia. So, if you are taking any drugs, always consult with your doctor before eating grapefruit.

Fruits such as açai berries, blackberries, blueberries, pomegranates, apples, grapes, cherries, plums and other berries contain *Vitamin C, bioflavonoids, carotenoids* and *other phytonutrients* that strengthen the immune system, prevent inflammation and provide protection from some cancers and cardiovascular disease. For example, raspberries, strawberries, cranberries, walnuts, pecans, pomegranates, and other plant foods contain ellagic acid. Ellagic acid may inhibit the growth of tumors caused by certain carcinogens by triggering apoptosis (cell death) in cancer cells, preventing the binding of carcinogens to DNA, and strengthening connective tissue, which may keep cancer cells from spreading.

Some vegetables and fruits such as grapefruit, apples, oranges, broccoli and Brussels sprouts contain *calcium d-glucarate*, a botanical extract that appears to protect against cancer and other diseases via a different mechanism than antioxidants such as Vitamin C and the carotenoids. These vitamin antioxidants work by neutralizing toxic free radical damage in the body. However, calcium d-glucarate works by using a detoxification process to combine toxins or carcinogens with water-soluble substances and removing them from the body. Early animal studies indicate that calcium d-glucarate may inhibit the production of the bad estrogen associated with prostate and breast cancers.

Medicinal mushrooms (such as shiitake and maitake) and other plant foods (such as aloe vera and fenugreek) contain some of the *essential monosaccharides* that help to support cell-to-cell communication and strengthen the immune system. This is very beneficial to a diabetic, whose immune system is weakened by the high glucose levels.

Note: These essential monosaccharides can also be obtained from a food-based glyconutrient (powder) supplement, but be wary of some of these glyconutrient supplements which contain mostly filler and very little nutritional value.

2: Filtered water comes from whole raw vegetables and fruits, raw juices, grasses, and tap water that has been filtered. Most tap water contains contaminants including bacteria, viruses, parasites, dissolved metals, pesticides, herbicides, waste, lead, asbestos fibers, fluoride, chlorine, and other chemicals. Of these, the most contaminating to the body are the heavy metals and chemicals such as pesticides, chlorine, and fluoride. Chlorine, which is used by your municipal water company to purify the water, is toxic to the thyroid and forms carcinogens when it combines with organic materials in the water. Exposure to chlorinated water (e.g. drinking, bathing, showering) may be linked with an increase in bladder and rectal cancers in the U.S, based on research conducted jointly at Harvard University and the Medical College of Wisconsin. There is also evidence indicating that chlorine damages protein in the body and may cause cells to mutate and cholesterol to oxidize. This disinfectant/bleach dries your skin, causes damaged and brittle hair, burns your eyes, and can make the following conditions worse: allergies, asthma, sinus conditions, diabetes, and skin rashes. Because of health issues associated with fluoride/fluorine (e.g. Alzheimer's, autoimmune diseases), many European countries have either reduced or discontinued their use of fluoride in their water.

Even if the municipal water supplies were pure at the treatment facility, the water has to travel through miles of pipes to reach your home, adding various pollutants and toxins. Consequently, it is imperative that you purify your water as best you can with one of three methods: (1) *Filtration*, which involves a carbon or ceramic filter that removes some contaminants, including chlorine, some heavy metals, pesticides, and odors, but, may not remove fluoride, which is difficult to remove; (2) *Reverse Osmosis*, which forces water first through a filter that removes sediment and then through a super-fine second filter that screens out microorganisms, asbestos, toxic chemicals and PCBs. Then, the water is passed through a reverse osmosis membrane and, finally, an activated carbon filter to provide a very tasty and pure water; or (3) *Distillation*, which heats the water to steam to remove almost all contaminants, but the water may have a poor taste with possibly damaged molecules.

Health impact: Water helps to hydrate the cells to transport nutrients throughout the body. Also, water is the medium that keeps tissues soft and permeable, helps to regulate body temperature and helps to ensure proper bowel movement. And, because water is so important to the proper functioning of all systems of the body, you want to provide your body with filtered water only. Given that many diabetics are dehydrated and have thick, sticky blood due to the high blood glucose levels, drinking filtered water is a necessity. But, do not get carried away with drinking too much water, which can cause frequent urination, depleting the body of important minerals such as magnesium and potassium. It is just as important to get water from the green, leafy and bright-colored vegetables and some fruits.

3: Lean protein includes fish (wild salmon, sardines, tuna, mackerel, tilapia), nuts, seeds, beans, lentils, whey protein, whole soy foods (tofu, tempeh, miso, soy protein powder); lean, organic beef, chicken breast without the skin, turkey breast without the skin; goat's milk, low fat plain yogurt; organic eggs, egg whites; low fat cheese, soy/tofu cheeses, blue-green algae (spirulina, chlorella); grains (amaranth, quinoa); wild game (venison, bear); organic seafood (shrimp, crab, lobster); and vegetables.

Health impact: These foods, when properly digested, provide the necessary amino acids without the high level of saturated fat, antibiotics and growth hormone that come from conventional animal meat. This increases the body's utilization of glucagon and insulin causing a decrease in the production of insulin, which leads to less fat storage and cholesterol production. These lean protein foods increase the production of growth hormones, stimulating the production of testosterone and muscle while burning fat. Some of these foods (beans, lentils, mushrooms) also provide fiber, which helps to slow down the amount of glucose that enters the bloodstream preventing a high rise in the blood glucose and insulin levels. In addition, the fermented foods such as yogurt, miso and tempeh help to improve the intestinal flora balance, build the immune system and generate new nutrients including Omega-3 fatty acids, digestive aids and the trace mineral GTF chromium. Wild salmon contains Omega-3 EFAs, high quality protein and the antioxidant astaxanthin.

Sardines (from the Mediterranean) contain Omega-3 EFAs, CoQ10, potassium, calcium, and, being small fish, they contain very little mercury. Lean organic beef and wild game provide the essential amino acids and conjugated linoleic acid (CLA), which may help to metabolize fat. *Raw* organic eggs from free-range chickens provide folic acid, choline and Omega-3 EFAs to help the cardiovascular system. Organic soy protein (with the isoflavones genestein and daidzein) can provide cardiovascular and anti-cancer health benefits, *but* soybeans, which contain hemaglutinins (that cause red blood cells to clump) and high levels of phytic acid, can increase the production of bad estrogen, leading to prostate and breast cancers.

4: Unsaturated fats include monounsaturated fat, Omega-3 polyunsaturated fat, and some Omega-6 polyunsaturated fat. Monounsaturated fat is contained in extra virgin olive oil, macadamia nuts, cashews, avocados, peanuts, walnuts, and almonds. Other foods/oils such as hazelnuts, Brazil nuts, sesame seeds, pumpkin seeds, pecans, and rice bran oil contain monounsaturated fat but have higher levels of saturated and polyunsaturated fats. *Monounsaturated fat*, which is considered to be the healthiest fat, contains large amounts of monounsaturated fatty acids (MUFAs), which are predominantly found in olive oil (73%) and macadamia nut oil (80%). Monounsaturated fat, which is not "saturated" with hydrogen, is heart-healthy, and has none of the adverse effects associated with saturated fats, trans fats or Omega-6 polyunsaturated vegetable oils. It is more resistant to oxidation, a process that leads to cell and tissue damage in the body. Olive oil and unrefined macadamia nut oil have a high oxidation threshold – that is, they remain stable at higher temperatures and do not easily become hydrogenated or saturated. Therefore, oils high in monounsaturates are better oils for cooking, although extra virgin coconut oil is even better under the heat.

Omega-3 polyunsaturated fat is another healthy fat that is contained in flaxseed oil, hemp oil, pumpkin seeds, walnuts and oily fish, such as wild salmon, sardines, tuna, mackerel, trout and herring. Plant-based foods such as flaxseed, nuts, and wheat germ contain one of the Omega-3 EFAs, alpha-linolenic acid (ALA). Marine crustaceans and oily fish such as wild salmon, tuna, sardines and mackerel contains the other two common Omega-3 EFAs, eicosapentaenoic acid (EPA) and docosahexaenoic acid (DHA). Other sources of Omega-3 EFAs include dark green vegetables such as seaweed, broccoli, spinach, kale; and, other green vegetables like spring greens, dark salad leaves, cabbage, Brussels sprouts, and parsley. Walnuts are the only nut that contains both monounsaturated fat and Omega-3 EFA.

Omega-6 polyunsaturated fat is contained in walnuts, sesame seeds, sunflower seeds, black currant seed oil, evening primrose oil and borage oil, which contain the Omega-6 EFAs, linoleic acid (LA) and gamma-linolenic acid (GLA) Use GLA to activate Omega-3 fatty-acids (via delta-6 saturase), ensuring absorption by the plasma cell membrane while inhibiting delta-5 desaturase (conversion to arachidonic acid).

Health impact: Monounsaturated fatty acids (MUFAs) and essential fatty acids (EFAs), especially the Omega-3 EFAs, are critical to cardiovascular and mental health but cannot be made in the body. For this reason, it is essential that we acquire these fats from vegetable and plant oils. MUFAs and EFAs are needed for heart and brain function, immune system support, healing, growth and development, bone health, joint health, muscle growth, stimulation of skin and hair growth, regulation of metabolism, control of inflammation, fat burning, and maintenance of reproductive processes. EFAs bring oxygen and vitamins to the tissues, repair cell membranes, keep cells supple, generate electrical currents, are crucial to the electrical reactions of cells, and are involved in generating the electric currents that maintain a regular heartbeat. EFAs act as solvents to remove hardened fat and are crucial for weight loss; and, appear to regulate chromosome stability. EFAs contain anti-inflammatory properties and do not clog the arteries or make the blood thicker like the oil or fat from animals or dairy products. These EFA oils lubricate the joints and arteries and keep the blood thin, preventing ailments such as arthritis and high blood pressure. They are also typically high in Vitamin E, providing antioxidant protection.

Since fats make up sixty percent of the brain and the nerves that run every system in the body, the higher the quality of the fat in the food, the better the brain and nerves will function. The brain sends chemical messengers throughout the body, telling each organ how to work. An important group of these chemical messengers are the prostaglandins (so-called because they were originally discovered in the prostate gland). Prostaglandins initiate the body's self-repair system. The body needs both Omega-3 and Omega-6 fats to manufacture healthy brain cells (the message senders) and prostaglandins (the messengers).

Specifically, the body uses the *Omega-3 EFAs* to make the beneficial Series 3 prostaglandins, which regulate platelet stickiness, arterial muscle tone, the inflammatory response, sodium excretion, and the immune function. All of these regulatory functions are reversing the fight or flight stress-related response in the body, so if the body is deficient in Omega-3 EFAs, it cannot wind down normally from the stress response, which may lead to anxiety, depression, or chronic fatigue – ailments that are prevalent in many diabetics.

ALA is the "parent" Omega-3 fatty acid that is the precursor to EPA and DHA. Your body converts ALA rapidly into EPA, and more slowly into DHA. Approximately 11 grams of ALA is needed to produce one gram of DHA and EPA. However, foods high in Omega-6 fatty acids (corn, sunflower, soybean or safflower vegetable oils) and refined foods can easily inhibit this conversion process, leading to increased inflammation.

EPA and *DHA* are better obtained from marine life (crustaceans known as krill) and from cold water fish such as wild salmon and tuna. Fish oil has been proven in many clinical studies to provide numerous health benefits to the cardiovascular, neural, joint, gastrointestinal, brain, skin, ocular, and immune systems.

EPA specifically protects the cardiovascular system by promoting normal cholesterol and triglyceride levels, increasing blood flow and enhancing immune function. *DHA* specifically supports the cell membranes of the eyes, nerves and brain, which is 60% fat and predominantly DHA fat. Because ocean-raised wild salmon feed on smaller fish that eat EPA-and DHA-rich algae, they are an excellent source of the EPA and DHA oils. (But, farm-raised salmon, which are fed grain and other contaminants, do not contain much of these oils).

Flaxseed delivers the full benefits of Omega-3 EFA (alpha linolenic acid), the Omega-6 and Omega-9 EFAs, plus all of the fiber, protein, lignans, vitamins, minerals and amino acids, which are important nutrients for overall good health. Lignans are a type of natural plant chemical contained within the cell matrix of the flaxseed that act as plant hormones. When bacteria in the digestive tract act on plant lignans, these compounds are converted into potent, hormone-like substances, known as a phytoestrogens. Research findings have concluded that the chemical release of these phytoestrogens is able to block the action of certain cancer-causing substances associated with breast, colon and prostate cancers.

Flaxseed helps to control the blood glucose level, and, therefore, helps to control appetite and cravings. Consuming the entire (ground) flaxseed with all of its nutritional components will leave you feeling satisfied for hours. Example: Two tbsp. of freshly ground flaxseed, 1 tbsp. wheat grass powder mixed in a 16-ounce container of raw vegetable juice, raw almond milk or yogurt will provide a complete breakfast. Flaxseed contains 98% more anti-cancer lignans and 97% more fiber (soluble and insoluble) than the flax oil; and, contains the flax oil in its freshest form. Eight ounces of wheat (or barley) grass juice provides most of the daily requirement of vitamins and minerals. The lignans, fiber, grasses and Omega-3 help lower cholesterol, control blood pressure, reduce weight, deter diabetes, and relieve PMS and menopause symptoms.

Researchers believe these plant hormones mimic the body's own estrogen type of cells and can block the formation of hormone-based tumors or growths. Unlike the hormones produced in the body, these plant hormones do not stimulate cancerous cells to grow. In fact, lignans boost production of a substance that fastens onto human estrogen and carries it out of the body. Lignans are also considered to be antioxidants; therefore, researchers believe they can protect healthy cells from free radical oxidative damage.

Similar to seeds, many *nuts* also provide the Omega-3 fats and quality fiber, which helps to slow down the body's absorption of the nut's carbohydrate content. But if you're trying to curb the carbs, the nut to avoid is the cashew. One ounce of cashews (about a handful) contains 9 grams of carbs, but only one gram of fiber. That's 8 net carbs, and no other nut comes close to that amount. The next highest in the carb category is the pistachio with 5 net carbs. Most of the others have only two or three net carbs. The pecan has the lowest number of carbs – 1 net carb per ounce. If you want more calcium, almonds are a good source. They also deliver magnesium, which helps the absorption of calcium. If you need to boost Vitamin E and potassium, then, eat hazelnuts. Brazil nuts provide selenium and zinc. The peanut provides good amounts of niacin, folate, and Vitamin E, but avoid the salty, roasted versions.

Concerning the Omega-6 EFAs, most people obtain an excess of linoleic acid from various foods. Linoleic acid can be converted to *GLA*, which is beneficial to the cardiovascular and nervous systems; and helps to increase absorption of Omega-3 EFAs. But, the linoleic acid is not converted because of metabolic problems caused by diets rich in sugar, alcohol, or trans fats, as well as smoking, pollution, stress, aging, viral infections, and other illnesses such as diabetes. Consequently, it may be necessary to supplement with GLA-rich foods such as borage oil, black currant seed oil, or evening primrose oil.

5: Organic whole grains include amaranth, quinoa, kamut, barley, oat, rice germ/bran, alfalfa. They provide vitamins such as the B-complex and Vitamin E; minerals such as chromium, magnesium, zinc, selenium, iron; and, insoluble fiber such as cellulose and hemicellulose. However, grain products that are labeled "multigrain", "stone ground" or "whole wheat" are not necessarily whole grain products – they are processed grains that cause glucose and insulin spikes. Check the ingredients carefully and look for "whole grain" as the first ingredient and at least 3 grams of fiber per serving/100 calories.

Health impact: Whole grains contain insoluble fiber (roughage), which helps to increase stool bulk, speeds the passage of stools through the bowel, and may help to prevent bowel cancer, diverticulitis, and irritable bowel syndrome. Insoluble fiber is also important in suppressing hunger since, with fluids, it helps to provide a feeling of fullness.

Whole grain oats, which are 55% soluble fiber and 45% insoluble fiber, provide glucose-lowering, cholesterol-lowering, blood-pressure-lowering and bowel regularity benefits. Oats contain beta glucan, a soluble monosaccharide fiber that stimulates the white blood cells to strengthen the immune system and binds with cholesterol to prevent its reabsorption. Oats also contain a type of antioxidant called avenanthramides, which prevent LDL cholesterol from oxidizing, one of the contributors to arterial plaque formation and heart disease. But only use organic whole grain oats, not the instant oats, to obtain these health benefits. Quinoa and amaranth provide a high quality protein and fiber, in addition to several minerals.

Because conventional bread is overly processed, removing most of the fiber and other key nutrients, it has a tendency to raise blood glucose levels. In fact, diabetics who may be sensitive to wheat/gluten should avoid grain, especially the traditional processed grains that many people eat for breakfast, e.g. cereal, toast, instant oatmeal, grits, wheat bread, muffins, and pancakes. As a result, sprouted grain bread has increased in popularity in recent years. Sprouted grain bread involves soaking the grain and allowing it to sprout. The sprouted seedlings are then mashed together and baked. Sprouting allows the enzymes in the grain to convert some of the carbohydrates and fats to vitamins, minerals, and amino acids. As a result, sprouted grain bread typically is higher in protein, fiber, and certain vitamins and minerals than traditional grain breads including wheat, rye, and oat. It is also less refined and processed than even stone ground wheat bread, so it has less of an impact on your blood sugar. Whole grain rye bread may also be a better choice than wheat bread for diabetics due to a lower insulin response, less gluten, and a higher fiber content.

These "live" super foods provide vital nutrients and exert less strain on the gastrointestinal system and other organs because they contain organically-active nutrients, good bacteria, antioxidants, fiber, amino acids, essential oils, enzymes, vitamins, and minerals. As a result, the body requires less energy to "break down" live foods and has the necessary energy and raw materials to strengthen the immune system and protect the body from oxidation, toxicity, acidity, inflammation, infection and the various systemic diseases such as heart disease, diabetes, and cancer. And, if you already have one of these diseases, these nutrients help to perform other biochemical functions that facilitate healing and reversing the disease in your body.

Coincidentally, most of the "live" foods are alkaline-forming foods that help the body to cleanse and initiate weight (fat) loss. All of the "dead" processed foods are acid-forming foods that cause a buildup of the toxins and acid waste in the body, leading to weight (fat) gain, and, the inability to burn fat and lose weight. Excess acid waste that accumulates in cells causes the cell walls to harden and inhibit their ability to absorb nutrients, which leads to cell starvation. Excess acid waste causes damage to the liver, which loses some of its ability to remove toxins. When the liver becomes overloaded with acid waste, it crystallizes bile and acid waste into gallstones. The gallbladder has difficulty releasing bile, which inhibits proper digestion and further slows peristalsis. As acid levels continue to rise, the liver becomes damaged, cells become depleted of oxygen, the other body organs become vulnerable to deterioration, and a degenerative systemic disease such as diabetes begins to settle in. In addition, some of the excess acid accumulates in the kidneys, causing damage that can prevent the kidneys from filtering toxins, leading to the formation of kidney stones and eventually to kidney failure.

When the body consumes too many acid-forming foods over a period of years, it leads to a gradual performance reduction in the liver, gall bladder, kidneys, and colon. When the body is unable to remove the accumulated waste, it tries to protect itself, for example, by retaining fluid and fat cells to help dilute these toxins. Unfortunately, this usually leads to digestive discomfort, headaches, joint pain, fat gain, elevated blood pressure, increased cholesterol production, or fatigue.

However, as long as you are eating more alkaline-forming foods than acid-forming foods, this will help to prevent your body from becoming a breeding ground for pathogenic bacteria and most systemic diseases. In general, you should eat 80% alkaline foods.
- Strongly alkaline foods: green leafy vegetables, tart fruits
- Mildly alkaline foods: fruits, vegetables
- Strongly acid foods: meat, dairy, soft drinks, processed foods
- Mildly acid foods: grains, legumes, nuts, fatty fish

Fiber

Fiber is not a major macronutrient, but it is one of the seven nutrient factors and it does help to control blood glucose levels. There are two types of fiber, soluble and insoluble.

Soluble fiber is very beneficial to diabetics because it slows digestion and the absorption of nutrients, resulting in a slow and steady release of glucose from accompanying carbohydrates. It also lowers cholesterol by soaking up excess bile acids found in the intestinal tract – the same acids that are converted into blood cholesterol. Soluble fiber can be helpful in people with Type 2 diabetes trying to achieve weight loss goals because it delays stomach emptying, triggering satiety (a feeling of fullness) and reducing appetite. Soluble fiber may also help to lower blood pressure. Soluble fiber sources include: oat bran, pectins of certain fruits/vegetables (e.g. blackberries, apples, artichoke), guar gum (e.g. beans, peas, nuts and seeds), psyllium husk, fenugreek seeds, and konjac.

Insoluble fiber (roughage) is beneficial because it acts as a regulator of gastrointestinal functions, removing waste and toxins to keep the colon clean. Insoluble fiber may prevent colon cancer as it decreases the amount of time that potential toxins interact with colon cells and enhances the colonic content of butyrate, a short chain fatty acid that keeps colon rectal cells healthy. Fiber may also help to prevent breast cancer as it decreases the amount of circulating estrogens in women. Insoluble fiber sources include: whole grains, apple skin, bran cereal, broccoli, kidney beans, pinto beans, pear skin, potato skin, and oatmeal.

Specific soluble and insoluble fiber-rich vegetable sources include broccoli, string beans, turnips, lima beans, Brussels sprouts, mushrooms, kale, collards, winter squash. Fiber-rich legume sources include black beans, garbanzo beans (chickpeas), kidney beans, lentils, pinto beans, split peas, navy beans, and yams. Fiber-rich nuts and seeds include almonds, cashews, chestnuts, filberts, flaxseeds, sesame seeds, sunflower seeds, walnuts. Fiber-rich fruits include avocados, dried figs, blackberries, prunes, raisins, apricots, apples (with skin), and pears (with skin). Other dietary fibers include inulin, oligofructose, and psyllium seed husk.

Most dietary fiber sources promote laxation by increasing colonic contents, which stimulates propulsion. Unfermented or incompletely fermented fiber and the accompanying moisture it holds are two contributors to this increased stool mass. Slowly or incompletely fermented fibers also contribute to stool weight by providing substrate for microbial growth.

Psyllium seed husk is a partially fermented dietary fiber that increases stool weight and promotes laxation by its presence in stool and by increasing the moisture content of stool. In various studies it was determined that the unfermented gel isolated from psyllium-containing stools functions as an emollient and lubricant. The greater ease of passage, gentleness, and softness reported by the subjects and the isolation of a very viscous fraction supports this hypothesis. Psyllium appears to increase stool mass more effectively than do other common laxative fiber sources including wheat bran fiber and oat bran fiber. Psyllium husk (7 to 10 grams per day) was shown in a short-term placebo-controlled study to lower total cholesterol and LDL cholesterol levels 5 to 10%.

Other fibers that provide gastrointestinal benefits include mucilage (which helps the body to get rid of pathogenic gut bacteria, clean the small intestine villi, and support beneficial intestinal microflora); konjac (which is a starch from the root of the konjac plant that grows in China and Japan); and, prebiotics (which is a non-digestible food ingredient that selectively stimulates bacteria in the colon). Food sources for mucilage include okra (gumbo), asparagus, flaxseed, psyllium husk, aloe vera, and slippery elm bark.

Sugar, Salt, Chocolate & Coffee Substitutes

Sugar, salt, chocolate, and coffee are four of the major foods/seasonings that everyone has questions about when they decide to make changes to their eating habits. Why? Because these four foods/seasonings drive many of our cravings and health issues.

Sugar

Prior to the turn of the 20th century, the average annual consumption of refined sugar was only 5 pounds per person. Today, the average American consumes more than 130 pounds of sugar annually with almost 20 percent of the daily calorie intake being some form of sugar. This is due to our addiction to sugar and not being aware of the many sources from which we get sugar. Sugar is found naturally in milk, fruit, vegetables and grains, but food manufacturers add sugar to many foods, especially "low fat", "fat free" and so-called "diet" products. The following is a list of some of the many disguises of refined sugar on the food label: brown sugar, corn sweetener, corn syrup, dextrin, dextrose, glucose, fructose, high fructose corn syrup, honey, lactose, malodextrin, maltose, mannitol, molasses, natural sweeteners, polydextrose, sucrose, syrup. Basically, refined sugar includes anything ending in "ose" on an ingredient label, including sucrose, fructose, and high fructose corn syrup, which increases hunger cravings and fat production.

Because refined sugar is absorbed very quickly causing the blood glucose level to rise, manufacturers developed sugar substitutes (artificial sweeteners) that do not cause this rise in the glucose level. However, studies have shown some health concerns with some of these sugar substitutes. Fortunately, there are natural sugars that do not raise these health concerns, including stevia, xylitol, and d-mannose.

Stevia is a non-caloric herb, native to Paraguay that has been used as a sweetener and flavor enhancer for centuries, but it may have an aftertaste. It comes in a powder or liquid form and can be found in most health food stores and some grocery stores.

Xylitol is a natural-occurring sugar in the body; and, is found in berries, plums, pears and in birchwood trees. More importantly, xylitol does not cause a rise in blood glucose levels because it is metabolized independently of insulin. Xylitol looks and tastes like sugar with the same sweetness level and has one third fewer calories than sugar. Xylitol has been used in Russia for many years as a useful sweetener for diabetics. However, the most beneficial aspect of xylitol is its effect on dental health. Normally, plaque bacteria in our mouth digest sugar, producing acid as a result. It is this acid which eats into tooth enamel to create cavities. Bacteria try to use xylitol, but they are unable, and consequently their growth is inhibited, lowering the incidence of tooth decay.

D-mannose is a natural sugar found in some fruits such as cranberry and is used to treat urinary tract infections.

Other sugar options include agave nectar (which is a natural fructose sweetener extracted from the Agave plant in Mexico); muscovado sugar (an organic brown sugar); demerara (a light brown raw cane sugar used in coffee), and sucanat (granulated cane juice). These unprocessed sugars are free of damaging chemicals used in white sugar processing.

Additional sugar options include organic spices such as cinnamon, vanilla, nutmeg, anise and mint, which add a sweet taste to foods without adding the sugar or calories.

Salt

The body does not need sugar or chocolate to live, but it does need salt. "Salt" is actually a chemical term for a substance produced by a reaction of an acid with a base. The terms "salt" and "sodium" are used interchangeably, but technically this is not correct. "Salt" is sodium chloride, or, in chemistry terms, NaCl. By weight, "salt" is 40% sodium and 60% chloride. Sodium is an essential nutrient, a mineral that the body cannot manufacture itself but is required for life and good health. However, due to the over-consumption of processed foods (which contain high levels of sodium) and the under-consumption of vegetables/beans (which contain high levels of potassium, magnesium, and zinc), the sodium-to-potassium ratio may be excessively high. Instead of strictly reducing salt intake, a better strategy may be to increase the intake of potassium-rich foods. This will trigger the cells to pump sodium out and potassium in via the "sodium-potassium pump". This pump is in the membranes of all body cells, and one of its most important functions is preventing cellular swelling. If sodium is not pumped out, water accumulates in the cell, causing it to swell and ultimately burst.

The sodium-potassium pump also functions to maintain the electrical charge within the cell, which is particularly important to muscle and nerve cells. During nerve transmission and muscle contraction, potassium exits the cell and sodium enters, which results in an electrical charge change. This change causes a nerve impulse or muscle contraction, so it is not surprising that a potassium deficiency affects muscles and nerves first. In an interesting study in Finland, researchers discovered that sodium/potassium pump activity increases with fitness. People who exercise regularly have more effective sodium/potassium pumps within their muscles. This means that a greater amount of nutrients are transported to their muscles than those of sedentary people.

According to the latest science, a proper balance of sodium, in addition to potassium and magnesium, is more important than severely reducing or eliminating sodium completely to achieve a healthy body. Sodium, potassium and magnesium help to regulate fluid balance in the body and allow nutrients and oxygen to travel to their necessary destinations within the body.

To provide a better balance of these minerals, use organic sea salt or a similar product, which contains magnesium and other nutrients and is not overly-processed and refined. Also, flavor your food with garlic, onion, peppers, herbs, and other organic spices. More importantly, eat potassium and magnesium-rich foods such as vegetables and beans to naturally reduce and normalize the sodium level in the body.

Also, avoid processed foods such as canned tomato juice, soups, and lunch meats because they tend to contain high levels of sodium. And, be wary of some salt substitutes that may contain too much potassium chloride, which can cause numbness, irregular heartbeat, low blood pressure (dizziness, weakness, fatigue), coma, and, even a heart attack.

Chocolate

Chocolate is made from tropical cacao beans, and is transformed by machines into a bitter, brown paste of cocoa butter and cocoa solids. The darker chocolate contains lecithin and flavonoids called epicatechins that act as antioxidants and modulators of hormone-like compounds in the body; and, also, contains oleic acid, a fatty acid that promotes normal cholesterol levels. However, chocolate contains caffeine and other stimulants that make it addictive, and, given its high fat content, excess indulgence can contribute to obesity and heart disease. Many women report particular chocolate cravings when they are pre-menstrual or pregnant. This is possibly because chocolate contains magnesium, a shortage of which can exacerbate pre-menstrual tension. Similar cravings during pregnancy could indicate mild anemia, which could be helped by the iron content in chocolate. Others crave chocolate because of the caffeine, sugar, or the fat.

There are very few good substitutes for chocolate, but, in general, if you choose the less-sweetened versions, you will be taking in less sugar. Some alternatives include the following.
- Carob: contains less fat and no caffeine; and, is used as a substitute by those who are allergic to chocolate.
- Dark chocolate: contains as much as 65% cocoa to provide the dark, rich color and the antioxidant benefits, and, the darker the better. White and milk chocolate have none of the benefits of dark chocolate because they are pure sugar and fat (empty calories).
- Unsweetened (semisweet or bittersweet) chocolate: contains the least amount of sugar; organic versions provide the most benefits.
- Cocoa: is similar to unsweetened chocolate, only it's in powdered form and has less cocoa butter. Don't confuse cocoa powder, which is bitter, with instant cocoa mixes, which are sweetened.

Note: Chocolate contains naturally occurring compounds such as phenylethylamine, theobromine and anandamine. These compounds trigger the release of endorphins in the brain that produce a mild feeling of euphoria, elevate mood, increase circulation and enhance sensory perception, mimicking the sensation of being in love.

Coffee

With over 400 billion cups consumed every year, coffee is the world's most popular beverage. Coffee contains natural antioxidants called flavonoids that are known as disease protectors. Caffeine acts as a mild stimulant to the central nervous system, that results in better memory, alertness, mood and sensorial activity. But, recent studies indicate that drinking more than 2 to 3 cups a day may have a negative effect on your health, e.g. high insulin levels, jitters, teeth stains.

Healthier alternatives to traditional coffee include but are not limited to: chicory, soy coffee, organically grown coffee with mushroom extract, roastaroma, and tea, which contain lower amounts of caffeine, and provide other health benefits. Chicory is an herb, the roots of which are dried, ground, roasted and used to flavor coffee. Chicory contains much less caffeine and is reported to help cleanse the blood and improve the health of the liver. Soy coffee is caffeine-free and is made from organic soybeans, which may provide cardiovascular and cancer-related health benefits. Organically grown coffee blended with the organically grown Reishi mushroom is reported to taste as good, if not better, than the best organic coffee from the health food store. Roastaroma is an herbal tea made from healthy grains and blended with selected spices to taste like coffee but without any caffeine. Green tea and white tea contain less caffeine and may provide anti-cancer benefits according to some studies.

Food Preparation

It is possible that even if you are eating the proper foods (e.g. vegetables, fruits, fish, plant oils, nuts), your body may not be acquiring the associated nutrients. This may be due to consuming the food in the wrong form, overcooking the food, or not preparing the food properly.

Many foods in their raw form offer the optimum level of nutritional value. And, as the food is processed at various stages, it loses more of its nutritional value. For example, an apple in its raw form is very nutritious, providing fiber, water, vitamins, minerals, enzymes, pectin, antioxidants and other nutrients. When that apple is processed to produce applesauce, it still provides most of these nutrients, but at lower levels. When that apple is further processed to produce apple juice, it contains very few of the original nutrients, especially the fiber and pectin.

Cooking may reduce the nutritional value of the food and rob it of essential vitamins, minerals, and enzymes needed for proper digestion. However, the following are some cooking guidelines to use to ensure that you are not killing all the nutrients in the food. Additional cooking tips are provided in the recipes chapter.

Cooking **vegetables** destroys their enzymes, and at high temperatures can deplete them of Vitamin C and the B-Complex vitamins by as much as 30 percent of their original value. If you boil these foods, more than 75% of the nutrients are lost. To minimize the loss of nutrients in vegetables, eat them raw; or lightly steam or stir-fry them. When steaming, ensure that the water in the pot does not touch the vegetables when the water starts to boil. When stir-frying, add in the vegetables last after the meat is almost done to prevent overcooking. If the vegetables look limp and discolored, then, they were overcooked. The vegetables should have a bright color and feel firm. In some cases, cooking actually increases the bioavailability and absorption of nutrients such as the folate found in spinach and the carotenoids found in brightly-colored vegetables such as carrots, broccoli, sweet potatoes, and yellow squash. Add onions, garlic, peppers, mushrooms, or organic spices to change the flavor and increase the nutritional value of the vegetables.

Cooking **meat** at the super-high temperatures involved in grilling and frying, can alter its properties, and turn it into a carcinogen. Meat and fish subjected to high heat may develop heterocyclic amines, chemicals that can cause cancer. And, although grilling meats can add extra flavor, components of the smoke can coat your food with carcinogens. Studies have shown that overcooking meat and fish transforms their protein, fat, and sugar into damaging compounds called advanced glycation end products (AGEs). AGEs are already known to inflame the coronary arteries of diabetics, and scientists strongly suspect that these AGEs can harm non-diabetics as well. To minimize your health risk, use the leanest possible cuts of meat and cook them for longer times over lower temperatures until they're done. When baking fish, chicken, or other meat, spray the pan with extra virgin olive oil to prevent any sticking or burning. You can also place a couple drops of extra virgin olive oil on top of the meat to prevent the meat from drying out. This is especially important for wild salmon, which can dry out quickly while baking. Use something such as the Foreman grill to cook chicken, beef or turkey to reduce the absorption of the animal fat/grease into the meat. Similarly, add onions, garlic, peppers, mushrooms, or organic spices to change the flavor and increase the nutritional value of the meat.

Cooking with various **oils**, even the good ones, can become harmful when they are overheated. They provide better nutrition when consumed in the raw form on top of salads or steamed vegetables, where they help the body absorb the vegetable's fat-soluble nutrients (e.g. carotenoids). When stir-frying, use olive oil, unrefined macadamia nut oil, or rice bran oil, which actually has the higher smoke point (490°F vs. 410°F, 325°F). Deep-frying creates compounds that oxidize cholesterol, causing it to stick to your arteries. And worst of all, studies have demonstrated that deep-frying can create carcinogens in the oil itself, especially when that oil has been re-used (as is frequently the case in restaurants). Deep-frying also destroys the nutrients in the oil, such as Vitamin E, which actually helps to prevent cholesterol buildup. So, when you do cook with oil, use olive, macadamia nut, or rice bran oil and use lower temperatures to keep the oil from smoking, which is the first sign of a dangerous oil heat. Do not cook with polyunsaturated oils such as safflower, corn, or soybean oil, which break down under heat. If you do decide to fry some food, always use a saturated oil such as virgin coconut oil, which can stand up to the heat. And, use a flash-fryer because it quickly sears the outside of the meat and prevents the oil from being absorbed into the meat.

Only use the **microwave** for thawing frozen food or to quickly heat a snack, but do not use the microwave to cook the food. Microwaving destroys many of the enzymes that are vital to the body being able to break down and absorb the nutrients from the food. Microwave cooking of food destroys some of the vitamins and minerals, and is believed to alter the molecular structure and taste of the cooked food.

A **blender** and a **juicer** are two utensils that will help you to more easily increase your intake of raw vegetables, fruits and fiber. A blender and juicer have benefits that warrant having one or both in the kitchen to prepare fresh nutritious beverages, especially for children and diabetics. Use a blender to mix vegetables, grasses and fruits to prepare a beverage that is full of nutrients and fiber – this is one of the easiest ways to get more fiber on a daily basis. Blenders tend to be more popular with people because they are easy to use and to clean. Use a juicer to extract the pulp and obtain pure raw juice. The "live" nutrients from the raw juice are absorbed very quickly into the blood, cells, tissues and organs.

Juicing

If eating raw vegetables, salads and soups are not appealing enough to acquire the minimum 6 to 9 cups (5 to 7 servings) of vegetables and fruits each day, then, juicing may be an effective addition to your nutritional program. Even as a diabetic, juicing can be very nutritious as long as you drink mostly green vegetables/grasses and avoid drinking too many of the fruits. Green juices have an alkaline reaction in the body and help protect against acid build-up as well as stimulate the body to manufacture hemoglobin. Green juices contain organic water, the purest most natural water available to us, and they cleanse the body of the waste within the cells and tissues. Green juices contain an abundance of chlorophyll, which is a molecule whose structure is almost exactly the same as the hemoglobin molecule of the human blood. Chlorophyll helps to repair tissue and is very important in helping to remove toxins from the body.

Juices are a perfect medium in which to mix and dissolve nutritional powders that will enhance their healing powers. The nutrients and herbs in powders are better absorbed than tablet forms of the same ingredients, and mixing them in juices enhances their solubility, digestion and absorption. The juices bring the healing nutrients to the cells in the surface of the mucous membrane of the gut in an easily absorbed form. This requires much less energy to assimilate than solid tablets, especially in people with inflamed mucous membranes in the intestines. Juices can be combined in so many ways to make them palatable and delicious. Their diverse colors and taste enable huge variety so that you will not get bored. For those who feel they need an extra boost there is nothing better than drinking 2 cups of raw vegetable juice everyday. It will brighten up your day by providing extra energy and endurance.

Raw juices are packed with living enzymes to assist the digestive process, which means your gut, liver and pancreas do not have to work very hard to extract almost 99% of the nutrients within the raw vegetables and fruits. This conserves vital body energy, which means that the body does not feel heavy or weighed down after drinking raw juices. For example, two cups of carrot juice (16 ounces) is approximately equivalent to eating one pound of raw carrots. Eating so many carrots at one time would be hard on the jaws and teeth and would take a long time to eat and digest. Juices are unique because they allow the gut to receive very concentrated amounts of phytonutrients that could not be obtained by eating a normal amount of raw vegetables and fruits.

Raw juices contain natural medicinal nutrients that provide antioxidant, antibiotic, and hormonal balancing benefits. For example, Brussel sprouts and string beans are known to contain insulin-like substances that can be beneficial to Type 2 diabetics, and especially Type 1 diabetics. In addition, phytonutrients needed by the pancreas to produce insulin are present in cucumber and onion juices; and, the phytonutrient properties of broccoli, carrot, celery, lettuce and spinach are also beneficial to diabetics. For example, broccoli is an excellent source of chromium, which helps to regulate insulin usage in the body. Fresh juices of garlic, onions, radish and tomatoes contain various antibiotic properties. Wheat/barley grass, celery, kelp, cucumber and cabbage juice are excellent to reduce acidity and blood pressure. Green, leafy vegetables such as spinach help to cleanse and heal the gastrointestinal tract. The phytonutrient properties of carrot are also beneficial to diabetics once they have their blood glucose level under control. Drinking as little as 3 cups of fresh vegetable juice each day will help the body detoxify and regenerate through the assimilation of the earth's life-giving nutrients.

The raw juice is obtained using a device called a juicer. It works by feeding raw vegetables, grasses and fruits into a chute that pushes the food into a high-speed rotating blade that shreds the food, extracting the juice from the pulp. This extraction process breaks down the cellulose barriers in the cells of the vegetables, grasses and fruits, allowing the release of powerful enzymes and other nutrients. Juicers are very powerful but are not as popular as blenders because they tend to be more difficult to use and to clean. Consequently, it is important that you purchase a juicer with fewer parts, a powerful motor and a wide chute. This will prevent you from spending a lot of time cutting up the vegetables/fruits to fit down the chute of the juicer. Depending on your needs and finances, purchase the appropriate juicer, e.g. twin gear press (vegetables and wheat grass), mastication, centrifugal ejection, single/dual auger (for wheat grass), or manual press (for fruits only).

Food Quality: Organic & Conventional

Food quality can be important, especially if your liver, colon, and kidneys are not functioning well enough to extract the toxins and chemicals from the pesticides and other pollutants that are in the food.

Organically grown vegetables, fruits and grains are free of pesticides and other chemicals and contain higher levels of key nutrients such as magnesium, potassium, chromium, and Vitamin C. Organic meat is free of the growth hormones and other chemicals that cows, chickens, and other animals are fed to support the high demand of meat consumption in America; and, is a safer choice if you're concerned about the bird flu. Organic food handlers, processors and retailers adhere to standards that maintain the integrity of organic agricultural products. The primary goal of organic agriculture is to optimize the health and productivity of interdependent communities of soil life, plants, animals and people.

Organic food is defined as "food produced without using conventional pesticides, fertilizers made with synthetic ingredients or sewage sludge, bioengineering, or ionizing radiation." However, read the labels to determine how much of the food is really organic. For example, a product made with 100% organic ingredients can be labeled as "100% organic ingredients"; and, a product with at least 95% organic ingredients can be labeled "organic".

Although there is a lot of controversy concerning the benefits of organic food, it does appear that organic foods are healthier because they contain more vitamin/mineral nutrients without the pesticides, hormones, antibiotics and other toxins. However, if financial considerations prevent you from purchasing organic food, then, do the best you can. For example, purchase fresh vegetables and fruits, and wash them thoroughly with an organic spray cleaner to remove most of the pesticides and chemicals. Concerning meat and dairy, try to purchase antibiotic-free or leaner versions of these foods from a local farmer's market. Because of the improvements in technology, frozen vegetables, fruits and some meats are just as nutritious as fresh – just check the label to ensure no preservatives or other chemicals have been added during the processing.

Sometimes if the frozen food is not prepared properly or the grocery freezer is not cold enough, the food may be frostbitten. If the food is frostbitten, return it to the store.

Some canned foods such as kidney beans and chickpeas are excellent because they retain their fiber content and contain few preservatives if any. Canned wild salmon and tuna in water are other excellent canned foods. However, canned fruits tend to have a lot of sugar, syrup, and high fructose corn syrup, which increases hunger and fat production. So stay away from these canned foods. For other canned foods, read the ingredients on the label to check the sodium level and other added chemicals. Avoid most frozen dinners, canned soups, canned vegetables, and dehydrated mixes for soups, sauces, and salad dressing because they tend to have a lot of sodium. Also, avoid most cured and processed meats such as hotdogs, sausage and luncheon meats because of the high amounts of sodium.

Food Phobias

During the mid-1980s in the United States, there was a shift to low-fat diets because of the health concerns that were raised concerning fat. This created a **fat phobia** that led to a reduced fat intake coupled with the over-consumption of refined carbohydrates, producing a nation of fat people. Although some people are now realizing this was a major mistake, we are still not consuming enough of the good fats from foods such as fish, nuts, seeds, and plant oils such as extra virgin olive oil and flaxseed oil.

During this "all fat is bad" period, another type of fat was also targeted as being very bad for our health – cholesterol. Cholesterol, which is manufactured in the liver and in most of the body's cells, is very critical to our health as it provides structural integrity to all the cell membranes. Cholesterol acts as a precursor to vital corticosteroids, hormones that help us deal with stress and protect the body against heart disease and cancer; and, as a precursor to the hormones androgen, testosterone, estrogen and progesterone. Cholesterol is also a precursor to Vitamin D, a very important fat-soluble vitamin needed for healthy bones, a healthy nervous system, proper growth, mineral metabolism, muscle tone, insulin production, reproduction and immune system function. Dietary cholesterol plays an important role in maintaining the health of the intestinal wall, preventing leaky gut syndrome and other intestinal disorders. Recent research shows that cholesterol surprisingly acts as an antioxidant by protecting us against free radical damage that leads to heart disease instead of today's belief that cholesterol causes heart disease!

As a result of this false belief, many people stopped eating one of the "perfect protein" foods that provides a rich source of choline, Omega-3 EFAs, selenium, Vitamin E, and folic acid, which are all important for our cardiovascular health – **the egg**. The egg has received a bad rap because it contains 190 mg of cholesterol and 5 g of fat. But, most of the fat is good fat (monounsaturated: 2.2 g, polyunsaturated: 0.8 g), while only 1.6 g is potentially bad (saturated) fat. And, the cholesterol is not the culprit that we all believe it to be – especially when it is part of a food that is comprised of mostly good fats. If you still have a concern with the cholesterol in the egg, then, eat the egg raw or just eat the egg white, which actually contains more protein than the yolk and contains no cholesterol. However, the yolk contains choline, which is responsible for the structural integrity and signaling functions of cell membranes and the breakdown of homocysteine to protect the cardiovascular system. It also contains lutein and zeaxanthin, which are yellow/orange carotenoids known as xanthophylls that provide health benefits to the eyes. You can reduce the health concerns with the yolk by eating the eggs *raw* or *soft-boiled* as heat damages the protein and other nutrients in the yolk.

In addition to cholesterol, saturated fat also received a bad rap as a "bad fat" that causes heart disease and cancer. This was primarily due to a major shift in how animals were raised – from being grass-fed to being corn-fed and given growth hormones and antibiotics. Actually, saturated fats are essential for body tissues as they are a major part of the phospholipid component of cell membranes and the structural integrity of all cells. Unfortunately, when animals are fed corn, growth hormones and antibiotics, this compromises the saturated fats. However, the saturated fats of animals that are wild or organic are healthier because these animals are grass-fed, are not given growth hormones, antibiotics, or other animal byproducts, and are not raised in confined areas. Of course, this does not mean that you can eat more saturated fat, since it does cause inflammation and a rise in several cardiovascular risk factors.

The food phobia has now shifted to include **carbohydrates**. And manufacturers are now providing "low-carb" foods to feed that phobia just as they did with "low-fat" and "low cholesterol" foods to feed the fat phobia. Unfortunately, we have not learned our lesson that the lack of any major macronutrient will lead to health problems in the long run. In this case, if we don't eat the good carbohydrates (vegetables, fruits, organic grains), our bodies will not acquire important vitamins, minerals, antioxidants, fiber, and other nutrients. This will lead to several nutrient deficiencies, which will eventually evolve into one or more systemic diseases such as heart disease, diabetes or cancer.

Despite the cardiovascular health benefits of Omega-3 EFAs and lean protein in fish, some people have a phobia about fish because of the concern about mercury contamination, which is very real. However, this concern can be reduced by eating fish less frequently, eating smaller fish, eating only fish such as wild salmon, sardines, haddock, tilapia, summer flounder, and not eating fish such as swordfish, farmed salmon, halibut, shark, king mackerel, and some canned tuna. Also, use herbs such as parsley and cilantro to help remove heavy metals such as mercury from the body.

It is interesting to note that the food phobias about eggs and fish have led many people to consuming less of these foods while losing their cardiovascular benefits. This aligns with two of the major health issues that continue to grow as the number one and number three killer diseases among men and women in the United States, namely heart disease and stroke. The best way to handle food phobias is to educate yourself about that specific food and the science behind why that food may or may not be good for you. In many cases the phobia is not well-founded, which leads to poor decisions concerning your health.

Scams & So-called "Healthy" Foods

Because of the number of so-called healthy foods and other products in the marketplace, always read the product labels and do your own investigation of these products. If it sounds too good to be true, it probably is too good to be true. Many so-called "health" foods contain high fructose corn syrup or other additives and chemicals that have nothing to do with proper nutrition. Examples of foods and other products that have become popular due to marketing gimmicks and misinformation include the following.

- **Artificial sweeteners:** contain chemicals that have been linked to Alzheimer's, cancer and other ailments. We are attracted to these sweeteners because of their low calorie count, but some of these sweeteners actually stimulate the appetite while other sweeteners are made by processing table sugar with chlorine. Xylitol (a natural sugar found in berries and birch bark) is a better choice, especially since it does not trigger rising blood glucose levels.

- **Aspirin:** is often recommended by doctors to reduce inflammation and protect against cardiovascular risks, but daily aspirin increases the probability of gastric bleeding in the stomach and brain, based on several studies. More effective and safe alternatives include fish oil, nattokinase and ginger.

- **Bottled juices:** contain refined sugar and high fructose corn syrup. Many bottled juices are marketed as "100% fruit juice", but the juice is "dead". This is due to using over-ripe fruits, which are pasteurized destroying most of the beneficial vitamins, minerals and enzymes. It is better to make your own fresh juice with a juicer or blender. Be wary of bottled beverages that claim to cure many diseases without any supporting clinical studies.

- **Bottled water:** may contain many of the contaminants found in tap water; plus, deterioration of the plastic container leaks contaminants into the water. A well-designed water filter (counter, console models) will provide a better quality of water.

- **Calcium supplements:** that contain calcium carbonate cannot be absorbed by the body to stop or reverse osteoporosis. In fact, the supplement can make matters worse because the body is unable to get rid of the extra inorganic calcium, which may lead to kidney stones or arthritis. Generally a person consumes enough calcium as it is one of the most widely occurring nutrients in our diet. It is more likely that lifestyle choices and nutritional habits are interfering with the body's ability to absorb calcium, e.g. drinking coffee, soft drinks; excess intake of protein, especially milk and meat.

- **Cereals:** have some of the best TV commercials but cereals are overly processed and fortified with synthetic vitamins. Most cereals are full of sugar and lack organic vitamins and fiber. And, when you combine it with milk, some sugar, and a cup of coffee, you basically have a "dead" breakfast that contains almost zero nutritional value. If you really like cereal, then, choose an organic whole grain version.

- **Dairy products:** are not the best sources of calcium for adults – this is a nutritional myth that dairy produce is a good source of calcium. Milk products do contain a fair amount of calcium, but, because of the calcium to magnesium ratio in these products, the calcium is not well absorbed. Eating dairy foods in excess can inhibit the absorption of magnesium and cause the body to produce too much mucous. And, as we get older, the body produces less of the lactase enzyme, which is needed to break down milk and other dairy products. Calcium rich foods such as kelp, seaweeds, sardines, nuts and other plants offer the best sources of bioavailable calcium.

- **Diabetic foods:** are primarily processed "dead" foods that may not contain sugar but contain other harmful food chemicals, e.g. high fructose corn syrup, hydrogenated oil, sodium. Technically speaking, there is no such thing as "diabetic food". This is a marketing gimmick trying to take advantage of a growing market of diabetic people looking for answers.

- **Diet foods, beverages:** contain partially hydrogenated oil or high fructose corn syrup, which make you hungrier and fatter. This is another marketing gimmick taking advantage of a growing market of overweight people looking for answers.

- **Diets (Low Carb):** will cause additional health issues because it does not distinguish between the good and the bad carbs. But, in the meantime, many commercials and diet books will be marketed and sold to the public.

- **Diets (Low Fat):** actually make you fat! Diets create a chemical imbalance that can cause fatigue, emotional imbalance, and illness; and, induce the loss of lean muscle tissue – that's one of the reasons why it becomes more difficult to lose weight the next time around. Also, diets assume that you are relatively healthy and never address your other health issues that always accompany being fat. That's one of the reasons why the weight eventually returns – the diet never addressed the other health issues.

- **Diet sodas:** contain aspartame, phosphorous, and other chemicals that make these drinks just as bad as the regular sodas. In fact, they contain chemicals that may trigger cravings causing you to eat more food. The ingredients in aspartame are aspartic acid, phenylalanine, and methyl alcohol. Methyl alcohol is a chemical that breaks down in high temperatures and turns into formaldehyde and diketopiperazine (DKP), two chemicals known to cause problems in the nervous system. When a small child drinks a 12-ounce can of diet soda he consumes almost twice the daily amount of aspartame that is considered safe.

- **Drugs:** provide instant relief from pain and other discomfort by suppressing the symptoms, but they don't really address the root cause of your pain or discomfort. Many of these drugs have serious life-threatening side effects but only a few have been recalled from the market. There is an increasing number of drug-related commercials that are promoted on TV every day to increase your level of self-medication.

- **Exercise equipment:** can be helpful, but be wary of infomercials about exercise equipment that targets a specific area of the body or promises a lot of weight loss with little effort. Instead purchase something that will exercise the entire body and will motivate you to exercise on a consistent basis.

- **Granola bars, energy bars, drinks:** contain a lot of sugar, fructose corn syrup and other chemicals to provide a "sugar rush". Instead eat organic granola bars or make your own energy drink.

- **Hormone Replacement Therapy (HRT):** has proven to be harmful, but women still ingest these hormones derived from the urine of a pregnant horse. Instead, consider using natural wellness solutions that include bioidentical hormones and supplements that contain phytoestrogens from plants such as black cohosh, red clover, and flax; and, soy supplements with the isoflavones genistein and daidzein to address hot flashes, night sweats and other related issues.
- **Infomercials on TV and radio:** advertise that (some) drugs, vitamins or other supplements will cause effortless weight loss or cure most diseases. There is no such "magic" pill that causes effortless weight loss or cures most diseases. If it sounds too good to be true, it probably is.
- **Low-carb, low-fat, low-cholesterol foods:** are processed foods that are either lacking nutritional value or contain chemicals that are harmful to your health. "Low carb" does not mean low calories. Low fat foods are dangerous because most of them contain refined sugar, which turns to fat in the blood and causes more insulin production, which in turn produces and stores more fat.
- **Milk:** contains calcium, Vitamin D, is very nutritious in its natural (raw) form, and has some of the best commercials, e.g. "Got milk?" But, pasteurization converts the fragile proteins in milk (especially casein) into harmful proteins; destroys valuable enzymes, vitamins (B6, B12); and, eliminates the good bacteria normally present in the milk, reducing the vitamin and nutrient content of this nutritious food. Homogenization keeps the milk from separating naturally and creates harmful molecules (xanthane oxidase) that increase oxidation stress, which contributes to the development of heart disease. This prevents the proper absorption of nutrients into the blood and restricts the elimination of the toxic waste from the blood, leading to the formation of mucous, congestion, colds, etc. In addition, cows are given antibiotics (to fight diseases) and growth hormones (to increase their milk production).

   Note: Low fat or fat-free versions of milk have fewer calories, but are virtually void of beneficial Vitamin D and calcium. Organic milk is a little better but it's still pasteurized. Raw milk is the best choice if you can find it at a local farm.

- **No Trans Fat:** on the food label does not necessarily mean the food product does not contain trans fat or partially hydrogenated oil. If the amount of trans fat per serving is 0.49 grams or less, the food can be advertised as having "no trans fat". Check the ingredients to ensure "partially hydrogenated oil" is not listed.
- **Pizza:** is one of the most popular foods, but it is a potential "triple-killer" because it's loaded with saturated fat from the cheese; saturated fat from the meat and other toppings; and, refined flour from the dough. You can still enjoy pizza while reducing its health impacts by using vegetable toppings, less cheese and organic flour.
- **Salmon:** is sold in grocery stores as farmed salmon, which is fed grain and filled with antibiotics, cancer-causing PCBs, pesticides, and other chemicals; and, injected with a synthetic dye that gives the salmon its pink color (to disguise an unappetizing pale gray). The dye contains canthaxanthin, an ingredient used in tanning pills. Farmed salmon contains two thirds less of the Omega-3 EFAs. Instead, eat ocean-raised wild salmon, which feed on smaller fish that eat EPA and DHA-rich algae. Wild salmon (canned, frozen) can be found in some grocery stores or can be ordered from some websites.
- **Shakes for breakfast, smoothies, meal replacement meals:** are full of sugar, high fructose corn syrup, additives and other chemicals.
- **Soda:** is a very popular beverage, with some of the best commercials. But, soda contains sugar and phosphorous, which blocks the absorption of calcium making the body very acidic. An average 12-ounce can of soda contains at least 10 teaspoons of sugar and over 120 calories.
- **Soy milk, soy foods:** are overly processed in some cases, removing the critical nutrients such as the isoflavones, and may contain high levels of refined sugar. These overly-processed soy products can trigger the production of the bad estrogen. Some soybeans may contain chemicals that cause red blood cells to clump together or block the absorption of key minerals. Ensure the soy is organic, contains the isoflavones genistein and daidzein, or is fermented. Fermented soy foods (e.g. miso, natto, tempeh) neutralize the phytates, which block the absorption of nutrients such as calcium.

- **Sugar-free snacks:** contain partially hydrogenated oil, other additives and hidden sugars that increase hunger, inhibit fat metabolism, or increase fat production and fat storage.
- **Sunscreens:** help to protect us from sunburn by blocking UVB rays, but, most do not block the more damaging UVA rays. Avoid chemical sunscreens that interact with the sunlight, increase the oxidation, and are absorbed into your skin. Use paraben-free, mineral-based sunscreens that contain zinc oxide as the only active ingredient. Since the invention of sunscreen years ago, skin cancer rates have actually gone up. However, in tropical countries (where the sun's rays are the strongest) the skin cancer rate is extremely low. **Sunshine is actually *good* for us** because it helps to metabolize cholesterol and produce Vitamin D, a potent cancer-fighter. Sunshine also causes the body to produce melanin, which is the pigment responsible for turning the skin brown when you tan while providing a natural protection against skin cancer. Using sunscreen blocks the production of melanin, depriving your skin of this natural protective ability. In addition, scientists have uncovered that sunscreen itself may cause cancer, because of parabens and other chemicals contained in the sunscreen. The following chemicals have been found to behave like estrogen and stimulate tumor-growth and cancer cells: octyldimethyl PABA, benzophenone-3, homosalate, octyl-methoxycinnamate, and 4-methyl-benzylidene camphor.
- **Vitamin pills:** are mostly "rocks" containing additives, fillers, binders, and other chemicals. Most of them provide very little nutritional value and fail to provide the necessary vitamin/mineral levels supported by the clinicals. Use wholefood supplements, food-based supplements or natural vitamins that are 100% additive-free.
- **Yogurt:** can contain a lot of sugar and fructose corn syrup, and, not enough "live" cultures – most are either killed during the pasteurization process or die by the time they reach the grocery shelves. Use the organic or low fat versions without the extra fruit and sugar, or consider making your own yogurt.

The key defense for protecting yourself from marketing gimmicks and scams is knowledge, so educate yourself about proper nutrition.

Nutritional Supplements

Nutritional *food*-based supplements have value, but only if you have a sound nutritional/exercise profile and the supplements are derived from food sources that align with nature's blueprint. Supplements do not work optimally if they are *chemical*-based (synthetic) or are taken in lieu of a sound nutritional and exercise profile. Also, supplements do not work optimally if they are modified such that they no longer resemble their structure in nature (e.g. food). Many people take vitamins and other supplements for the wrong reason – to "cancel out" the negative effects of poor nutrition and a sedentary lifestyle. But, this type of supplementation strategy does not work especially if you are fighting a major disease.

If you have a disease such as diabetes, live or work in a highly polluted environment, or have a very stressful job, you can benefit from proper nutritional supplementation as long as you eat nutritious meals most of the time – to establish a sound nutritional foundation that will help combat the disease, the stress, and the environment.

In general, there is enough nutrition in raw organic foods, raw juices and super foods to prevent a disease that is due to vitamin/mineral deficiencies – as long as you are eating these foods on a consistent daily basis. But, if you have a disease like diabetes, then, you are already not getting enough nutrients to successfully fight the disease. Having a disease is like being in a deep dark pit. Each time you eat properly, you take one step up out of the pit. Each time you take a (proper) supplement, it ensures that you don't slip down a step, but it doesn't help you to step up out of the pit. To ensure that you are taking the proper supplements, refer to Chapter 8 for a list of the key selection criteria.

Author's Personal Note: In my case, I was able to reverse my diabetes with very little nutritional supplementation because I maximized my consumption of several nutritious meals and snacks each day. I wanted to ensure that I was doing everything reasonably possible with my meals before I started taking too many supplements. For a list of higher quality supplements, review the Resource List on page 374.

Types of Cravings

One of the major challenges that diabetics (and non-diabetics) face is appetite control and food cravings created by the excess consumption of "dead" processed foods, which are full of the chemicals that trigger the cravings. In order to reduce and eliminate the cravings for these "dead" processed foods (refined flour products, sweets, salty foods, processed meats, snacks), it is important to understand what triggers the cravings and how to prevent the triggers in the future.

People with food cravings or strong appetites usually have a neuro-chemical/hormonal imbalance due to a toxic buildup that triggers a hunger/craving and creates a vicious cycle that never seems to end. For example, the hunger/craving for something sweet is usually due to low blood sugar. Once you eat something sweet, your blood sugar and serotonin levels rise quickly causing a "sugar rush" that makes you feel good. But, a couple hours later, you're hungry again because of the crash that occurs when your blood sugar level goes too low. Then, the cycle repeats itself when you feed the hunger with more refined carbohydrates and sweets. Eating foods rich in fiber, antioxidants and Omega-3s will stop this cycle, while helping to reduce the internal inflammation and the buildup of toxins that are driving the food craving or strong appetite.

A craving is also a signal from your body trying to tell you that your cells are starving and lacking key vitamins, minerals and other nutrients – a nutrient deficiency. Unfortunately, this signal is misunderstood as a craving and once the craving is fed, the signal returns indicating the cells are still starved.

There are basically two types of cravings:
- **Emotional craving**, which is usually due to a stressful situation triggered by an emotion such as sadness, depression, or anger; and usually comes upon us very quickly.
- **Physical craving**, which is usually due to a biochemical imbalance; and, usually comes upon us gradually.

Emotional craving
The following is a list of countermeasures that you can take to reduce and eliminate different types of emotional cravings.

Stress eating is one of the most common reactions to dealing with stress because it boosts the production of cortisol, a hormone that facilitates your fight or flight response. According to a recent study, participants with higher cortisol levels tended to eat more in stressful situations.

Countermeasure: No matter how hectic your schedule, devote a few minutes a day to giving yourself a breather. Step outside the office or house and take a walk around the block. Do something – anything – that removes you from the rat race, even if it's only for a few minutes.

Anger eating is the No. 1 eating trigger for women, according to a study from the University of Wurzburg in Germany. Because anger resembles stress in terms of how the body reacts physiologically, cravings for sweet, high-fat foods such as ice cream and chocolate can increase.

Countermeasure: Reaching for fat, sugary foods such as ice cream is a natural reaction to anger, since fat and sugar boost serotonin, our brain's feel-good hormone. But sugary foods also flood the bloodstream with glucose, which releases the hormone insulin, making blood sugar levels momentarily spike, then drop. When blood sugar falls, so does serotonin, leaving you feeling worse than you did before. Instead, take a few deep breaths when you feel angry. Collect your thoughts and try to articulate them in a calm, coherent manner. Sometimes, just letting go of the emotion can release you from its hold. If you still want the ice cream, mix some fresh blueberries and walnuts in the ice cream to slow down its absorption into the bloodstream.

Sadness or depression often makes us seek solace in the cookie jar or container of ice cream. The reason comes down, again, to serotonin. Many of the most popular antidepressants alleviate depression by boosting the availability of serotonin in the brain.

Countermeasure: Talk to a friend – sometimes just talking releases the sadness. Or, get moving. Numerous studies indicate that exercise decreases mild depression as effectively as psychotherapy. A Duke

University study stated that only 14 minutes of walking reduced negative feelings by 82 percent. In addition to the 20-30 minutes of daily aerobic exercise (e.g. walking, swimming, biking), include at least 15 minutes of weight-resistance exercise three or four times a week. If you think you're suffering from clinical depression, consult your doctor.

Happy feelings occur during celebrations such as weddings, birthday parties, family picnics, reunions, graduations, anniversaries, holidays, or a night out on the town to celebrate that hard-earned promotion. And, we celebrate many of these happy occasions with big meals, cakes, and other goodies.

Countermeasure: Enjoy the celebration! Don't spend your time looking over your shoulder and miss all the fun! Try to eat as many "live" super foods as possible with your meals and snacks the day before the celebration. This will reduce your capacity to overeat. Even if you overeat, just make certain that your next two meals at home are full of fiber and water to help remove the waste from the body as soon as possible. Increasing the duration of your next two exercise sessions will also help to reduce the impact of the celebration and help to remove the toxins and waste out of the body.

Stress, anger, sadness or happy feelings can also trigger the need for alcohol and/or recreational drugs such as marijuana and cocaine.

Countermeasure: Find another food/drink alternative or ask your doctor for the name of a local support group that can help you, e.g. Alcoholics Anonymous (AA), Narcotics Anonymous (NA).

Physical craving
The following is a list of countermeasures that you can take to reduce and eliminate different types of physical cravings.

Low blood sugar is the most common physical/biochemical craving that triggers the need for bread, pasta, French fries, sweets and other refined carbohydrates. Once the need is satisfied, within two hours, the craving returns creating a vicious cycle.
Countermeasure: Add more fiber and Omega-3s to breakfast (e.g. spinach, broccoli, whole-grain cereal, wild salmon, whole fruit). Add a tablespoon of ground flaxseed or wheat grass powder to your breakfast drink or cereal. Drink a glass of raw vegetable juice (or V-8 juice) instead of bottled juice, which is full of refined sugar and high fructose corn syrup. Also, **avoid your food triggers**, e.g. driving past a fast food place.

Low fat intake causes a craving for cheese, animal meat, pizza, and other foods with a high fat content.
Countermeasure: Ensure all your meals including your snacks contain some fat, preferably the good fat found in fish, plant oils, lean organic meats, nuts and other plant foods.

Low salt intake causes a craving for potato chips, pretzels, French fries.
Countermeasure: Ensure all your meals including your snacks contain some sodium, but more importantly, eat enough foods that contain water and potassium, e.g. green, leafy vegetables, legumes. This will reduce the craving. If you find that you must have some potato chips, then, try baked tortilla chips with some guacamole (mashed seasoned avocado); or, organic potato chips, which contain more flavorful organic spices, less sodium and no hydrogenated oil. Use organic sea salt.

A mineral deficiency causes a craving for a food that contains that specific mineral. For example, a craving for chocolate may be due to a mineral deficiency in magnesium.
Countermeasure: If you have a craving for chocolate, eat the pure cocoa kind and stay away from the milk chocolate, which has more fat and more sugar. Review your blood work over the past two years with your doctor to ensure that you do not have any major mineral deficiencies.

Chapter 7. The Super Meal Model

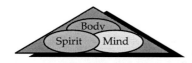

The Most Important Key

Most people are aware that nutrition, more than any other factor, is the key to successfully managing and controlling diabetes. However, many diabetics are not aware that nutrition is also the key to reversing diabetes. The primary reason for diabetes (and other systemic, degenerative diseases such as heart disease and arthritis) is nutritional imbalance. Nutritional imbalance can be characterized in two ways: (1) **toxic buildup/congestion** – eating too many "dead" foods full of chemical toxins that cannot be processed and eliminated by the body; and, (2) **nutritional deficiency** – eating too many "dead" foods that lack vitamins, minerals, amino acids, saccharides, fatty acids, enzymes, fiber and water. Both of these imbalances interfere with the body being able to function properly and successfully defend itself against any disease.

Most diabetics are either not aware of the right nutritious foods to eat or are not willing to change their eating habits, leading to congestion and nutritional deficiency. This, in turn, progresses to increasing insulin and glucose levels, insulin resistance, inflammation, weight gain, fatigue, cravings, increasing blood pressure and cholesterol levels, and eventually a serious disease such as diabetes. And, all of this is primarily due to the diet (nutritional profile) of most diabetics being full of common mistakes, some of which are made knowingly, some unknowingly. This chapter will define the proper nutritional profile for diabetics – the Super Meal Model. This model will help diabetics to better control their insulin and blood glucose levels and trigger their bodies' internal healing mechanisms.

The Super Meal Model

Most nutrition and diet books provide good descriptions of foods, vitamins, minerals and other vital nutrients. But, because those descriptions are seldom done in the context of a "model" (picture), it is difficult to understand and remember all the specific foods that are good or bad for your health. Even if you know what foods are good for you, it is still not clear what combinations of these foods will provide optimum health or help to fight a disease like diabetes. And, even if you know the right combinations of foods, counting calories can be very tedious and frustrating. All of this makes it difficult to design a program that is enjoyable, flexible, inexpensive and easy to remember, implement, and modify on a consistent basis to suit your health needs. Bottomline, if it's not enjoyable or easy to implement, then, you will eventually return to your old eating habits.

As engineers, we design and develop products and solutions, based on an architectural design model that is supported by a set of engineering principles that meets the needs of the customer. As a result, it is easier to design a successful product that will work properly according to those engineering principles and customer needs.

Similarly, I felt that it would be easier to design a healthy meal if I had a set of sound nutritional principles that aligned with the body's needs. And because of my own frustration and ignorance with trying to figure out how to identify the right foods and design meals that would work for me, I felt that a simple model (picture) of what my meal plate should look like every time I ate would be easier to remember than counting calories. And, if that model is based on what my body requires biochemically and hormonally to fight the primary root causes of systemic degenerative diseases (e.g. nutritional deficiency, toxic overload, oxidation, inflammation, and hormonal imbalance), then, the model should work to optimize my health and fight any disease, including diabetes.

Since I was not much of a cook, I decided to design a simplistic model based on the body's physical structure at the cellular level, e.g. water, fat, protein, saccharides, etc. And, modify that model, based on information from several clinical studies about nutrition (listed in the Clinical References section of the Appendix). I initially started with approximately 65% carbohydrates and gradually lowered it to 40 to 45% (based on my *post-meal glucose testing*), while increasing the quality of the carbohydrates from processed to plant, the protein from land animal to plant and fish; and, the fat from animal and processed to plant. Refer to the following diagram, which depicts the contents of a typical super meal and what a typical meal plate should look like as a starting point.

- From a physical viewpoint, at least half of the plate should contain green, leafy and other bright-colored **vegetables** such as spinach, broccoli, red/yellow peppers, mushrooms, onions; a quarter of the plate should contain **lean protein** such as wild salmon, tuna, sardines or other cold water fish; and, depending on your health needs, the other quarter of the plate should contain a **legume, a whole grain or another vegetable** such as cauliflower, black beans, chickpeas, or organic brown rice. And, add a tablespoon of a **plant oil** such as extra virgin olive oil on top of the vegetables for the good fat.

- From a calorie perspective, approximately 40% to 50% of the total calories should be allocated for the **carbohydrates** such as **vegetables**. The percentage depends on your daily activity level and the amount of daily exercise. In general, if you have low activity and low exercise levels, as most diabetics tend to have, you should decrease your intake of carbohydrates to the low end of the range. And, because everyone is different, *increase your post-meal blood glucose testing* to determine the specific amounts of carbohydrates and other macronutrients that are best for you.

- Approximately 20% to 30% of the total calories should be allocated for the **proteins**, depending on the type of exercise (amount of weight-resistance training), the amount of land animal protein and how well your body metabolizes proteins. If most of the protein that you consume is conventional land animal protein, you should decrease your intake to the low end of the range. If you are eating mostly plant protein or performing a lot of weight-resistance training to build muscle, you should increase your intake of protein to the high end of the range.

- Approximately 25% to 35% of the total calories should be allocated for the **fats**, with the majority of that fat (90%) being allocated to fish and plant-based oils versus land animal-based fat. Increasing the amount of quality fat (and meal frequency) will be crucial for most diabetics to reduce the internal inflammation, obtain a feeling of satiety, metabolize old fat, and increase the absorption of the vegetable's fat-soluble nutrients (e.g. carotenoids).
- In general, 6 to 9 cups of **filtered water** should be consumed daily, including the water from the vegetables and fruits. But, don't get carried away with drinking too much water. In fact, if you are eating enough vegetables and fruits throughout the day, you may only need to drink 5 to 6 cups of water each day.

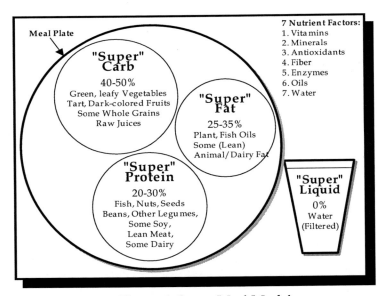

Figure 6. Super Meal Model

Since this Super Meal Model is *not* a one-size-fits-all model, these percentages will vary from person to person and should only be used as a guideline. These percentages will vary depending upon your activity and stress levels as you progress through your recovery.

Note: More importantly, ensure your super meals include foods that suit *your* taste/texture preferences, e.g. salty, sweet, bitter, buttery, crunchy, etc. Otherwise, you will not stick with the program!

For a typical meal of 500 calories, the gram and calorie counts would be:

- Carb   50 grams   200 calories
- Protein   37.5 grams   150 calories
- Fat   16.7 grams   150 calories
- Liquid   16 ounces   0 calories

Note: If you add a juice or similar beverage to the meal, don't forget to include its calories as part of the carbohydrate total. To maintain the balance of carbohydrates, protein, and fat, you can add a tablespoon of ground flaxseed or a protein/fiber powder supplement to the beverage.

If each meal consists of small, proportioned balanced amounts of these four macronutrients every time you eat, this will prevent the biochemical and hormonal imbalances such as glucose/insulin spikes, fat storage, inflammation, and dehydration that occur with traditional meals. These meals tend to be carb-heavy, fiber-deficient, water-deficient, and nutrient-deficient. If the four macronutrients come strictly from the group of 5 "live" (super) foods, your meal will qualify as a super meal. Ideally, your meal plate will physically look similar to the diagram in Figure 6, where most of the plate is bright-colored vegetables, a quarter of the plate is lean protein, and a small portion is allocated for the healthy (liquid) fat, which can be placed on top of the vegetables.

As you consume more of these super meals on a consistent basis (4 to 6 times a day), this will turn on the body's cleansing and healing mechanisms to gradually improve your health. On the other hand, the consistent consumption of the 5 "dead" foods will deteriorate the body leading to poor health and disease. Refer to Chapter 17 for some recipes of super meals and super snacks.

Whether you are a diabetic or not, you will notice an increase in your energy level if you can maintain the momentum of eating super meals consistently. If you are a diabetic you will notice a decrease in your average fasting blood glucose level within two to three weeks; and, more importantly, a decrease in your post-meal blood glucose level.

Nutritional Protocol: Attributes of Super Meals

The nutritional protocol, or attributes, of a super meal are similar to those of the Mediterranean diet, which includes fresh whole foods -- vegetables, fruits, fish, whole grains, nuts and olive oil -- that are high in fiber, Omega-3 fatty acids and low in refined carbohydrates. The super meal is designed to provide optimum nutrition to prevent and fight diabetes and other systemic, degenerative diseases/ailments such as heart disease, stroke, and obesity. These attributes specifically nourish, protect, cleanse and repair the body's cells by addressing the major root causes of Type 2 diabetes: insulin resistance (hormonal imbalance), inflammation, oxidation, nutritional deficiency, and toxic overload. Implement these attributes over a period of time, based on your current state of health, your health goals, lifestyle, exercise regimen and food preferences.

Smaller meal size (350-700 calories): This will reduce the production of insulin and prevent the body from storing fat. Too much insulin in your blood also depletes the body of specific vitamins and minerals, e.g. Vitamin B-complex, Vitamin C, chromium, potassium, magnesium.

Minimum daily quantities of foods: If you don't like to count calories, then, the minimum daily quantities must be met and distributed across 4 to 6 daily meals/snacks to ensure the body is acquiring enough of the proper nutrients throughout the day to repair the trillions of defective cells:

- 5 to 7 cups of bright-colored raw/lightly-steamed **vegetables** and 1-3 cups of **fruits**, including raw juices; 8-16 oz. wheat/barley grass juice; ideally at least 1-2 vegetables with each major meal.
- 3 to 4 tablespoons of a **plant oil** such as extra virgin olive oil or some other good plant oil such as macadamia nut oil; ideally 1 to 1½ tablespoons with each major meal.
- 5 to 7 cups of **filtered water**; approximately 2 cups with each meal.
- 2 to 3 cups/servings of **lean protein** (legumes, organic/fermented soy foods), fish, lean meat, low fat dairy.
- 1 to 2 cups of organic whole grains, including 1 to 3 slices of sprouted grain bread.

More frequent meals (4 to 6 times/day): This increases the thermogenic mechanisms, speeding up your metabolism. This also reduces the production of insulin, cholesterol, homocysteine, and triglycerides leading to the reduction in the thickness of the blood and a lower blood pressure.

Author's Personal Note: This was difficult for me because I didn't like to eat snacks and my schedule made it difficult to eat more frequently. But, I was able to find some healthy snack foods that made it easy to eat more frequently and more healthy. For example, a handful of nuts/seeds, some grapes and a glass of water are actually a balanced super snack because it contains the 4 major macronutrients: a carbohydrate (the grapes), a protein/fat (the nuts/seeds), and a liquid (the water). Apples, strawberries, pears, bananas, pulse food, and organic fruit juice were some of the other carbohydrates that I ate/drank as part of my snacks. Black bean soup, canned wild salmon, tuna, skinless chicken breast, ground flaxseed, soft-boiled eggs, whey protein powder, and soy protein nuggets were some of the other proteins and fats.

Meal balance of "live" super carbohydrates, proteins, fats and liquids: This reduces the production of insulin and prevents the body from storing fat. For a typical (smaller) meal of 400-500 calories, the gram and calorie count should be similar to the following:

Macro-nutrient	% Calories	No. of Grams	No. of Calories
Carbohydrate	40-50%	40-62.5 grams	160-250 calories
Protein	20-30%	20-37.5 grams	80-150 calories
Fat	25-35%	11.1-19.4 grams	100-175 calories
Liquid	0-15%	16-24 ounces	0-75 calories

Figure 7. No. of Calories & Grams in a Super Meal

- **Super carbohydrates** include:
  - Bright, colorful and green, leafy (raw, lightly-steamed) vegetables such as Brussel sprouts, stringbeans, spinach, broccoli, cauliflower, kale, sprouts, and greens (collard, beet, mustard); sea vegetables (chlorella, spirulina, sea plankton, kelp); and, grasses (wheat, barley)
  - Other (raw, lightly-steamed) vegetables such as carrots, celery, cucumbers, peppers, squash, zucchini, and tomatoes.
  - Dark, colorful fruits such as berries, cherries, apples, and grapes.
  - Organic whole grains such as amaranth, quinoa, barley, oat; and sprouted grain bread.
  - Other plant foods such as onions, mushrooms (shiitake, maitake)
- **Super proteins** include:
  - Cold-water fish such as wild salmon, trout, sardines, tuna.
  - Nuts/seeds such as walnuts, almonds, macadamias; flax, sesame.
  - Organic whole soy products such as tofu, soy protein, soy cheese.
  - Dairy such as organic eggs, egg whites, low fat cheese, yogurt.
  - Meats such as lean, organic beef, poultry, wild deer.
  - Organic seafood such as shrimp, lobster, crab.
- **Super fats** include:
  - Monounsaturated fats such as extra virgin olive oil, macadamia nut oil, avocados, almonds.
  - Omega-3 EFAs within flaxseed oil, nuts and seeds which provide alpha linolenic acid (ALA); and, within krill and fish to provide eicosapentaenoic acid (EPA) and docosahexaenoic acid (DHA).
  - Omega-6 EFAs within borage oil, evening primrose oil and black currant oil, which provide gamma linolenic acid (GLA).
  - Saturated fats such as extra virgin coconut oil.
- **Super liquids** include:
  - Filtered water
  - Raw vegetable/fruit juice (with the pulp/fiber extracted)
  - Raw, blender-mixed vegetable juice, wheat/barley grass juice; blender-mixed fruit juice (whole vegetables/fruits with the fiber)
  - Green, white teas and herbal teas (e.g. chamomile, hibiscus)
  - Some organic bottled juices with fiber pulp and less sugar

High fiber content requires at least 32 to 35 grams of fiber daily. Soluble fiber sources include: oat bran, pectins of certain fruits/vegetables (e.g. blackberries, artichoke), guar gum (e.g. beans, peas, nuts, seeds), psyllium and konjac. Insoluble fiber (roughage) sources include: whole grains, apple skin, bran cereal, broccoli, kidney beans, pinto beans, pear skin, potato skin, and oatmeal.

Note: The average person consumes less than 15 grams of fiber daily, which is at least 15 grams below the minimum daily requirement. If necessary, use freshly ground flaxseed or a quality fiber supplement with each meal to increase your daily fiber intake.

Fermented foods (probiotics), such as organic yogurt, sauerkraut, miso, and kefir, promote the growth of friendly intestinal bacteria, which aid digestion and support immune function, including an increase in B vitamins, Omega-3 fatty acids, chromium, digestive enzymes, lactase and lactic acid, and other immune nutrients that help to heal the gastrointestinal tract and fight off harmful bacteria and cancer cells.

- Unprocessed fermented foods boost the immune system by increasing antibodies that fight infectious disease.
- The flora in living cultured foods form a "living shield" that covers the small intestine's inner lining and helps inhibit pathogenic organisms including E.coli, salmonella and an unhealthy overgrowth of candida (yeast).
- Some fermented foods create antioxidants (glutathione and superoxide dismustase) that scavenge free radicals, which are a cancer precursor.
- Fermenting transforms hard-to-digest lactose from milk to the more easily digested lactic acid. It neutralizes the anti-nutrients found in many foods including the phytic acid found in all grains and the trypsin-inhibitors in soy.
- Fermentation generates new nutrients including Omega-3 fatty acids, digestive aids and the trace mineral GTF chromium, which increases the insulin cell receptor sites causing an increase of insulin usage.
- Foods and substances that decimate intestinal flora are: antibiotics, commercial meats containing antibiotic residues, chlorinated water, alcoholic beverages and a diet high in processed and packaged foods.

Nutritional food-based supplementation: includes wholefood, food-derived vitamins, minerals, super foods, glyconutrients, and herbs. But, supplementation should only be considered once a sound super meal program is in place. Some of the nutrients within supplements include:

- **Antioxidants:** alpha lipoic acid, CoQ10, N-acetylcysteine, Vitamin C, Vitamin E; selenium, mixed carotenes; shiitake mushrooms; flavonoids (cranberry, green tea, grape seed); l-carnitine; aloe vera.
- **Enzymes:** amylase, protease, lipase, lactase, especially if you have trouble digesting food or you eat less than 50% raw vegetables.
- **Fats/Oils:** Omega-3 EFAs in fish, krill and flax help repair cell membranes and improve glucose control and fat metabolism.
- **Fiber:** insoluble fiber (such as psyllium), primarily for temporary relief from constipation; soluble fiber (such as oat bran and flaxseed) helps to lower cholesterol.
- **Glyconutrients:** contain saccharides that help support the immune and endocrine systems to provide protection and hormonal balance.
- **Herbs/plants:** for cardiovascular health and increased glucose uptake.
  - o   Hawthorne berry, raw/aged garlic: for cardiovascular system.
  - o   Plant sterols, policosanol, fenugreek: for high cholesterol.
  - o   Banaba leaf, gymnema sylvestre, bitter melon, cinnamon cassia bark extract, garcinia cambogia: for insulin, glucose control.
- **Minerals:** magnesium, potassium, calcium for electrolyte and pH acid-alkaline balance; vanadium, chromium for carbohydrate metabolism and insulin/glucose control.
- **Probiotics:** acidophilus, bifidophilus, organic yogurt, sauerkraut, miso, tempeh, tofu -- especially after taking antibiotics.
- **Super foods:** grasses (wheat, barley), sea vegetables (plankton, chlorella, spirulina, kelp), royal jelly, aloe vera, rice germ help increase absorption of nutrients and the strength of the immune system.
- **Vitamins:** B-complex for carbohydrate/protein/fat metabolism, energy production, body functions, cell health.

Periodic cleansing/detoxification (one to four times a year, depending on your health needs) helps to keep waste, toxins and other chemicals from accumulating in the body.

Calorie Planning

Calorie counting can be tedious and frustrating. However, you can use calorie counting as a tool or guide to help you design your daily/weekly meal program. And, once you become familiar with the physical size and calorie counts for various foods, you will not have to spend a lot of time counting calories at each meal.

In order to accomplish this, first, you need to determine the amount of calories you require on a daily basis to maintain your current weight – this is known as your maintenance calorie count. You can determine this by using one of the calculators on any of the many diet-related websites – just google with "diet calculator". For an example, let's use 2250 calories as the maintenance calorie count.

If the overall goal is to lose weight, specifically, fat, then, you need to set a target calorie count that is at least 20% below your current maintenance calorie count of 2250:

2250 – (20% of 2250)= 2250 – 450 = 1800
So, 1800 calories would be your daily target calorie count.

Next, using 40%-30%-30% as a starting point, the calories would be distributed as follows:

Carbohydrates: 40% of 1800 = 720
Protein: 30% of 1800 = 540
Fat: 30% of 1800 = 540

Since there are 4 calories in each gram of a carbohydrate, 4 calories in each gram of a protein, and 9 calories in each gram of a fat, the number of grams for each of these macronutrients would be:

Carbohydrates: 720 divided by 4 = 180 grams
Protein: 540 divided by 4 = 135 grams
Fat: 540 divided by 9 = 60 grams

Next, to determine the number of grams (of each macronutrient) for each meal/snack, you need to divide each of the gram numbers by the number of meals/snacks that you plan to have each day. For this example, let's assume that you are going start with a total of 4 meals/snacks each day. That means each meal/snack will have the following distribution of grams and calories:

Carbohydrates: 180 divided by 4 = 45 grams
Protein: 135 divided by 4 = 33.75 grams
Fat: 60 divided by 4 = 15 grams

If you assume that the snack is much smaller in size and calories, let's say by 50%, then, it will contain 22.5 grams of carbohydrates, 16.9 grams of protein, and 7.5 grams of fat. As a result, each of the three major meals will have the following distribution of grams and calories:

Carbohydrates: 45 times 3 plus 22.5 divided by 3 = 52.5 g, 210 cal
Protein: 33.75 times 3 plus 16.9 divided by 3 = 39.4 g, 157 cal
Fat: 15 times 3 plus 7.5 divided by 3 = 17.5 g, 157 cal

These numbers may appear small initially, but, once you begin eating more "live" foods and more frequent meals, your body chemistry will make the proper adjustments and you will actually find it difficult to eat 1800 calories every day – unless you consume a lot of "dead" food or exercise more than 60 minutes a day. If you are not familiar with the number of grams and calories for different foods, obtain a nutrition or diet book that provides this information.

Note: This is a simplistic model that does not take into account the addition of lean muscle tissue as a health goal. That would require a higher target calorie count and at least five if not six or seven meals/snacks each day.

Note: If you need help with your meal planning and shopping, contact our wellness center or visit our website at www.DeathToDiabetes.com.

Nutritional Profile

So, how do you go about designing a set of meals that meet the criteria for super meals and fits into your busy schedule? There are basically two ways, depending on the level of detail that you prefer:

Physical look ("eye-ball"): If your plate contains mostly colorful super carbohydrates, with a quarter portion of your plate containing a super protein and super fat, then, your meal will qualify as a super meal. For example, the following is a good example of a super meal (for dinner):

- Super carbohydrate: 1 ½ cups steamed spinach and 1 cup broccoli
- Super protein: 4-5 oz. baked wild salmon
- Super fat: 1 ½ tbsp. extra virgin olive oil (add on top of vegetable after steaming)
- Super liquid: 16-24 oz. filtered water
- Optional (addition): 8 oz. raw carrot juice, with 1 tbsp. of freshly ground flaxseed or 1 tbsp. wheat/barley grass powder

Nutritional profile (calorie calculations): If the total number of calories, grams of fiber and other nutrient measurements fit within the super meal guidelines, then, your meal will qualify as a super meal. The following is a profile example of one of my breakfast super meals.

Food	Carb (calories)	Protein (calories)	Fat (calories)	Total Calories	Fiber (grams)
1 cup Broccoli	120	24	0	144	4
1.5 oz. Baked Salmon	0	48	30	78	0
1 Tbsp. Olive Oil	0	0	115	115	0
2 Tbsp. Protein Powder	0	62	4	66	4
8 oz. Carrot Juice	84	9	3	96	2
16 oz. Water	0	0	0	0	0
Total Calories	204	143	152	499	10g
Calorie Percentages	41%	29%	30%		

Figure 8. Nutritional Profile of a Super Meal

Dining Out Guidelines

The Super Meal Model and nutritional profile will work very well because you have total control of what you buy at the grocery store and what meals you prepare at home. However, today more than 60% of Americans consume meals and snacks away from home on any given day. This accounts for approximately 50% of one's daily caloric intake. Even the educated consumer has difficulty controlling carbohydrates, fat and calories, when eating out, due to the large portion sizes and the hidden fat, sodium, and other chemicals in foods. While maintaining good eating habits when dining out may be difficult, it is not impossible.

The following are some guidelines to help you when dining out:

- If possible, limit the number of times that you dine out to once or twice a week – at least until you have better control of your blood glucose level.
- Avoid restaurants that do not accommodate special dietary requests. Don't be hesitant to call ahead and make special requests. Most restaurants are willing to accommodate your dietary needs when possible.
- Take the time to examine a menu carefully. Never be hesitant about asking a waiter how a food is prepared and whether it can be prepared to suit your needs. Most restaurants will be more than happy to accommodate your requests.
  - o Look for these words indicating low fat preparations: baked, broiled, grilled, garden fresh, in its own juice, poached, roasted, steamed.
  - o Watch out for these words indicating high fat/high calories: au fromage, au gratin, basted, butter sauce, braised, béarnaise, casserole, cheesy sauce, creamed, creamy sauce, crispy, escalloped, fried, hash, hollandaise, marinated (in oil), parmesan, pastry crust, potpie, prime, sautéed, stewed, stir-fried, stuffed.
  - o Watch out for these words indicating hidden sodium: au jus, broth, cocktail sauce, cured, pickled, smoked, soy sauce, teriyaki, tomato baste.

- Avoid entrées that are fried or sautéed. Order entrées that are baked, broiled, grilled or poached because they are normally lower in fat. To avoid getting a lot of hidden fats in your meal, inquire about the butter, margarine, cream or oil that is used in preparing that item.
- Order at least one lightly-steamed green vegetable and another bright-colored vegetable instead of rice, pasta, mashed potatoes, or French fries.
- Because portion sizes served in most restaurants are very large, automatically cut your plate in half and place half the meal in a doggie bag to take home and enjoy with a later meal; or, share it with a friend. Keep your portion of lean animal meat to the size of a deck of cards (3 oz.). If you're eating fish, you can eat a larger portion (5 oz.).
- Select foods prepared by baking, broiling or boiling rather than frying. If you're not sure how your food will be prepared, ask.
- Ask for foods to be prepared with less fat. Trim off visible fat from meats.
- Avoid dishes with sauces, or preparations that include breaded, deep fried, sautéed, or have creamy in their name.
- Order condiments such as salad dressing, butter, sour cream, sauces, seasonings and gravies on the side and use sparingly.
- Avoid coffee, but if you plan to have a cup, ask for low fat or skim milk for your coffee instead of cream or half and half.
- At Oriental restaurants, start with hot and sour soup; eat half portions of chicken, fish or lean meat stir-fried with vegetables; order plain rice instead of fried rice.
- At Italian restaurants, choose pasta with tomato-based sauces. Avoid sausages, fatty cuts of meat and limit the amount of cheese.
- At delis, order sliced turkey, ham or lean roast beef. Skip the cheese and replace mayonnaise with mustard. Ask for coleslaw, tomatoes, or a pickle instead of fries or chips.

Fast Food Restaurants

Although fast food restaurants are now providing healthier choices, dining out at a fast food restaurant can be very challenging. Use the following guidelines to help reduce the negative impacts to your health:

- Try to limit the number of times that you eat at fast food restaurants to once or twice a week. Studies show that if you eat fast foods more than twice a week, it increases your insulin resistance and weight gain.
- Choose grilled chicken or turkey sandwich with lettuce, tomatoes, and mustard instead of a jumbo cheeseburger (or hamburger).
- Choose baked potato instead of French fries.
- Choose low sodium pretzels or baked potato chips instead of regular potato chips.
- Choose vegetarian pizza instead of regular pizza or meat lovers.
- Choose water (with or without lemon), unsweetened ice tea, skim milk, flavored non-calorie sparkling water, juice spritzer (half fruit juice and half sparkling water), low sodium V-8 juice, or low sodium tomato juice instead of soft drinks, diet sodas, coffee, milkshakes, punch, whole milk, 2% milk.
- Healthier choices for Breakfast fast foods:
  o Beverage: water, fresh fruit or juice
  o Grain: whole grain bread, cereal, bagel, oatmeal
  o Dairy: skim milk; egg substitute or egg white omelets; nonfat yogurt (add fruit or cereal)
- Healthier choices for Lunch and Dinner fast foods:
  o Appetizers: steamed seafood, fruit, garden salads with lemon juice, or low fat vinaigrette dressings
  o Entrée: baked, broiled, steamed, or lightly sautéed lean meats
  o Side Dishes: steamed vegetables, pasta with red sauce or with vegetables (primavera); mustard, salsa, spices, nonfat sour cream, or nonfat yogurt instead of sour cream or butter; garden salad made from 100% fresh vegetables (go easy on toppings such as deli meats, bacon, eggs, cheese, and croutons); low-fat, lemon juice-based, and vinegar-based dressings on the side; go easy on the bread and butter
  o Dessert: fresh fruit, fruit sorbet

Chapter 8. Nutritional Supplementation

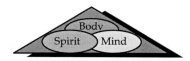

Nutritional Supplementation Strategies

An estimated 40 percent of the U.S. population uses nutritional and dietary supplements on a regular basis while 70 per cent uses supplements occasionally. Vitamin E and Vitamin C are among the most commonly used supplements.

So, are nutritional supplements really necessary? In today's fast-paced, hectic world, it is very difficult to eat nutritiously all day long every day. So, the short answer is "yes". If you are relatively healthy and you are eating four to six super meals/snacks with primarily raw organic foods and superfoods every day, you may not need any nutritional supplementation until you get older. On the other hand, if you are ill with a disease like diabetes, this should tell you that you are not consuming and absorbing enough of the proper nutrients. Because your body is very depleted in terms of nutrients, you need to supplement the super foods that you've begun to consume with some food-based nutritional supplements to help accelerate the body's healing process.

You may find it difficult to obtain all the necessary nutrients from the food you eat due to the loss of soil quality, water quality, picking vegetables/fruits in unripened state, and how animals are fed and raised. But, as long as you are predominantly eating the "live" (raw) foods instead of the "dead" foods, you will be successful. If finances are not an issue, you can buy organic food to ensure you are receiving the best quality foods, but for the most part this is not necessary. I did not eat organic food during my recovery. **The reduction and elimination of eating the "dead" processed foods will have a more dramatic positive effect on your health, more so than any other single factor.**

Because it may be difficult to eat four to six super meals consistently each day due to your work life, family, or lifestyle, some type of nutritional supplementation is necessary. In fact, medical institutions, such as the American Medical Association (AMA), agree that nutritional supplementation is necessary today.

In order for a nutritional supplementation plan to be effective, **you must have a sound nutritional meal program as a foundation.** An effective nutritional supplementation plan must accomplish the following three objectives to optimize your health: (1) nourish/balance; (2) protect/defend; and (3) cleanse/detoxify the body's cells and tissues. There are basically three major strategies to employ for nutritional supplementation, depending on your personal needs, preferences and financial resources:

Take a wholefood or food-based multivitamin/mineral supplement.
This is probably the easiest and most economical option for most people and requires the least amount of knowledge about nutrition and supplements. However, you should ensure that the nutritional supplement is *food*-based so that the nutrients within the supplement will be *recognized*, *absorbed* and *utilized* by the body! To help you select better nutritional supplements, use the criteria in the next section.

Take specific wholefood supplements and specific food-based vitamin and mineral supplements, based on your health need.
This may be the more optimum solution, but may not be as economical for some people. This option also requires a better knowledge of the benefits and the quality of each type of supplement and how that supplement addresses your health needs.

Take a combination of a wholefood supplement, a food-based multivitamin and multimineral supplement, and/or specific vitamin, mineral, fiber, enzyme, and plant extract supplements.
This option provides the most flexibility and the best of both worlds: a simple strategy to ensure a minimum level of nutritional supplementation, plus the ability to add new supplements based on specific health needs.

Natural vs. Synthetic Vitamins

Most vitamins and other supplements sold in a pharmacy, health food store, or grocery store are made synthetically with chemicals, coal tar and oil derivatives, and, as a result, are inexpensive. Vitamins and other supplements that are made from plants and other whole foods (e.g. nutriceuticals, food-based) are more expensive and are not as readily available in a pharmacy, health food store, or grocery store. In general, it is better to select natural vitamins over synthetic vitamins. *However*, in many cases it is difficult to determine whether the vitamin comes from a natural *food-based* source or a synthetic *chemical-based* source. And, because of the FDA's loose definition of "natural", there are many so-called "natural" vitamins and supplements that come from natural sources that include rocks and coal tar!

In most cases, a supplement from a *true food-based* natural source is 100% additive-free with no fillers, binders, dyes, preservatives, sugar coating, or other chemicals. It contains co-factors that are part of the vitamin in food (nature) and help to increase its absorption by the body – because the body recognizes it as food! For example, bioflavonoids are a co-factor of Vitamin C that helps its absorption. A synthetic vitamin with filler and binders uses heat, pressure, and chemicals that destroy the health benefits of the vitamin and create a foreign substance that the body expends energy trying to metabolize.

Natural forms of *Vitamin C* are those that contain rose hips, acerola, bioflavonoids, rutin, and other important co-enzymes. Synthetic forms of Vitamin C only contain ascorbic acid or calcium ascorbate, one of the non-acidic forms of synthetic Vitamin C. The non-acidic forms, which have less of a tendency to upset the stomach, include calcium ascorbate, sodium ascorbate, magnesium ascorbate, and Ester-C. At a minimum, ensure that the synthetic Vitamin C contains the bioflavonoid co-factor. The fat-soluble form of Vitamin C, which is called ascorbyl palmitate, may be better absorbed, but is harder to find and is more expensive.

Natural forms of *Vitamin E* are those that contain all four tocopherols and tocotrienols: alpha, beta, delta, and gamma. However, most Vitamin

E is sold containing only *one* of the four tocopherols, d-alpha tocopherol. Some Vitamin E is sold as dl-alpha tocopherol, which is the synthetic form of d-alpha tocopherol, and has very little if any nutritional value. *Gamma* tocopherol, not alpha tocopherol, is more effective at fighting nitrogen free radicals, which are the major culprits in arthritis, multiple sclerosis and Alzheimer's. Also, *gamma* tocopherol appears to be more potent than alpha tocopherol in increasing the activity of the antioxidant enzyme, superoxide dismutase (SOD), in plasma and arterial tissues. Tocotrienols and, in particular, gamma tocotrienol, suppress the production of the HMG-CoA reductase enzyme involved in cholesterol production, resulting in less cholesterol being produced by the liver.

Natural forms of the *B-Complex vitamins* are those that contain all of the B vitamins in balance with its co-factors to facilitate the biochemical reactions that support the nervous system and the metabolism of carbohydrates, proteins and fats to generate energy. Wholefood sources include organic eggs, raw milk, organic yogurt, wheat germ, Brewer's yeast, barley, organic brown rice, oily fish; extracts from spinach, cabbage, cauliflower, beets, other green leafy vegetables; and, lean protein from nuts and grass-fed, antibiotic-free beef and poultry.

Natural forms of the various *minerals* should come from wholefood sources such as bean curd, dark green vegetables, and nuts and seeds. Otherwise, use a *multi*mineral supplement to avoid the imbalances of individual mineral supplements; and, ensure it is a food-based liquid or a finely ground powder in a pharmaceutical-grade capsule with no fillers, binders or other additives. Unfortunately, the majority of mineral supplements is made from rocks, coral or seashells; and, usually contains other contaminants such as lead. The most common form of calcium supplements, calcium carbonate, is difficult for the body to absorb because it depends on stomach acids, which tend to decrease as the body ages. So the calcium accumulates in the body's joints and tissues and can eventually lead to arthritis or kidney stones. Various scientific studies have shown that organic calcium sources such as calcium citrate outperform inorganic sources such as calcium carbonate with regard to their relative bioavailability. Some studies indicate that calcium carbonate absorption may be as low as 22%. In addition, there are other calcium supplements that clinical studies indicate are as good or even better than calcium citrate. Calcium hydroxyapatite, for example, is the form of calcium found in our bones. This form contains a wide array of other minerals that occur naturally in bone. Calcium hydroxyapatite is quickly emerging as a quality calcium that may rival the absorbability of calcium citrate and may even be able to rebuild bone. A significant British study was carried out on post-menopausal women with accelerated bone loss and severely impaired calcium absorption. The results showed the group supplementing with calcium hydroxyapatite had a notable 12% increase in bone thickness, while the group supplementing with calcium carbonate had no change. Numerous studies have demonstrated that calcium hydroxyapatite supplementation is an excellent way to help reduce the risk factors of osteoporosis.

Natural forms of *Coenzyme Q10 (CoQ10)* are derived from a yeast fermentation process involving a bacterial culture of beet, with the majority of natural CoQ10 produced by a company in Japan. CoQ10 is a powerful antioxidant that exists in every cell of the body to provide the "spark" for cellular energy, especially in the heart, brain, lungs, liver, and kidneys – the hardest working organs in the body. CoQ10 also recycles Vitamins E. However, due to the popularity of CoQ10, manufacturers are producing a synthetic form that is derived from tobacco leaves. Unfortunately, the synthetic form is not as powerful and beneficial to your health.

The natural form of *Alpha Lipoic Acid (ALA)* is known as R-lipoic acid. ALA is known as the "universal" antioxidant because it is able to function in both aqueous (water-soluble) and lipid (fat-soluble) environments. The R-lipoic acid is more biologically active than the synthetic form of alpha lipoic acid. R-lipoic acid has antioxidant-recycling properties and energy-production properties by improving adenosine triphosphate (ATP) synthesis. R-lipoic acid also provides neuroprotective benefits and can aid in preventing cataracts and their complications by recycling or increasing levels of glutathione, Vitamin C, Vitamin E, and certain protective enzymes in lens tissues. Unfortunately R-lipoic acid supplements may be less stabile, and, therefore, less effective than the S-lipoic, or alpha lipoic acid version.

Wholefood Supplements vs. Isolated Vitamins

Wholefood supplements are comprised of foods (not extracts, but entire foods) that have been concentrated into supplemental form. Wholefood supplements are those that have been carefully processed and unaltered in any way that would change the molecular structure or biochemical combinations and actions of the vitamin, mineral and enzyme complexes. Isolated supplements and some natural supplements are singular or groups of individual vitamins, minerals and/or amino acids. Whole foods contain vitamins, but isolated vitamins never contain the rest of the whole-food "complex".

In general, it is better to select wholefood supplements over natural or synthetic isolated vitamin supplements. Many biochemical researchers, nutritionists and herbalists have noted that without the wholefood complex, the body will never achieve whole nutrition, as a synthetic vitamin supplement lacks its co-factors. In fact, as noted by several doctors and biochemists, isolated vitamins eventually lead to biochemical imbalances and consequential nutritional deficiencies, as the body is forced to surrender its stores of nutrients in order to make any isolated vitamin work. The use of isolated synthetic vitamins amounts to the practice of "chemistry", whereas the use of wholefood supplements translates into the practice of "biochemistry". Whole foods are live organic substances with enzyme activity, while isolated vitamins are dead inorganic substances that lack enzyme activity. Isolated vitamins do not resemble foods, but they resemble parts of the chemicals in the food.

Nutrition relates to nourishment by whole foods, not isolated chemicals. Whole foods work biochemically and harmoniously, while isolated vitamins run the risk of creating biochemical imbalances. Taking isolated vitamins/ minerals, even in a multivitamin/mineral supplement, is a biochemical risk, especially if you are already ill. Too much magnesium or phosphorus may imbalance calcium; too much copper may imbalance Vitamin C; too much zinc can lead to copper deficiency, and so on. Because nutrients in foods are balanced within the food complex, the risk of imbalance or toxicity is very low.

Nature's design is a safer choice due to its inherent intelligence in providing a variety of nutrients with its co-factors. Consequently, when using wholefood supplements, it is important to realize that the *quality* of the food complex is more important than the quantity of individual vitamins and minerals.

Selection Criteria for Nutritional Supplements

Since more than 60% of the U.S. population takes some form of a nutritional supplement and more than 65% have some type of illness, it would suggest that some nutritional supplements are not working. So, if you choose to use nutritional supplements, how can you reap the benefits they offer without risking your health and wasting your money? The following criteria will help you select a quality nutritional supplement that aligns with your health needs and financial constraints: source, content (nutrients, dosage level), physical makeup, packaging, delivery system, cost, documentation, manufacturer, and performance.

Source: Ideally, you want wholefood supplements or natural supplements created from whole foods and processed in a manner that keeps the nutrients in their natural form, intact with their co-factors, instead of a synthetic form made in a lab. Most synthetic vitamins contain artificial colors, sweeteners, preservatives, binders, and fillers with a sugar or chemical tablet coating; and, use extreme heat, pressure, or possibly toxic solvents; and, in most cases, are made in a laboratory setting from coal tar derivatives. You can sometimes tell this by the *chemical smell* of some tablets. In general, supplements that are 100% additive-free are much more likely to have come from natural sources.

For herbal supplements, be wary of some "standardized herbs", which only contain one or two of the herb's active ingredients. Herbs contain many compounds that work together to produce a specific effect. Other factors that influence the herb's efficacy include the soil, when the herb was harvested, and how it was processed. This is why many consumers are disappointed with herbal supplements. Only use herbs that are 100% organically-grown, tested for efficacy and do not conflict with your drug therapy.

Content (Nutrients): For a wholefood supplement, check the ingredients on the label for additional nutrients/foods that may support your specific health needs, e.g. sprouts, probiotics, barley, spirulina, chlorella, other grasses. Also, look for terms such as organically-grown, pesticide-free, not genetically-modified, and unheated (to preserve enzyme activity). Be wary if the label states that the supplement's formula is proprietary and fails to disclose the ingredients. For a multivitamin/mineral, look for a comprehensive list of vitamins and minerals, including the necessary co-factors to increase the supplement's bioavailability. For example, for Vitamin C, look for bioflavonoids as an ingredient to increase its absorption. For Vitamin E, make sure it's a mixed set of the four tocopherols and four tocotrienols.

For calcium supplements, be wary of large calcium tablets that are difficult for the body to metabolize and absorb – look for a capsule form with very fine granules of calcium citrate or hydroxyapatite. Check to see if the calcium is certified as pure and not high in lead and other metals especially coral and bone meal. Ensure the supplement contains magnesium and boron to help with absorption of the calcium. Also, be wary of eating too many foods high in phosphorous, which inhibits the absorption of calcium, e.g. soda, milk, corn, biscuits, ice cream, yogurt.

Content (Other Nutrients): Besides Vitamin C and Vitamin E, check for other key ingredients such as antioxidants, e.g. lutein, lycopene, selenium, zinc, green tea. Ensure there is no Vitamin A (due to the concern with osteoporosis if consumed over the long term). Instead, check for the precursor to Vitamin A (mixed carotenes), which can be converted to Vitamin A by the body. For older adults, ensure there is no iron in the vitamin (unless you're anemic).

Content (Dosage Level): For the wholefood supplement, check the dosage level of each nutrient contained within each scoop. For the multivitamin, check the dosage levels of Vitamin C and Vitamin E within a multivitamin. A good multivitamin will provide at least 500 mg of Vitamin C and 400 IU of Vitamin E. For fish oil, look for a balance of EPA and DHA. Many of the traditional multivitamins are single pills ("rocks") that do not contain the required levels of vitamins and minerals that the body requires as specified by the clinical studies. For example, most multivitamin/multiminerals provide less than 100 mg of Vitamin C and less than 60 IU of Vitamin E; and, most clinical studies require much higher dosage levels in order to provide the specified health benefits.

Content (Additives, Fillers, Binders, Dyes): Check the ingredients label for fillers, binders, and additives that may upset your stomach and reduce the bioavailability (absorption) of the nutrients. Be wary of supplements with fillers, binders and other chemicals such as color dyes, sucrose and acids that add no nutritional value. Many vitamin/ supplement manufacturers use color dyes because they have determined that you, the consumer, prefer bright-colored pills covered with sugar or chocolate. So, their focus is on how the pill looks and tastes, not what's in it, which should be your primary concern. In general, if the supplement contains these additives, then, it is not a "natural" sourced supplement. Also, be wary of marketing ploys such as "carb-assist" vitamins – most of which contain carbohydrates such as glucose, sucrose, and starch and other unnecessary additives.

Content (Physical Makeup): For the wholefood supplement, look for some type of food-based powder/extract that can easily be dissolved in a drink; or, a food-based liquid that uses liposomal encapsulated technology. For the multivitamin, look for a supplement that provides a food-based liquid or a very fine powder in a set of pharmaceutical-grade capsules that can be taken throughout the day – to better distribute the vitamin/mineral dosage, especially the water-soluble Vitamin B-complex and Vitamin C. If the multivitamin/ mineral consists of a single tablet, it will be difficult to digest and, more than likely, it will not contain the proper levels of the key nutrients such as Vitamin C and Vitamin E.

Packaging (Protection): For the wholefood supplement, look for a container that is vacuum-sealed for extra protection. For the multivitamin, look for a supplement that is contained in a dark (opaque), vacuum-sealed bottle or is packaged as a set of capsules in a dark cellophane package for protection from light, air, and moisture and to ensure a more potent supplement. For flaxseed oil, check the expiration date and ensure it is organic and refrigerated.

Delivery system (liquid, powder, capsule, tablet): For the wholefood supplement, look for a liquid, small tablets or a powder that is easy to add to a drink, salad or other food/beverage. For the multivitamin, look for a supplement that is easy to swallow, e.g. a liquid or a small capsule to accommodate the narrow throats of most women and children. This is important because it ensures a consistent daily use of the supplement, which enables a more optimum level of health. Consequently, stay away from the hard tablets and large pills, which are difficult for the body to break down and extract the nutrients. For Vitamin E, saw palmetto, fish oil, Omega-3 EFAs and other oil supplements, look for a pharmaceutical-grade capsule that offers maximum protection to ensure its potency. Be wary of the conventional soft football-shaped capsules because they allow in air, light and moisture, which oxidizes the oil reducing its potency and causing rancidity.

Cost: Once the manufacturing processes are set up, it is very economical for the vitamin manufacturer to mass-produce synthetic vitamin pills. That is part of the reason why they can sell vitamins so cheaply. Think about it for a minute – why are you able to buy something so valuable for pennies? If vitamins are so valuable, shouldn't the cost reflect that to some degree? On the other hand, an expensive vitamin doesn't necessarily guarantee that it's any better. That's why these criteria are important.

Manufacturer: Ensure the manufacturer is not just a distributor and has the technical background, experience, documentation, and integrity backing up their supplement. Unfortunately, more than 80% of the vitamins manufactured are controlled by a few companies, which are connected to the pharmaceutical companies, making it more difficult to find a reputable manufacturer that values your health instead of making money. Many of these manufacturers make unfounded medical claims about their supplements; and, most people trust that these manufacturers and their distributors (drugstores, health food stores, websites, consultants) are selling them quality supplements that support those medical claims. Because of information provided by drugstores, TV, radio, dietitians, and doctors, most people believe that the vitamin products and other supplements work as advertised. Most people are unaware of the manufacturing process used to mass-produce these vitamins and other supplements. Most people assume that if a bottle says "Vitamin C" or "Vitamin E" that it must contain that nutrient, as it exists in food and nature. But, in most cases, it exists in synthetic (inorganic) form, which is not effectively absorbed by your body.

Performance: This is the ultimate criterion, although in most cases, it is difficult to measure appreciable serum level differences from one blood test to the next. It may be more important to track your blood tests over a period of time and look for any major trends or shifts to determine whether your body is obtaining any health benefits. Some people believe that they feel better after taking vitamins, but it's impossible to measure a feeling with a blood test. Also, since most vitamins primarily function as catalysts, they can only work well if they have the necessary raw materials to work with in the first place. So, if you are not consuming the proper "live" foods, it will be difficult to achieve a maximum health benefit from the vitamins.

Another Accident
About nine months after my coma incident, I accidentally mis-programmed my VCR to record a TV show on one of the home shopping networks. When I realized my error, I started to remove the tape when I heard the speaker mention something about vitamins. Initially I thought this was just another one of those infomercial scams about the next great "magic pill" that will cure everything for $19.95. But, the more I listened, the more I realized that the person talking was not a salesperson, but a biochemist who truly understood vitamins and how they really worked in the human body. His presentation was very educational, and led me to perform in-depth research into vitamins and other supplements. This led me to define the aforementioned criteria to objectively evaluate vitamins and other supplements. This has proven to be invaluable because I have been able to recognize inferior vitamins and scams from various TV infomercials, vitamin companies and salespeople. And, this is all due to the information I received accidentally from this biochemist, and my follow up research. Maybe one day I'll be fortunate enough to meet this biochemist from Nevada (Andrew Lessman). I would really like to pick his brain!

Supplements that Nourish, Protect & Cleanse

Nutrients from the food and nutritional supplements must meet three objectives in order to be comprehensive enough to prevent and reverse disease in the body:

- Nutrients must **nourish** the body – by providing vitamins, minerals, enzymes, co-factors, saccharides, amino acids, water, and oils to feed the cells, tissues, and blood. This nourishment enables the body to *repair* its sick, defective cells and *rebalance* hormone levels. As the cells get healthy, the amount of insulin resistance is reduced, enabling the cells to increase their glucose uptake and reduce their insulin levels.
- Nutrients must **protect** the body – by providing antioxidants and anti-inflammatories to *protect* the healthy cells and fight free radical oxidation and inflammation. These nutrients help to *strengthen* the immune system to fight pathogenic bacteria and other invaders. This is important for diabetics because their bodies are under a tremendous amount of oxidative stress and their immune systems are very weak.
- Nutrients must **cleanse/detoxify** the body – by providing herbs, fiber, enzymes, water and other nutrients to help the body *remove* waste and toxins, including excess glucose. This, in turn, helps the body to *repair* its sick and defective cells, and reduce the internal inflammation.

Based on biochemical and hormonal imbalances driven by nutritional deficiencies, most diabetics either lack specific nutrients or are consuming too many of the wrong chemicals and toxins due to poor eating habits and lifestyle choices. The following is a list of the key nutrients that most diabetics require in order to properly nourish, protect, cleanse and detoxify the body. Ideally, diabetics should try to obtain the majority of these nutrients from eating more raw, unprocessed foods, and use quality food-based supplements to close the nutritional gap.

Note: If you need help with selecting quality nutritional supplements while saving your hard-earned money, contact our wellness center or visit our website at www.DeathToDiabetes.com.

> **Nourishment:** The following is a list of nutrients that nourish the body, improve insulin/glucose levels, support hormonal balance, and stimulate the body's internal healing resources for repair.

Vitamins

- Vitamin B-complex: (B1 thiamine, B2 riboflavin, B3 niacin, B5 pantothenic acid, B6 pyridoxine, B9 folic acid, B12 cyanocobalamin, and H, biotin) for carb metabolism to provide energy; and, protein/fat metabolism to aid the functioning of the nervous system, cell health, and muscle tone in the intestinal tract. Brewer's yeast is a rich source of the B-Complex vitamins and chromium.
- Vitamins B6, B9, B12: enables the breakdown of homocysteine. Food sources include eggs, Brewer's yeast, green vegetables, legumes, whole grains for B6, B9; and, fish, poultry, cheese for B12.
- Vitamin C: supports tissue repair and cholesterol reduction. Food sources include fruits and vegetables.
- Vitamin D: produced via sunlight to metabolize cholesterol; may help pancreas produce insulin. Sources: sunlight, cod liver oil, dairy.
- Vitamin E: helps to support better insulin utilization, glucose uptake and control. Food sources include oils, whole grains, nuts and seeds.
- Omega-3 EFAs: contain DHA and EPA, which help to repair cell membranes to lower glucose in the blood; and, support the heart, brain, nerves, and joints. Food sources include nuts, fish, krill, plants.

Minerals

- Chromium: is sometimes called glucose tolerance factor (GTF) and in its biologically active form, it works better than the synthetic forms. Chromium is called the master regulator of insulin, preventing glucose levels from going too high or low and increasing the insulin cell receptor sites. It is a potent metabolic hormone involved in protein, carbohydrate and fat metabolism. Chromium helps to reduce fat storage, maintain lean muscle mass, reduce sugar cravings and convert sugar into energy. Food sources include broccoli, oysters, salmon, turkey, liver, onions, whole grains, bran cereals, eggs, tomatoes, seafood, beans, mushrooms, and Brewer's yeast.

Note: Various clinical studies have shown that chromium lowers fasting blood glucose levels, improves glucose tolerance and lowers insulin levels – but *only* if your body is deficient in chromium.

- Magnesium: provides better insulin utilization and muscle relaxation. Food sources: beans, vegetables, whole grain cereals.
- Potassium: provides electrolyte balance by naturally lowering the sodium level. Food sources: vegetables, fruits, beans.
- Vanadium: as vanadyl sulfate, normalizes blood glucose levels and supports carbohydrate/fat metabolism. Vanadium is found in mushrooms, seafood and soybeans.
  Note: Increasing research indicates that vanadyl sulfate improves blood glucose levels for both Type 1 and Type 2 diabetics. In a study involving Type 2 diabetics, fasting blood glucose were reduced an average of 20%. In a similar study, Type 1 diabetics required less insulin for blood glucose control.

Herbs, Glyconutrients, Other Food-based Supplements

- Banaba leaf extract: contains corosolic acid, which stimulates the transport of glucose into cells to lower blood glucose levels and reduce cravings for refined carbohydrates.
- Bitter melon: is an herb that contains insulin-like peptides and alkaloids that help to lower the blood glucose level. Bitter melon contains polypeptide p (or p-insulin), which helps to reduce glucose tolerance and glycosylated hemoglobin A1C.
- Carnosine: is a di-peptide that provides antioxidant, anti-glycating, and metal chelating actions in order to protect and extend the functional life of the body's key building blocks: cells, proteins, DNA, lipids. Carnosine helps to generate nitric oxide which dilates blood vessels. Studies show that carnosine is effective against forms of protein modification including oxidation, carbonylation, cross-linking, glycation and advanced glycation end product (AGE) formation, all of which figure prominently in some of the familiar signs of aging, e.g. cataracts, neuro-degeneration, skin wrinkling.
- Cinnamon: contains a water-soluble polyphenol compound called MHCP (methylhydroxychalcone polymer), which mimics insulin, based on a study done in Pakistan. MHCP makes cells more

responsive to insulin, increasing insulin sensitivity and glucose uptake into the cells, so that blood glucose levels fall. Recent studies have shown that 1000 mg (daily) of this cinnamon (cassia bark) increased glucose metabolism, reducing blood glucose levels 18% to 29%.

- Flaxseed: provides Omega-3 oils, fiber, lignans, vitamins, and minerals. The powerful combination of the oils and fiber promote healthier cholesterol levels and a stronger immune system. Freshly ground flaxseed can easily be applied to salads or beverages.
- Glyconutrients: provide nourishment that support cell-to-cell communications and the immune/endocrine systems. Food sources include mushrooms, seaweed, aloe vera, gums, herbs, and seeds.
- Gymnema sylvestre: is an herb that has been used for centuries in the traditional Indian system of Ayurvedic medicine. It contains gymnemic acid, tartaric acid, gurmarin, betaine, and choline, which improve the uptake of glucose into cells by increasing the activity of the glucose utilizing enzymes, and prevents adrenaline from stimulating the liver to produce glucose. It also helps to raise insulin levels, due to the regeneration of the beta cells in the pancreas that secrete insulin. But, ensure that the herb has been organically-grown and tested for efficacy to obtain optimum benefits.
  - o Gymnema sylvestre, which is known as gurmar in its native India and is called the "sugar destroyer", reduces sugar cravings and may be the most powerful herb for improving blood glucose control. Clinical studies have demonstrated that gymnema has therapeutic value for both Type 1 and Type 2 diabetics. In a study involving Type 1 diabetics, average insulin requirements dropped by almost 30%. In another study of Type 2 diabetics, A1C levels were reduced from 12% to 8.5%.
  - o Based on recent research at the University of California, there is evidence that the pancreas continues to form the insulin-producing beta cells, but the immune system kills them faster than the pancreas can produce them. However, this would imply that this herb might be very beneficial for some Type 1 diabetics.

> **Protection:** The following is list of key nutrients that protect the body from oxidative damage by absorbing free radicals (which provoke more inflammation) and from foreign invasion by strengthening the immune system.

Antioxidants

- Alpha lipoic acid (ALA): provides free radical protection within the water and lipid (fat) portions of cells throughout the body, especially the eyes, kidneys, and nerves; recycles other antioxidants.
- Carotenoids: are contained within the bright-colored pigments of fruits and vegetables and include alpha-carotene, beta-carotene, cryptoxanthin, lutein, lycopene, and zeaxanthin. A study conducted by the Centers for Disease Control found that people with low levels of carotenoids were often diagnosed with Type 2 diabetes.
- CoQ10: provides energy and antioxidant protection in the mitochondria of all the cells, and helps to improve insulin sensitivity.
- Glyconutrients: are plant saccharides that provide several essential monosaccharides, which combine with proteins and fats to create glycoforms that coat the surface of cells in order to support the immune system (for defense against invading bacteria) and the endocrine system (for hormonal balance). Food sources include mushrooms, seaweed, aloe vera, gums, herbs, and seeds.
- L-carnosine: has anti-glycating properties.
- Mushrooms: contain saccharides that strengthen the immune system.
- Selenium: works synergistically with Vitamin E to provide protection.
- Vitamin C: provides protection within the aqueous portions of cells.
- Vitamin E: provides protection within the lipid portions of the cells by preventing the peroxidation of fat.
- Anti-inflammatory foods: help to reduce the internal inflammation of a typical diabetic body. These foods, which contain Omega-3s, anthocyanins, quercetin, curcumin, isoflavones, and salicylic acid, include: cold water, oily fish (wild salmon, sardines), fish oil, virgin olive oil, flaxseed, flax oil, walnuts, pumpkin seeds; blueberries, strawberries, cranberries, cherries; apples, onions, red wine, green tea; turmeric; tofu, berries, plums, apricots, cantaloupe, grapes, broccoli,

spinach, artichoke, beans, peppers, ginger root, cayenne pepper, cinnamon, nutmeg, oregano, rosemary, sage, thyme.

- Other antioxidants include green tea, white tea, curcumin, zinc; aloe vera; cranberry; grape seed extract, pine bark extract; artichoke, and shiitake mushrooms. But, avoid foods that cause inflammation, e.g. potatoes, wheat, rice, bread, cereal, refined grains, cheese, and pork.

Note: Antioxidant supplements should be taken together to leverage their recycling capabilities and maximize their protection. For example, Vitamin C and CoQ10 recycle Vitamin E, glutathione recycles Vitamin C, and alpha lipoic acid recycles all the other antioxidants.

Note: Antioxidants with a high **O**xygen **R**adical **A**bsorbance **C**apacity (ORAC) rating destroy more free radicals and provide more oxidative protection. ORAC is a scientific method developed by Tufts University in Boston to measure the level of antioxidant protection in a food or supplement.

Probiotics

Note: Probiotics are live bacteria that help to maintain a delicate balance between the gastrointestinal tract and immune system. Food sources of live bacteria include organic or homemade yogurt, sauerkraut, and fermented soy products (miso, tempeh, tofu, natto).

- Lactobacillus acidophilus, bulgaricus: help the intestines absorb more nutrients by forming colonies on the intestinal walls. They also help set up colonies on the intestinal walls.

  Note: This is the same type of bacteria used in yogurt and other fermented milk products.

- Bifidobacterium bifidum, longum: promote bacteria balance in the large intestine and help digest milk/dairy products by synthesizing lactase. They also scavenge and neutralize many everyday toxins found in the gut, keep the large intestine acidic to discourage the growth of other bacteria, help the body break down carbohydrates; and, keep bowel movements healthy.

- Most of the bacteria in probiotic supplements are dead by the time they reach store shelves, and, therefore, are not as effective as the food sources listed above.

> **Cleansing/Detoxification:** The following is a list of nutrients that help to cleanse/detoxify and rebalance the body by removing toxins, acid waste, cholesterol, fecal waste and other contaminants.

Herbs, Other Nutrients

- Bentonite clay, charcoal, pectin: help to remove compacted fecal waste, intestinal parasites and toxins.
- Flaxseed: contains Omega-3 EFAs and fiber, which help to metabolize old fat and remove cholesterol and fecal waste.
- Garlic: kills bacteria, fungi, and other harmful pathogens, and helps to increase intestinal microflora.
- Ginger, senna: strengthen the colon muscle and increase peristalsis.
- Peppermint leaf: reduces and moves gas that is created during a deep intestinal/bowel cleanse. It also helps to reduce spasms.
- Plant sterols, policosanol; guggulipid, fenugreek: help to reduce the production of cholesterol.
- Psyllium seed, marshmallow root: help to prevent inflammation and irritation of intestinal walls.

Super foods

- **Super greens:** are chlorophyll-saturated dark green plants that contain all the essential building block nutrients to support the immune system and provide nourishment. In the oceans and lakes these super foods are called spirulina, chlorella, sea plankton, and kelp. On land, these foods are the young spring time sprouts or shoots of the seed producing grasses such as barley grass, wheat grass and alfalfa grass. *Spirulina* helps to restore the acid-alkaline balance and acts as a heavy metal detoxifier. *Chlorella* reduces absorption of some dietary carcinogens and is a rich source of age fighting RNA and DNA. *Barley grass* is considered the most nutritional of the green grasses with a potassium content that helps to lower blood pressure.
- **Royal jelly, Bee pollen:** support the immune system; and, contain B vitamins (to provide energy), amino acids (to support the immune system), and proteins, lipids, and carbohydrates. They also contain aspartic acid, which aids in cellular health.

Chapter 9. Cleansing/Detoxification

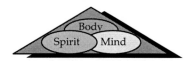

The Need for Cleansing/Detoxification

After some people have started eating properly and exercising on a consistent basis, they find that they reach a "wall" and either are unable to lower their blood glucose level below a certain point or lose more weight. In most cases, this is due to the body's toxic load preventing metabolism and energy production. For the people who are not eating properly and exercising on a consistent basis, their toxic load is definitely affecting their health and preventing metabolism and energy production.

Cleansing/detoxification is a set of normal biochemical processes performed by the body to prevent and fight disease on a continual basis and to keep the body as healthy as possible. This cleansing/detoxification is optimized when we eat healthy foods the majority of the time. However, in our fast-paced world it can be difficult to find the time to prepare healthy meals, especially, given the easy availability and accessibility of convenience and fast foods. Unfortunately, our bodies pay a heavy toll for eating unhealthy convenience foods, fast foods, and processed foods. To compound the problem, our bodies are also bombarded with chemicals and pollutants on a daily basis from the air, water and environment. Under this heavy barrage of toxins, the cells become sick and the human body eventually reaches a point where it is no longer capable of flushing toxins and acid waste on its own. As the toxins and acid waste accumulate in the cells, blood, tissues, and organs, they trigger an increase in inflammation, the formation of pathogenic bacteria, fungus and mold, and lead to a state of poisoning commonly referred to as toxicity.

Common symptoms of toxicity include headaches, fatigue, increased allergy symptoms, overall aches and pains (particularly joint pain), and digestive discomfort. These symptoms occur when the body has become so clogged with toxins that it can no longer perform necessary functions effectively. Toxins are generally acquired in one of three ways: through things we ingest (such as foods, drinks, drugs, etc.); through external sources (such as the air we breath, radiation, environmental chemicals, etc.); and, internally by the body's own metabolic processes. Over the past decade, extensive research has found that if the body's detoxification system is sluggish, toxins will accumulate, slowing down cellular energy production and increasing the number of tissue-damaging free radicals. In addition, pathogenic bacteria continue to multiply faster than the immune system can kill them and remove their debris, creating an overloading and clogging of the lymphatic system and various organs. This can eventually lead to various systemic diseases/ailments such as chronic fatigue, weight gain, high blood sugar, high blood pressure, high cholesterol, heart disease, cancer, fibromyalgia, and Alzheimer's. In the meantime, the body's detoxification and excretory organs (e.g. colon, kidneys, liver, gallbladder, lymphatic system) struggle to effectively remove the toxins, excess glucose, and acid waste.

The **liver** is the primary organ that performs the detoxification. The liver accomplishes this by using specific enzymes to transform the toxins into intermediate chemicals; and, other enzymes to transform the intermediate chemicals into harmless water-soluble substances that are then excreted in the bile or urine. But, if the liver becomes sluggish, clogged, or impaired, these toxins can begin to accumulate in the body's tissues and blood. Consequently, it is very important that the liver is kept as healthy as possible. Ironically, when we don't feel well, we take an over-the-counter or prescription drug, which is toxic and only puts more stress on an already deteriorating liver and suppresses the symptoms, making us think we're okay.

The **colon** (or large intestine) is important to cleansing and detoxification because it removes the unwanted fecal waste and other toxins. Discomfort in the colon usually manifests itself as something such as diarrhea or constipation. Unfortunately, our response to this is usually a drug, such as a laxative, to "force" the elimination of the fecal waste. But many of the other toxins are left behind and reabsorbed into the bloodstream attacking the tissues and organs, and producing their own pathogenic bacteria that attack the body's weakest points. These attacks manifest themselves in the form of aches and pain in the back, joints, stomach, and head, and, then onto the other tissues and organs. This leads to more discomfort and more drugs, followed by more diseases, stronger drugs, hospital visits, and eventually death – unless the toxins are removed.

The **kidneys** are important to cleansing and detoxification because they filter the blood (210 quarts a day) by eliminating toxins and waste materials from the blood, and for maintaining the electrolyte balance by selectively eliminating some electrolytes while retaining others, according to the body's needs. Electrolytes include sodium, potassium, magnesium, calcium and chloride. These electrolytes are important because they are used by the cells to maintain voltages across the cell membranes and carry electrical impulses (e.g. nerve impulses, muscle contractions) across themselves and to other cells. The kidneys also help regulate other bodily functions by secreting the hormones renin, erythropoietin, and prostaglandin. Renin helps control blood pressure, erythropoietin stimulates the body to produce more red blood cells, and prostaglandin helps control blood pressure, muscle contractions, and inflammation.

The high levels of glucose in the blood and the accumulation of acids in the kidneys cause the formation of kidney stones and ultimately cause kidney cells to die. Because kidney cells cannot be regenerated or repaired, the remaining cells have to work that much harder to filter substances from the blood. To help with the filtering process, the heart increases the flow of blood plasma to the kidneys, which in turn elevates blood pressure. As the kidney cells continue to die, the risk of kidney failure increases dramatically.

The **lymphatic system** is also important to cleansing and detoxification. As the blood circulates, providing nutrients and oxygen to all parts of the body, the lymphatic system accumulates dead bacteria and toxins that need to be removed. Lymphatic vessels are situated intricately alongside blood vessels, relying upon body movement to move the lymph fluid around to collect and drain away toxins and dead bacteria through the lymph nodes and skin (pores).

If the colon, liver, kidneys, lymphatic system, and other body systems are working properly, the body will cleanse and detoxify itself to get rid of the toxins. And, as long as the body is provided with the proper nutrients, the body will continue to cleanse and detoxify itself.

However, if you have a systemic degenerative disease/ailment such as diabetes, high blood pressure, high cholesterol, heart disease, indigestion, or constipation, then, your body and its cells are sick and full of toxins, and are unable to cleanse and detoxify properly. Consequently, you will need to eat "live" super foods to help your body with the cleansing and detoxification until your body is healthy enough to perform the cleansing and detoxification on its own.

If you want to further accelerate the detoxification process, you should drink at least 2 cups of raw vegetable juices (with 1 tbsp. ground flaxseed or wheat grass powder), followed by 2 cups of filtered water at least 2 times each day. Within a few days you should notice an increase in your regularity (bowel movements) and a better texture of your fecal waste. Then, depending on your health state, within two to three weeks you should notice an increase in your energy level and a reduction in your cravings for the "dead" processed foods. These are indicators that your body is cleansing and detoxifying itself and initiating the healing process. To further accelerate this healing, and depending on the severity of your health state, it may be necessary to use wholefood supplements and organic herbal products to nourish the colon, liver, gall bladder, lymph nodes, and kidneys while protecting them from oxidative damage during the cleansing/detoxification process.

Why is cleansing/detoxification necessary? Let's take a car that has not had an oil change or engine tune-up and has been running on cheap fuel for several years. If you switch from the cheap fuel to a higher-octane "super" fuel, the car may run a little better, but it will still run sluggish. Once you change the oil and air filters and tune up the engine, the car will run even better. The same principle applies to the human body – if you clean the filters (the kidneys and liver), then, this will help them to remove the buildup of toxins and waste and kill the pathogenic bacteria and parasites so that the body will run better.

If you are overweight by more than 20 pounds, more than likely, you are carrying as much as ten pounds of fecal matter packed in your colon. If you are also struggling with high cholesterol or high blood pressure, then, your body is carrying extra fluid/waste in your cells and tissues. Consequently, cleansing the liver and kidneys, your body's primary filters, will help the body to better release this extra fluid/waste. This will thin out the blood, hydrate cells, break down fats, absorb protein, convert glycogen to glucose, turn on the body's natural healing mechanisms, and, in most cases, lower blood pressure, inflammation, cholesterol, glucose levels, and body weight.

Types of Toxins

Toxicity (poisoning) of the body occurs gradually over a period of years and goes unnoticed, due to the liver, colon, kidneys, and other excretory organs being able to remove most of the toxins. But, eventually, one or more of these excretory organs begins to break down, primarily due to the environment and poor nutrition causing higher-than-normal accumulated levels of these toxins in the body. The major types of toxins are metals, organic chemicals, food additives, internal metabolic waste products, and negative emotions.

Metal toxins include lead, mercury, cadmium, arsenic, aluminum, fluoride, chlorine, bromine, barium, copper, iron, manganese, selenium and other elements. Some of these metals such as copper, iron, and manganese are needed in small amounts by the body. Others, such as lead, mercury, cadmium and arsenic, have no known function in the body. Heavy metal pollution is mainly due to industrial processes, car exhausts and pesticides. These not only contaminate the air, but are also absorbed by the crops and water supplies. We are therefore eating and drinking, as well as breathing, these toxins. Other sources include the lead solder in tin cans, mercury fillings, fluoride in the water, contaminated fish (particularly near the coast), antacids, aluminum pans and cosmetics. The main effects of heavy metal toxicity are on the brain and central nervous system, affecting mental ability, co-ordination and behavior.

Organic chemicals include pesticides, herbicides, insecticides, solvents, household cleaners, detergents, formaldehyde, petrochemicals, adhesives, perfumes, dental materials other than metals, toxic substances on fabric, in building materials, furniture, plastics, residues in drinking water, air, packing materials, most food additives; gases and fumes from cars, factories, paints; and, chemicals formed in cooking (i.e. from pans, oils and the burning or frying of food); and drugs of all kinds, including prescription, over-the-counter, recreational, e.g. pain medication, aspirin, alcohol, tobacco. These substances often impair the liver's ability to detoxify, but may impact the kidneys, brain, immune system, energy production and other organs and body systems.

Food additives include thousands of chemical substances that are added to food for flavor, color, shelf life, growth, disease protection, texture and other reasons. There are growth hormones and antibiotics given to animals every day; agricultural and inorganic contaminants added to the farmland; plus more than 3,000 additives used in our food today. The largest group of food additives is the flavoring agents, which are synthetic chemicals. Another group of food additives is coloring agents, and most of these are also synthetic chemicals. Most of these food additives are usually made from petroleum or coal tar products. Other food additives include preservatives (such as hydrogenated oil), refined sugars, bleaching agents, emulsifiers, texturizers, humectants and ripening agents, such as ethylene gas, which is sprayed on bananas to make them ripen faster. The main effects of these toxins are on the nervous system and liver, but many of them also have an effect on the endocrine system and respiratory tract, and most of them are carcinogenic (cancer-forming).

Metabolic waste products include natural toxins (by-products of metabolism and energy production); intestinal putrefaction byproducts such as mercaptan (a natural substance released from decaying matter) and hydrogen sulfide (from the breakdown of sulfur-containing proteins in the intestinal tract); exotoxins from E. coli and various infections in the bladder, mouth, lymphatic system, etc.; and, other metabolic end-products such as accumulated lactic acid due to impaired oxygenation, hydration or circulation.

Emotional toxins include exposure to negative, violent, fearful, angry, envious, selfish or devious thoughts from the people in your life. Emotional toxins are produced by toxic relationships, which occur within dysfunctional families, work environments, co-dependent relationships, friendships, educational environments, community endeavors and other environments. Studies indicate that negative feelings trigger stress hormones such as cortisol, leading to poor eating habits and eventually poor health. This can lead to problems with weight gain and the cardiovascular system (constricted arteries, overworked heart muscle), causing a heart attack or stroke.

Nutrients for Cleansing/Detoxification

The following sections provide the key nutrients that you should look for when purchasing any herbal cleanser, detoxifier, or wholefood supplement. Most of the nutrients are based on information from clinical references and the key molecules associated with the organs responsible for cleansing and detoxifying the body. For example, phosphatidyl choline is identified as a nutrient for the liver because it is a key building block of the liver cells and other cell membranes.

Use wholefood, natural and herbal products that contain a synergistic blend of these nutrients instead of purchasing them separately. Work with an experienced herbalist or other knowledgeable healthcare professional to ensure you select high quality products. As a precaution, review the ingredients of any product that you consider purchasing with your doctor and pharmacist. If the product does not provide a detailed list of its ingredients, do not purchase it.

Note: If you are unable to find quality wholefood, natural and herbal products, consult a nutritionist or consumer lab, or talk to your (healthy) friends for reliable resources. If necessary, search on the web if you know what you're looking for or refer to the Resources section (page 374) in the Appendix as a starting point for reliable manufacturers.

Colon/Gastrointestinal System

If the colon is backed up (e.g. constipation) when the liver empties its toxins into the colon for removal, the liver deposits the toxins into fat cells, and the toxins are retained in the body. Consequently, colon cleansing/detoxification can provide relief from the buildup of these toxins and illnesses such as colds, flu, constipation, diarrhea, breath and body odors, fatigue, headaches, sinusitis, allergies, hemorrhoids, weight problems, digestive difficulties, back and muscle aches, knee pain, poor eyesight, poor memory, stress, etc. The human body cannot expect to have a quick mind or vitality for living when it is polluted with waste. Benefits from colon cleansing include a dramatic relief of aches and pains in the back, chest and joints; a dramatic increase of energy and mental awareness; overwhelming joy, incredible insight, and even better sex. Proper colon cleansing/detoxification can promote improved assimilation of food and nutrients leading to improved health.

The following is a list of the key nutrients that help to cleanse, detoxify and nourish the colon.

- Bentonite clay, charcoal, apple pectin, psyllium husk: provide needed bulk fiber for removal of compacted fecal matter, mucosal plaque, intestinal parasites and toxins. Bentonite clay acts as a bulk laxative by absorbing water to form a gel. It binds toxins such as pesticides and heavy metals and helps to carry them out of the colon, preventing them from being reabsorbed in the colon.
- Chlorella: contains high levels of chlorophyll, which is one of the greatest nutrients for cleansing the bowel and other elimination systems, such as the liver and the blood. Chlorella contains amino acids, enzymes (including pepsin for digestion), vitamins, minerals, carbohydrates; and, RNA and DNA, the building blocks of life. Chlorella is marine algae comprised of a fibrous, indigestible outer shell that has been proven to actually bind with pesticides like PCBs and heavy metals like mercury. Chlorella helps to remove metabolic wastes in tissues and provides support to the liver.
- Flaxseed, psyllium seed, slippery elm bark, marshmallow root: reduce inflammation and irritation of intestinal walls to facilitate healing. Ground flaxseeds absorb water and expand in the colon, allowing

toxins and mucus to be removed. In addition, flaxseed has been found to help lower cholesterol and blood pressure levels.

- Garlic (raw/aged): provides microflora balance to the gastrointestinal tract and strengthens the immune system.
- Herbs effective in killing parasites: include garlic, black walnut hulls, clove stems, cranberry extract, grape seed extract, fennel, goldenseal, pumpkin seeds, sage, thyme, and wormwood.
- Oxygen-based colon cleanser: uses specialized ozonated magnesium oxides to reduce the solid toxic mass into a liquid or gas form. The best way to melt away compacted matter is through an oxidation reduction reaction. Oxygen therapy removes old, impacted fecal matter as it detoxifies and cleans the entire colon. By thoroughly cleansing the intestinal tract, it allows room for a normal bowel process.
- Peppermint leaf: helps to reduce and move gas that is created during a deep intestinal/bowel cleanse. It also reduces spasms.
- Probiotics: help to replenish the population of friendly bacteria in the colon after cleansing.
- Senna, ginger: help to strengthen the colon muscle and increase peristalsis.
  Note: Colonic hydrotherapy also strengthens the colon as it helps to remove the accumulated fecal waste and other debris, but it should only be performed by a licensed and experienced healthcare professional.
- Whole foods: include green, leafy vegetables, dark-colored fruits, and organic whole grains that contain fiber to help eliminate toxins and other waste products.
- *Note:* Stop taking laxatives, and other similar products that do not stimulate the normal peristalsis action, but create a dependency for their use and fail to help cleanse and detoxify the body properly.
- *Note:* These herbal nutrients should not be used too frequently – to prevent any dependency or harm to your gastrointestinal system, including your intestinal villi.
- *Note:* The colon is surrounded by a layer of fat called the omentum, which stores fat and can become very large in overweight people.

> **Toilet sitting:** To facilitate proper removal of fecal matter from the colon, you should use the squatting position, but our modern-day toilets make this difficult by elevating the lower part of our body too high above the ground. Either elevate the legs slightly by placing them on a foot stand to simulate the squatting position or purchase a squatting platform that can easily be added to your toilet. This may seem to be a minor point, but, you will be surprised how much easier it will be to get rid of the waste as well as the amount of waste that will be removed during your initial cleansing/detoxification!

Liver/Gall Bladder

Liver cleansing/detoxification can provide relief from ailments such as high cholesterol, high blood pressure, blood clots, thick sticky blood, constipation, diarrhea, fatigue, allergies, weight problems, digestive difficulties, stress, and low sex drive. Liver cleansing/detoxification helps to purge old fats, old cholesterol deposits, gallstones, poisons, drug residues, and toxic waste from the liver while regenerating and healing liver cells.

The following is a list of nutrients that help to cleanse, detoxify and nourish the liver. Use only 100% organic, additive and toxic-free herbal and nutritional foods/supplements that contain these nutrients.

- Apple juice (organic): contains mallic acid, which weakens adhesions between solid globules and softens/dissolves gallstones.
- Alpha lipoic acid (ALA): protects the liver from potentially harmful cell changes and assists it in flushing toxins from the body. ALA is effective in minimizing liver toxicity following exposure to poisons such as heavy metals (including lead) and toxic industrial chemicals such as carbon tetrachloride.
- Amino acids: including l-taurine, l-glutamine, and l-methionine, help the liver neutralize ammonia and remove heavy metals and toxins. The liver must be able to neutralize anything that produces ammonia in the body. Two of the biggest ammonia producers are animal protein and over-the-counter drugs such as pain relievers, diuretics, and sedatives.

- Aloe vera: contains polysaccharides, enzymes, glycoproteins, amino acids, vitamins and minerals that help to support the immune system and detoxify the digestive system.
- Artichoke: contains potent polyphenols (bioflavonoids, caffeoyl-quinic acids) that work to cleanse the liver and provide antioxidant protection while it releases accumulated toxins. Artichoke increases the production of bile in the liver to aid in the digestion of fats, which can relieve bloating, gas and other uncomfortable symptoms of indigestion. Artichoke is an excellent source of fiber, and contains magnesium, folate and Vitamin C.
- Barley/wheat grass, dandelion root, wormwood: contain nutrients that increase bile and help to clean the liver and bile ducts to allow excess cholesterol to leave the body. They help to flush fat deposits from the liver and prevent the formation of gallstones.
- Cilantro: is known as Chinese parsley, and refers to the leaves of the coriander plant. It is a cooling herb and puts out excess flames in the stomach and generally enhances digestion. In recent years, modern science has discovered that cilantro is a natural chelation agent that is very helpful in removing heavy metals such as lead, mercury and aluminum from the body.
- Dandelion root: is one of the two major herbal liver tonics (with milk thistle) that helps to increase both the production and the flow of bile. It also prevents liver congestion by helping to flush out fat deposits.
- Epsom salt: contains magnesium sulfate, which serves to relax and dilate the bile duct so that larger stones can pass through during a liver flush. The Epsom salt also serves to evacuate the small and large intestines of feces.
- Extra virgin olive oil, barberry: stimulate the liver, the gallbladder and the production of bile. Extra virgin olive oil specifically stimulates the gallbladder and bile duct to contract and expel its contents.
- Garlic: kills bacteria, fungi, and other harmful pathogens, and helps to increase intestinal microflora. Also, binds with cadmium, mercury, and lead and removes these metals from the body to prevent cancer. Aged garlic has shown to provide even better health benefits.

- L-carnitine: protects the liver from the harmful breakdown products of everyday fat metabolism. It helps to detoxify lactic acidosis and ammonia, both of which are very toxic to the liver; and, it helps in the metabolic breakdown of alcohol.
- Liver flush: stimulates a sluggish liver and promotes bile production. Use a 100% organic, additive-free supplement that contains many of the aforementioned nutrients. Ensure that you have the guidance of a professional, licensed herbalist (or naturopathic doctor) who can show you how to prepare and administer your own liver flush.
- Methionine, choline and carnitine: are lipotropic factors that help to reduce fatty infiltration of the liver. Methionine is involved in producing sulphur-containing compounds, which bind onto various toxins, making them more easily transported from the liver.
- Milk thistle: is the other major liver tonic (with dandelion root). It contains silymarin, a bioflavonoid antioxidant that provides protection and healing of the liver by strengthening the structure of the liver membrane to prevent the penetration of toxins; and, increasing protein synthesis to stimulate the regeneration of damaged liver cells and the generation of new healthy liver cells. Milk thistle supports the production of the liver's own powerful antioxidant enzymes, such as glutathione.
- Phosphatidyl choline: supports the physical structure and health of the liver in its processing and excretion of chemical waste products. Just as calcium is important to the physical structure of the skeleton, phosphatidyl choline is important to the liver.
- Protein foods: include nuts, seeds, organic free range meats, organic eggs (from free-range chickens), wild salmon and other cold water fish, providing the essential amino acids, especially the sulfa-based amino acids that support the liver.
- Turmeric: contains essential oils and the powerful active ingredient curcumin, which is a strong anti-inflammatory and antioxidant that protects the liver. Curcumin increases the secretion of bile by stimulating the bile duct. Curcumin also protects the liver from detoxification, stimulating the gall bladder and scavenging free radicals. In conjunction with the adrenal glands, curcumin inhibits both platelet aggregation and the enzymes that induce inflammatory

prostaglandins. Curcumin also helps to break down fats and reduce cholesterol.

- Stop drinking alcohol because the alcohol, which is metabolized by the liver, damages and scars the liver tissue.
- Stop eating foods that contain trans fat (partially hydrogenated oil) because their toxic nature interferes with bile production and detoxification; and, increases the production of bad estrogen (estradiol) as people get older.
- Stop smoking because of tobacco carcinogens, which are toxic to the liver, lungs, and brain.
- Stop taking drugs including recreational, over-the-counter drugs, and prescription drugs (with your doctor's approval), especially cholesterol-lowering statins (e.g. Lipitor, Zocor), acetaminophens (e.g. Tylenol), NSAIDs (non-steroidal anti-inflammatory drugs) and blood pressure drugs because they damage the liver and other organs.
- Stop high doses of a Vitamin A (retinol palmitate) supplement greater than 15,000 IUs daily, because it places stress on the liver. A dose of 7,500 IUs of beta-carotene is preferred.

Kidneys

Cleansing/detoxification of the kidneys can provide relief from ailments such as high blood pressure, fatigue, urinary tract infections, and kidney stones. The following is a list of the key nutrients to cleanse, detoxify and nourish the kidneys.

- Apple cider vinegar (organic): contains nutrients that dilute the toxins in the bladder; and; help to remove acid crystals that collect in soft tissues and the joints (causing arthritis). Take a mixture of 2 tbsp. organic apple cider vinegar, 1 tbsp. raw honey and 1 cup of filtered water 4 times daily during a weekend so that the crystals can be flushed out of the body by the kidneys and other organs.
- Cranberries: contain phytonutrients that help to fight urinary tract infections. Specifically, cranberries contain concentrated tannins known as proanthocyanidins that prevent Escherichia coli (E.coli) bacteria from adhering to walls of the urinary tract. They also contain Vitamin C, which inhibits the growth of some bacteria by acidifying the urine.

Note: Avoid bottled cranberry juice, which contains refined sugar and high fructose corn syrup.

- Dandelion leaves: provide diuretic effects in treating urinary disorders and fluid retention without depleting the body of as much potassium as other diuretics.
- Goldenrod: increases the production of urine without reducing levels of important electrolytes.
- Horsetail: contains potassium and manganese along with several bioflavonoids, which cause the diuretic action, while the silicon content exerts a connective tissue strengthening and anti-arthritic action.
- Juniper berries: support the urinary system to maintain proper fluid balance.
- Lemons/limes: contain phytonutrients that help to flush the kidneys, relieving some of its workload. They contain Vitamin C, which inhibits the growth of some bacteria by acidifying the urine. Drink a glass of warm lemon water every morning.
  Note: A tablespoon of organic apple cider vinegar in a glass of warm water will provide a similar benefit.
- Parsley: supports eliminating wastes from the blood and tissues of the kidneys; prevents salt from being reabsorbed into the body tissues; helps improve edema and general water retention, fatigue and scanty or painful urination; and, aids in the dissolving of kidney stones and gall stones.
- Uva ursi leaves: contain the glycoside arbutin, which kills bacteria in the urine. Arbutin is water-soluble so it is easily carried via the blood to the kidneys.
- Vegetable juices (raw): such as celery, cucumbers, parsley, lemons, limes, and cranberries are very beneficial to the health of the kidneys and the urinary tract. Optional: wheat/barley grass juice.
- Water (filtered): helps to cleanse the urinary tract of bacteria and dilute the concentrated toxins in the bladder. Water also increases urine flow to reduce the exposure time of the toxins in your bladder and prevent bladder infections.

Lymphatic System
Cleansing of the lymphatic system removes the toxins, dead bacteria and waste material, thereby allowing, oxygen and vital nutrients to flow freely through the bloodstream. This starts the rejuvenation, healing and rebalancing processes within the body. Cleansing of the lymphatic system can help address the following health problems: ear problems, edema, fatigue, headaches, high blood pressure, frequent infections, lupus, multiple sclerosis, obesity, puffy eyes, excessive sweating, and acceleration of the aging process. The following is a list of the key nutrients to cleanse, detoxify and nourish the lymphatic system.

- Echinacea: stimulates macrophage activity, which in turn helps to maintain a healthy lymph flow. Macrophages located in the lymph nodes help to destroy viruses and foreign invaders in the lymph fluid.
- Exercise: is key because the lymphatic system is powered by muscle movement. One of the more effective forms of exercise is jumping up and down (carefully) on a small trampoline (with a handle bar) because it stimulates movement of the lymph fluid. Diaphragmatic deep breathing is also helpful.
- Protein: is critical to immune health and the ability to heal. The best protein sources for immune response are those with plenty of EFAs, e.g. wild salmon, sardines, fresh tuna, sea vegetables and green superfoods such as spirulina, barley grass and sprouts.
- Red clover (blossom): cleanses the blood and the lymph by promoting urine and mucous production, improving circulation, and stimulating the secretion of bile. Red clover improves the blood's hemoglobin levels and the size and number of blood platelets.
- Saunas: help to increase the blood circulation and are deeply relaxing.
- Spicy foods: boost a sluggish lymph system and reduce mucous congestion, e.g. natural salsas, cayenne pepper, horseradish, ginger.
- Stop consumption of caffeine, sugar, dairy, alcohol: because they contribute to lymphatic stagnation and inhibit white blood cell activity, weakening the immune system.
- Vegetables (green): such as green onions, zucchini, celery, parsley, mustard greens, turnip greens, cabbage, green peppers, spinach, lettuce, broccoli, and homemade vegetable broth provide potassium, magnesium, chlorophyll, water, and other key nutrients.

Pancreas

Cleansing of the pancreas supports the production and rebalancing of insulin and glucagon. The following is a list of the key nutrients to cleanse, detoxify and nourish the pancreas and the endocrine system.

- Beta glucan: contains soluble fibers that help to improve insulin sensitivity and reduce the elevation in blood glucose levels by delaying gastric emptying so that dietary sugar is absorbed more gradually. Beta glucan is found in the cell walls of baker's yeast, grains (e.g. oat bran, barley bran, oat/rye sprouts) and mushrooms (e.g. maitake, reishi, shiitake).
- Broccoli, onions, oysters, salmon, whole grains: contain biologically-active chromium to support insulin regulation and increase insulin usage by increasing the number of insulin receptor sites within cells.
- Cedar berries: improve insulin sensitivity.
- Dandelion root: contains trace minerals, inulin (a pre-biotic), and beta-carotene for the digestive system, especially the liver, gall bladder and pancreas.
- Enzymes (plant-based): ensure proper absorption of food for digestion of proteins, carbohydrates, and fats. Lack of enzymes can possibly manifest as a food allergy or acid reflux.
- Glyconutrients: are plant saccharides that support the endocrine system to provide hormonal balance. Food sources include mushrooms, seaweed, aloe vera, gums, herbs, and seeds.
- Goldenseal root: supports the function of the liver and the pancreas.
- Gymnema sylvestre, bitter melon, cinnamon cassia bark extract: help to increase glucose uptake, reducing the blood glucose level.
- Juniper berries: support the pancreas, adrenal glands, digestive system.
- Licorice root: helps with hypoglycemia, and supports the adrenal glands and immune system.
- Uva ursi leaves: support the pancreas and urinary system.
- Vegetable juices (raw): such as Brussel sprouts and stringbeans are believed to contain specific phytonutrients that stimulate the insulin receptors increasing insulin sensitivity and lowering insulin resistance.
- Avoid refined carbohydrates and excess conventional animal meat consumption, which put a strain on the pancreas.

Cleansing/Detoxification Guidelines

You should work with a healthcare professional that has experience in the use of nutritional supplements and herbs for cleansing and detoxification to design and tailor a procedure that fits your health needs and budget. As a precaution, review the procedure and products with your doctor, especially if you are taking any drugs/medications.

Caution: These procedures should only be performed under the supervision of a trained healthcare practitioner. If you have never performed this type of procedure, discuss this with your doctor, nutritionist, herbalist or other healthcare professional familiar with proper cleansing and detoxification. Ensure that the healthcare professional has experience in the use of nutritional supplements and herbs for cleansing/detoxification – especially if you are taking any kind of drug/medication that may interact with the nutritional supplement/herbal product. Also ensure that you acquire top quality herbal products from a reputable, licensed and experienced herbalist or other related professional, preferably someone who has had vast experience in the use of these products.

Cleansing/Detoxification Guidelines

1. If you need additional help with cleansing and detoxification, contact our wellness center or visit our website at www.deathtodiabetes.com.
2. Ensure that you have the following kitchen equipment/utensils: blender, juicer, and steamer.
3. Ensure that you have the following foods: extra virgin olive oil, garlic cloves, onions, cayenne powder, flaxseed, filtered water, fresh/frozen vegetables, wheat/barley grasses, and fruits.
4. Purchase 100% organic wholefood nutrition and herbal-based cleanse/detox supplements. Obtain these products from a reputable nutrition/wellness-related website, with the help of a healthcare professional. Ensure that these cleanse/detox products contain the majority of the nutrients listed on the previous pages 152-160.

5. Walk through the procedure with your healthcare professional. Review any areas of concern in detail. If possible, ensure that someone is home with you before you perform your first cleansing/detoxification.

6. Set aside a restful period of time on the weekend, when you will be indoors. Plan to rest (lay down) for most of the first day so that your body's energy is focused on healing.

7. Follow the instructions of your healthcare professional. In general, perform the cleansings in the following order to maximize the benefits: colon, kidney, and liver.

Colon cleanse
You want the colon to be functioning properly to remove all the waste products. If the colon is compacted, the waste products from the cleansing/detoxification will be backed up and may spill over into your bloodstream, causing you to experience headaches or stomachaches during the first few hours. This is one of the reasons why it's important that you conserve your energy by resting during the day. But, if the headaches continue, you may want to stop and contact your doctor.

Kidney cleanse
You want your urinary tract and bladder working properly before trying a liver cleanse, which can be more intense. Avoid acidic drinks such as coffee and soda during a kidney cleanse. Also avoid tap water and drink filtered water and fresh raw juices, especially juices made with lemons and limes.

Liver cleanse
Now that the colon and kidneys are working, this will put less stress on the liver. Cleansing will remove the sludge, toxins, and other contaminants and enable the liver to do a better job at detoxifying, cleansing and thinning the blood. This will also help the function of the lymphatic system and the gall bladder. If you have had your gall bladder removed, your liver is working overtime. Consequently, the cleansing of the liver becomes even more important and critical to your health.

- Drink fresh, organic apple juice every 2 to 3 hours for 2 days before performing a liver flush. The mallic acid found in the apple juice helps to dissolve and soften gallstones.
  Note: If you are a diabetic, dilute the apple juice with one-third filtered water – unless you have achieved better glucose control (less than 120 mg/dl) for the past month.

- Eat a no-fat breakfast and lunch such as a steamed vegetable, cooked cereal with fruit, organic fruit juice (no butter or milk). This allows the bile to build up and develop pressure in the liver. Higher pressure pushes out more stones.

- Purchase or prepare your liver flush. Immediately after drinking the liver flush, lie down and try not to move for at least the first 20 minutes to allow the gall stones to move through the ducts.
  Note: The unrefined olive oil in the flush stimulates the gallbladder and bile duct to contract and expel its contents; and, you may experience abdominal cramps the morning after the liver flush. When you sit down on the toilet, you may feel pressure building in the intestines, leading to an explosive expulsion of 10 to 50 little green, slimy balls.
  Note: Since the gall bladder does not hold enough bile to neutralize all of the liver flush that you have ingested, the empty gallbladder signals the liver to empty all of its available bile together with stones, gravel and crystals to condition (treat) the bile using the potent liver cleanse solution.
  Note: Epsom salt contains magnesium sulfate, which serves to relax the tubules to enable the passage of larger stones. The Epsom salt also serves to evacuate the intestines of feces.

- **Warning:** The liver flush may be unsafe for some people, especially those who have gallstones. The large amount of oil causes the gallbladder to contract, making it possible for a gallstone to become lodged in the narrow opening of the gallbladder and necessitate emergency gallbladder surgery. Since the absence of gallbladder-related symptoms does not mean an absence of risk, this procedure should *only* be done under the supervision of a trained health practitioner.

8. Perform a periodic cleansing/detoxification 1-4 times a year, depending on several factors, including your overall health, lifestyle, living environment, work environment, spiritual health, nutrition, and exercise regimen.

9. Perform a cleansing/detoxification after taking any major drugs/ medications for an extended period of time; or, after spending an extended period of time in the hospital or out of the country.

10. Use one or more of the following metal detoxifier nutritional supplements to enhance your cleansing/detoxification. But, ensure that they do not contain fillers, binders, and other contaminants. And, use bentonite clay in conjunction with most of these detoxifiers to prevent reabsorption of the metals in the colon.

   • Aloe vera: contains enzymes, glycoproteins, amino acids, vitamins, minerals, and polysaccharides (acemannan) that facilitate the destruction of many pathogenic organisms -- by interjecting itself into the cell membranes. This increases the fluidity and permeability of the membranes, allowing toxins to flow out of the cell more easily and nutrients to enter the cell more easily. This helps to improve cellular metabolism and energy production, while healing the intestinal tract.

   • Alpha lipoic acid: is an excellent metal detoxifier, particularly for mercury, lead and cadmium, which it binds to and neutralizes for excretion. It also helps to remove excessive copper and iron.

   • Cilantro: helps to remove heavy metals, especially mercury.

   • Garlic (raw/aged): is a powerful heavy metal detoxifier because of its high selenium content; and, is also a powerful detoxifier of nitrates and nitrites.

   • Glyconutrients: consist of several monosaccharides, which surround all cells and help the cells to remove toxins and absorb nutrients, and to identify and interact with one another to strengthen/modulate the immune system.

   • N-acetylcysteine (NAC): can detoxify heavy metals such as mercury, lead and cadmium. NAC is also a powerful antioxidant that helps in supporting the immune system.

   • Vitamin C, chlorophyll, herbs (red clover, echinacea, cayenne): help with detoxification and strengthening the immune system.

Other Cleansing/Detoxification Methods

If time, finances or a concern with side effects is preventing you from cleansing/detoxifying your body, then, consider other alternative therapies that may not be as time-consuming, expensive or risky in terms of possible side effects. In addition to food and herbal-based therapies, there are other therapies available to cleanse and detoxify the body.

- Colonic hydrotherapy: helps to cleanse and remove congestion within the colon, reducing inflammation and increasing the cleaning capabilities of the body. Many health issues can be attributed to a compacted colon.

- Exercise therapy: that consists of long duration, medium to high intensity exercises helps to mobilize the lymphatic system, and helps to remove toxins via sweating.

- Juicing therapy: helps to provide "living" nutrients to cleanse/repair the cells, when juicing with chlorophyll-rich wheat/barley grasses and various vegetables.

- Lymphatic detoxification: uses physical massage of the lymph nodes or a lymphatic footpad that is believed to help draw out the body's toxins. However, buyer beware since there are no clinical studies to substantiate these claims at this time.

- Sauna therapy: helps to increase metabolism and circulation while removing toxins via sweating. It is also beneficial for relaxation and stress reduction.

- Spiritual therapy: comes in many forms, e.g. prayer, guided meditation, concentrative meditation, transcendental meditation, transformational meditation, motion meditation (i.e. Tai Chi, Qi Gong), energy therapy (i.e. Reiki), and other forms of meditation and enlightenment. Spiritual therapy is very powerful as it helps to remove the emotional toxins that deteriorate the physical body. Also, forgiving others for the wrongs they have done to us is an important step in the healing process. However, ensure that you forgive the most important person – you!

- Other therapies: clay baths, chelation, foot detox patches.

Chapter 10. Exercise

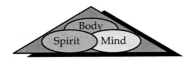

The Next Most Important Key

Most people are aware that exercise is important, but many of us either do not like to exercise or have the time to exercise. To further compound matters, some people exercise incorrectly and for the wrong reasons. Consequently, people stop exercising after becoming bored, frustrated or discouraged due to the lack of progress in their health, weight loss or other health objective. Actually, exercise may be the closest thing to a "fountain of youth". By taking yourself from a sedentary state you can, in effect, reduce your biological age by ten to fifteen years. Researchers who have conducted extensive studies on fitness and mortality have concluded "moderate levels of physical fitness and exercise are protective against early mortality." Exercise imparts vigor and activity to all organs and maintains the healthful integrity of all their functions by improving the tone and quality of muscle tissue and stimulating the processes of digestion, absorption, metabolism, and elimination. Exercise also strengthens the blood vessels, lungs, and heart, resulting in improved transfer of oxygen to the cells and increased circulation of the vascular and lymph systems. In addition, studies indicate that physical activity promotes the growth of mitochondria (the cell "energy factories"), leading to increased adenosine triphosphate (ATP), the molecule that transfers energy between living cells; and, this increase in cellular energy can trigger fat burning.

Years ago, the physical activity from farming, steel mills and other labor industries served many purposes, including stress reduction, removal of food congestion and toxins, and the slow down of the aging process. But, when our society shifted from this industrial state to more of a service state (office work, computers), our level of physical activity and our children's level of physical activity decreased dramatically. According to Mark Fenton (the walking guru), "We are living in an epidemic of physical inactivity and improper nutrition." Interestingly, exercise is a form of physical activity that was "created" to address this loss of physical activity. It was discovered that the loss of physical activity led to early deterioration of the body and its parts, and eventually degenerative diseases/ailments such as backaches, constipation, headaches, chronic fatigue, high blood pressure, obesity, heart disease, stroke, cancer, diabetes, arthritis and osteoporosis.

In general, aerobic exercise is important for improving your cardiovascular health. *However*, **anaerobic** exercise (weight-resistance training) as part of a circuit-training regimen that includes aerobics is the *optimum* form of exercise that provides the maximum health benefit. Unfortunately, many people overdo the aerobic exercising to try to lose weight, and they end up losing lean muscle tissue, which lowers their metabolism rate, making it even more difficult to lose weight.

But, if you have been living a sedentary lifestyle, walking is the easiest form of exercise to get your body acclimated to moving again. You will need to initiate a gradual training regimen to prevent any unwanted injuries that many beginners experience due to their overcompensating for not exercising in years. Consistency and low-to-moderate intensity exercise are the ways to introduce your body to exercise and fun; and, you can grow from there by finding other forms of exercise (e.g. gardening, sports, bicycling, skiing, swimming, dancing, trampoline jumping) that you may enjoy and actually not see as just exercise.

Types of Exercise & Variables

There are three major types of exercise: stretching, aerobic, and anaerobic.

Stretching Exercise
Stretching exercise is performed to passively or actively elongate soft tissue and muscles to improve the range of motion (ROM), reduce unnecessary muscle strains and tears, and provide flexibility. Exercise examples include: light stretching, inversion table, yoga, and Pilates.

Aerobic Exercise

Aerobic means oxygen. Aerobic exercise is continuous rhythmic movement of the major muscles groups without intermittent rest periods such that the muscles are working in an oxygen-rich state, which can cause the body to produce fat-burning enzymes under the right circumstances, e.g. after your body has burned off most of the glucose. Examples of aerobic exercise include: walking, step aerobics, running, swimming, other water exercises, bicycling, dancing, skiing, jumping, cardio kick-boxing, and rowing.

Anaerobic Exercise

Anaerobic means lack of oxygen. Anaerobic exercise consists of short bursts of body movements with some resistance such that the muscles are working in an oxygen-deprived state, which causes the body to produce glucose-burning enzymes. Because you are expending energy faster than the body can replace it by metabolizing oxygen, intermittent rest periods are required during the exercise session. Anaerobic exercise puts the body into an anabolic state that builds lean muscle tissue and burns fat. Muscles that are already conditioned rely less on glycogen (stored glucose) and more on fat for fuel, so the muscles of a trained individual burn more body fat than those of people who do not exercise. Examples of anaerobic exercise include: weight/resistance training, interval strength training, water exercise, and weight lifting.

Exercise Variables

There are three major variables that you can adjust to customize your exercise program, based on fitness level, health, age, personal health goals, risk factor profile, medications, behavioral characteristics, and individual preferences.

- Duration: is the amount of time that you spend during an exercise session. In general, you should start with a low duration of 10 to 15 minutes and gradually work up to 30 to 60 minutes, depending on your age, health state and health goals.
- Frequency: is the number of times that you exercise on a weekly basis. In general, you should start exercising on alternate days (4 times a week) and gradually work up to exercising on a daily basis (5 to 6 times a week).

- Intensity: is related to the amount of work and calories expended during the exercise session. The higher the amount of work and the lower the duration, the higher the intensity. For example, walking one mile in 30 minutes has a much lower intensity level than running four miles in 20 minutes. In general, you should start out at a low intensity level such that you are able to speak comfortably while exercising; and, gradually work up to moderate to moderate-high intensity, where it is difficult to talk. When you are exercising at a higher intensity your cardiovascular system is under such a significant amount of stress that the mere act of talking makes you unable to provide your body with enough oxygen. However, if you cannot talk at all, then you have gone too far and need to decrease the intensity. In general, the intensity level should be between 50% and 90% of your maximum heart rate.

Increasing the duration, frequency and/or intensity causes the body to burn more calories (energy), more glucose and eventually more fat. However, at some point the law of diminishing returns sets in such that increasing duration, frequency and/or intensity can lead to the break down of muscle tissue causing the body's metabolism to slow down.

Benefits of Exercise

Beyond reducing your biological age, there are many physical, emotional, and spiritual benefits associated with exercise.

Stretching Exercise
- Increases blood flow to muscles to prepare them for exercise.
- Improves ability of muscles to stretch and elongate (to increase range of motion) and develop functional mobility.
- Increases muscle tone and firmness.
- Increases balance and coordination.
- Increases metabolism.

Aerobic Exercise
- Improves cardiovascular endurance, strengthens the heart and bones.
- Increases oxygen intake, due to more deeply breathing causing oxygen to be received fully into the lungs and, into the blood stream.
- Makes the lungs better conditioned so that activities (e.g. climbing stairs) will not leave you breathless.
- Helps the lymphatic fluids to drain and circulate properly to increase immunity.
- Promotes sweating which helps to detoxify the body via the skin.
- Stimulates the immune system, putting more white blood cells including T-helper cells (made in the thymus gland) and macrophages (from arterial walls) into circulation.
- Helps to lower the total cholesterol, and, may increase the HDL (good) cholesterol, lowering the risk of heart disease.
- Helps to lower blood pressure by increasing the production of nitric oxide, which relaxes the artery walls.
- Helps to release enzymes (e.g. hormone-sensitive lipase) to mobilize fat in adipose tissue
- Helps to increase insulin sensitivity so that glucose enters the cells and is burned as fuel.
- Helps to trigger the release of brain chemicals called endorphins that help improve mood, relieve stress and make you more productive.

Anaerobic Exercise
- Multiplies muscle strength, tone, and firmness.
- Helps tone the body by increasing muscle strength while burning fat.
- Reduces belly fat; also, reduces body fat, re-shaping the body.
- Develops strength of tendons and ligaments.
- Increases bone density and strength.
- Increases metabolism and intensifies fat loss (especially *belly* fat).
- Makes muscle cells more sensitive to insulin, increasing the uptake of glucose into the muscle cells to provide more energy.
- Boosts stamina, energy, and endurance.
- Develops functional mobility to improve day-to-day quality of life.
- Increases balance and coordination.
- Enhances mental clarity; improves attitude.

Exercise Guidelines

Utilize the following guidelines to optimize your exercise program based on your health goals.

1. Ensure that you are exercising for the right reasons. For example, some people exercise to compensate for overeating. This may work for a while, but eventually, this will stop working; and, you will become discouraged with exercising. The key message here is that you must provide the body with the proper fuel in order to reap the maximum benefits of exercise; otherwise, exercise can be counter-productive and damaging to your health.

2. Increase your daily physical activity – don't sit around all day and expect 30 minutes of exercise to reap any major benefits. Wear a pedometer to keep track of your daily physical activity and to provide motivation to increase your overall physical activity each week.
    Note: 2000 steps equal one mile, 100 calories for a 150-pound person.

3. Initiate a consistent, low-intensity exercise program as soon as reasonably possible, with the consent of your doctor. Try to exercise 4 times a week – once a week for 2 hours on the weekend is harmful.
    Rationale: Consistent exercise will reduce your insulin resistance, your blood glucose and stress levels. The majority of the research shows that women derive a greater proportion of their energy expenditure from fats during low to moderate intensity exercise, relative to men. Thus, this will improve fat metabolism, particularly for women.

4. Take a 10 to 15-minute low-intensity walk an hour or so after dinner. This will burn off some of the meal, provide energy and induce a deep sleep that night. The following morning you will awaken refreshed and full of energy because you will be well rested.
    *   In general, walking 2-3 mph burns 250-300 calories per hour.
    *   Depending on walking speed, 1000 steps equates to about 10 minutes. You can personalize this by determining exactly how many steps you take in 10 minutes while wearing your pedometer. Then just multiply this number by 3 to 6 to find out how much you might want to increase your daily walking, depending on your personal schedule and goals.

- When you start to exercise you may wake up the next morning with that sore, aching feeling, especially if you haven't exercised in a while. That pain or soreness is called delayed onset muscle soreness, or DOMS. Most people's first reaction is to stop exercising, because they don't want to wake up sore every morning. But, according to a new study from the University of Ohio, the best way to get rid of that soreness is to stay physically active. The University of Ohio researchers found that muscles get stronger the more frequently they are exercised. DOMS occurs when tiny skeletal muscle segments called sarcomeres pull apart as a muscle lengthens. Contractions that lengthen muscles are particularly damaging to sarcomeres. And these contractions occur all the time in humans – when we sit down, walk, run, or even lower heavy objects. The findings also suggest that there will be less post-exercise pain after later workouts.
- If walking is difficult, try an exercise that you can perform while sitting down, e.g. using a rowing machine, resistance bands, tension cord/rope or flex-bar.

5. Gradually, move to a low intensity/medium duration regimen; and, depending on your health goals, gravitate to a medium intensity/medium duration regimen to burn more calories. Use an exercise tracking worksheet to record your progress and provide motivation.

6. Incorporate some weight-resistance or interval strength training with higher intensity for a shorter period of time at least 3 times a week.
   Rationale: Resistance training causes the muscles to increase their glucose uptake, which is exactly what insulin does. As a result, eventually, this may reduce the body's need for insulin. In addition, as intensity increases, the absolute amount of energy derived from fat is increased, for both men and women.

7. Incorporate various modes of training, referred to as cross-training.
   Rationale: Cross-training prevents the body from getting overly fatigued and from overuse of the same muscles in the same movement patterns. This helps to prevent muscle stress, muscle soreness and injuries. Therefore, a person will be able to safely do more exercise, more frequently, which equates to higher total energy and fat expenditure and much better glucose control.

8. Design a consistent exercise regimen with the following 3 major components:
    - **Stretching/Balancing:** Use yoga, Pilates (2-4 times a week)
    - **Cardio warm-up/Stretching:** (5-10 min)
    - **Strength training (Upper/lower/core body training):** Anaerobics (10-20 min) on alternate days
    - **Cardio training/Cool-down:** Aerobics/anaerobics: (15-30 min)
9. Once you design your initial exercise program, vary the workouts every other week or at a frequency that meets your needs.
    Rationale: Varying the workouts provides a new stimulus to the body's cardiovascular, muscular, skeletal and respiratory systems, preventing muscle fatigue, soreness, and boredom.
10. Measure/check your blood glucose before and after each exercise session.
    - If your blood glucose (BG) is greater than 300, do not exercise. Contact your doctor, if necessary.
    - If your BG is less than 90, eat a snack before you exercise.
    - Know the signs of low blood sugar (hypoglycemia) and how to treat it. For example, if you feel weak, dizzy, sweaty, or have the shakes, you may be experiencing a hypoglycemic episode (low blood sugar). Eat something immediately to raise your blood glucose level. Do not attempt to exercise.
11. Consume adequate fluids and foods that provide key antioxidants, vitamins, minerals, and other nutrients that are needed to perform exercise. And, since exercise increases the production of toxins in the body, it is even more important to replenish the body with these critical fluids and super foods – to facilitate removal of the toxins and to nourish the body and prepare it for the next exercise session.
    Important Note: If you do not eat properly, your muscles will not be properly nourished and will remain sore and not recover after exercise. Consequently, you will become discouraged with exercise and eventually stop exercising.
12. **Warning:** Measure your blood glucose level *before* you exercise. If your blood glucose is too low (e.g. below 90 mg/dl), eat a small sandwich before you exercise.

Exercise Regimen

Cardio Warm-up/Stretching

1. Spend 5 to 10 minutes walking as an easy way to first warm up the body, muscles and joints.
2. Perform balancing activities such as standing on one foot 2-4 times a week, or use yoga or Pilates.
3. Perform flexibility stretching exercises to further warm up the body, muscles and joints.
   Caution: Do not stretch cold muscles without first warming them up by walking for several minutes! This is a common source of injury.
4. Do not bounce during stretching – maintain good form and hold your stretch in a static position.
5. Stretch the muscles: quadriceps, hamstrings, calfs, back, arms.
6. If necessary, work with a health coach or go to your local YMCA/YWCA to get going in the right direction.

Strength Training (Core & Upper/Lower Body)

1. If your health goals include building lean muscle tissue to change your body composition, perform some form of weight-resistance or interval strength training (anaerobics). It can be something as simple as carrying a small can of corn or other small object in each hand and slowly moving your arms up and down as you walk.
   Rationale: This combination of aerobics and anaerobics will multiply the benefits of both. Strength training will maintain and build lean muscle mass, which starts to decrease one pound every two years after the age of 35. Also, lean muscle mass increases the metabolism and enables the body to burn more calories.
2. To burn maximum glucose and to increase your metabolism, ensure that you are exercising with proper core, shoulders and hip alignment to engage more muscles during your exercise.
3. Perform strength training exercise after the cardio warm-up for 10 to 20 minutes. Otherwise, work different muscle groups every 2 to 3 days to allow recovery time and prevent injuries to the muscles.

Note: If anaerobic and aerobic exercises are being performed on the same day, this enables the body to burn up the glycogen in the muscles, so that the body will burn fat during the aerobic exercise.

4. Perform 8 to 12 repetitions at least three times before moving to the next body part – a total of 24 to 36 resistance motions for the same body part. Strength for bones and muscle is gained by the amount of resistance and the intensity, but straining is not necessary or beneficial.

    • Perform exercises that support an increase in spinal elongation, lean muscle tissue, core strength and the range of motion without causing injury, e.g. Pilates.

    • Perform the repetitions until the muscle fails if the objective is to build muscle mass.

5. For upper body training, use one or more of the following: weights, resistance bands, wrist weights.

6. For core and lower body training, use one or more of the following: stair climbing, squats, use of resistance bands, use of ankle/thigh weights, trampoline jumping.

Cardio Training (including Cool-Down)

1. Finally, perform aerobic exercise for 15 to 30 minutes, low to moderate depending on current health state and your health goal.

    a. Exercise at 50% to 80% of your maximum heart rate (MHR), based on general health and endurance. Use of the MHR is only a guideline – you may need to exercise at a different level, depending on your health state and your health goal.

       • To calculate your MHR, subtract your age from 220. For example, if you are 50 years old, your MHR will be 220 – 50, or 170 beats per minute.

       • To calculate the range of 50% to 80%, multiply the MHR by 0.5 and 0.8. For this example, the range would be 170 x 0.5 to 170 x 0.8 or 85 to 136 beats per minute. Verify these numbers with your doctor, especially if you have any heart problems.

    b. Start slow. Work up to 20 to 30 minutes over several weeks/months.

       Rationale: This will improve your cardio health; and, can also help to burn excess fat.

    c. Integrate some form of weight-resistance training during this portion of your exercise regimen to exercise the muscles in your arms, shoulders, legs, chest, and abdomen – especially, if you do not perform the Strength Training portion of this exercise regimen. This can be accomplished in many different ways, e.g.:

- Use resistance bands or a flex-bar.
- Wear wrist weights and/or ankle weights.
- Wear a weight vest.
- Carry a three to five-pound weight or object in each hand while walking.

    d. *Caution:* Do not make the mistake of running too much just because you have the extra energy. Excessive aerobic exercise (with no anaerobic weight-resistance exercise) may enter the body into a catabolic state causing some loss of lean muscle tissue during exercise. This change in body composition, in turn, can lead to a reduction in the basal metabolic rate (a slowdown in metabolism) and make it difficult to lose weight (fat). Instead use the extra energy to perform some weight-resistance exercise.

2. Spend 3 to 5 minutes to warm down by walking and stretching.
   Rationale: This prevents "pooling" of the blood in the muscles. It also helps to remove lactic acid from the muscles, which in turn reduces muscle soreness.
3. Do not over-exercise! Excess exercise decreases growth hormone, testosterone levels and thyroid output. It also increases cortisol and insulin levels.
4. Replenish the body with water and a well-balanced super snack.
5. Update your exercise tracking worksheet and modify your nutrition and exercise plans accordingly to provide any personal motivation.
6. Optional: Utilize an elliptical exercise machine to reduce the impact on joints, knees, and the lower back and provide an upper body workout in addition to the lower body workout.

Motivational Tips for Exercising

If you are like most people, you do not like to exercise, especially if you have not exercised for more than a few years. And, once you decide to start exercising, many people will drop out within 6 weeks, half will quit within 6 months and less than one third of those who began an exercise program will still be exercising by the end of their first year. The following are some tips to get you started and keep you going for the long term.

1. Schedule your exercise sessions on your calendar as if they were any other important appointment. This way, you will be able to balance your exercise program with family, work and social activities. Again, you will be more successful if you fit exercise into your current lifestyle. A little is always better than none.

2. If possible, try to build your exercise/physical activity into your daily activities, e.g. going to work, shopping, house chores, etc.

3. Don't work out too hard or too fast at the beginning. If you do, you will end up sore and uninspired. It's better to work out 2-3 days a week for life than to work out 6-7 days a week for a couple of weeks. Consistency is the key.

4. When you feel like skipping a workout, get yourself to do some form of exercise for at least 10 - 15 minutes. Most people struggle during that initial 5 minutes, but once they get past that 5-minute mark, they are actually able to complete their entire workout. (If you don't, don't worry about it – 10 minutes is still better than nothing).

5. When you get bored or unfocused, change your exercise routine a bit by adding a yoga, aerobics, Pilates, swimming or dancing class. If you don't care to join a gym, there are many wonderful classes at the local recreational centers. Try a new exercise video or machine, or, try an outdoor activity such as bicycling or a beach walk.

6. Give yourself a little leeway - if you miss a workout or even an entire week, get back on track as soon as possible. Setbacks and challenges are normal. The sooner you get back on track, the sooner you will reach your goals. Remember - fitness is not about being perfect, but about a series of healthy choices that you make consistently. It is not an all or nothing proposition.

7. If possible, work out in the morning. You will feel more energized all day and will avoid "life" getting in the way of achieving your exercise and health goals.

8. If possible, get in the habit of taking a 5 - 10 minute walk after lunch and/or dinner, especially if the weather is nice. Walk with your partner or a friend. You will be amazed how well you feel physically and emotionally.

9. Keep a pedometer and a fitness journal to chart your progress and accomplishments, and provide motivation.

10. Try to limit the number of times that you use the weight scale to once a month or once a week at the most. As you get fit, lose fat and gain muscle, you will actually drop inches and pants/dress sizes and not move the scales that much.

11. Evaluate your progress every 6 - 8 weeks and increase the duration, frequency or intensity of your workouts to stay challenged and inspired.

12. If you need help, ask a fitness professional or instructor for suggestions and advice on how you can most effectively achieve your goals. There are also a variety of other resources on health and fitness available on the web.

Exercise Excuses/Countermeasures

Here are the most common excuses for skipping exercise along with ways to combat them.

I don't have time: This is by far one of the most common excuses that people use. People that use this excuse are actually saying that exercise is not enough of a priority to make it on their daily or weekly to-do list. If you fall into this category, then it's time to review your daily priority list. Certainly there is something less important that you are doing for 10-15 minutes every day that can be replaced with exercise. After all, exercise is one of the most important things you can do for yourself and your family to ensure that you live a high quality life. Try to increase your daily physical activity and integrate exercise into your daily life.

I'm too fat (or out-of-shape): Unless your doctor has forbidden you to exercise, then it's very unlikely that this excuse has any validity. If you are extremely out-of-shape, then you simply need to start with baby steps. Walking is always a great place to start. You may have to start with just five minutes. That's okay. You can gradually add more time each week. If walking is not an option, then you could try some pool exercises. There are many beneficial strength training exercises you can do while sitting with a resistance band, flex bar, resistance chair or a rowing machine.

I'm too tired: This is a common excuse, especially with diabetics, overweight people and people who have insulin resistance – all because of poor nutrition. Without proper nutrition (fuel), the body cannot produce the necessary energy for exercise, leading to fatigue. This excuse also creates a vicious circle because the more sedentary you are then the more tired you become; and, the more tired you are then the less appealing exercise sounds. Exercise can actually make you feel more revived then a nap because it stimulates your lymphatic, immune, and cardiovascular systems – especially if you provide your body with the proper nutrition. Regular physical activity increases your energy level. In addition, consistent exercise helps you to fall asleep faster and sleep better, which allows you to feel rested every day.

I really don't like to exercise: This is usually due to the boredom that you feel during exercise or the fact that your body not only feels achy after exercising but the fact that it aches for the next couple days. Many people still have the old "no pain, no gain" mentality and think that in order for exercise to be worthwhile you have to be miserable doing it. This just isn't true. Some people don't like to exercise because they don't like to sweat. Actually, you don't have to work up a big sweat every time you exercise – it's all about just getting the body moving. Consider things that you really like to do. If you prefer competitive situations, then consider joining a recreational sports team. If you are a social person, join an exercise group or take an exercise class with your friends. If you enjoy spending time alone, then try yoga or evening walks. And, don't over do the exercise – that is part of the reason for the sore muscles.

I've tried and failed in the past: It's true that it can be difficult to get motivated to exercise after you've failed before, but isn't your health worth another try? If you've been unsuccessful in the past, then re-evaluate what went wrong. Did you try to do too much, too quickly? It's very common to be overzealous when starting out and end up either burning out or getting injured early on. Did you set unrealistic goals for yourself? Try to establish small goals that are truly achievable, for example, that you will workout three times a week for the next month.

I'm too old to get started: It may sound cliché, but you are never too old to get started. Everyone can benefit from exercising. Even if you are a senior citizen you can reap many rewards from starting an exercise program. Okay, so maybe you won't be a marathon runner or a bodybuilder, but you'll be able to carry your groceries, walk the stairs easier, play with your grandchildren, improve your balance, and improve your glucose control if you're diabetic. And, more importantly, you'll enjoy your meals because you realize that the meals are providing the extra energy you didn't have in the past.

The inconsistent weather makes it difficult, or I don't have any exercise equipment: Nice try, but you can exercise indoors and get your heart pumping without any fancy exercise equipment. Don't underestimate what you can do with things that are already in your house. For example, if you have a flight of stairs then you have an awesome way to get your heart rate up by walking or running the stairs. Grab a couple of soup cans to emulate dumbbells for strength training exercises.

I can't afford a gym membership: You don't have to spend a single dollar for a gym membership in order to get fitter. Just walking outside is a great place to start. Also, home fitness equipment has become very affordable and accessible. For as little as $35 you can buy some great home equipment that will really challenge your body. A resistance band, a couple of small hand weights and an exercise ball allow you to work every muscle group and even obtain a good cardiovascular workout.

I don't know what exercises to do: There are literally dozens of ways to learn what exercises will help you. There are hundreds of books, websites, television shows and videos that offer advice and tips. If you have the money, another way to ensure your workouts are most effective is to hire a personal trainer or an online personal trainer. They can guide you every step of the way so that you don't waste any time doing exercises the wrong way.

I just can't get motivated or I don't want to change: Keep in mind that most of us are resistant to change. So, find something that will motivate you to exercise. For me, initially, it was the fear of dying. Later, it was the feeling I got from a good exercise session. For you, it may be your spouse, your children, your grandchildren, the quality of your life, or it may be financial (less expenses for drugs, doctors and hospitals).

To help you get started, set small, short-term goals. Start with a promise to just take the stairs instead of the elevator, for example. Then you might move onto scheduling 10 minutes of activity a couple of times per week. Also, make a list of all the positive benefits exercising has on your life. Your list might include giving you more energy, reducing your health ailments and more. The list should be pretty long. Post it somewhere that you will see it regularly and it can serve as a reminder to you as to why you need to workout.

Another option is to take a yoga or T'ai Chi class. They are two great ways to get the physical activity you need and learn the techniques of proper breathing and relaxation. Yoga is a physical way of life emphasizing the harmony of the body and mind, and a philosophical way of life that is based on Eastern metaphysical beliefs. T'ai Chi is an ancient Chinese art of exercise and self-defense with an emphasis on relaxation, both physical and mental, which leads to developing internal strength. T'ai Chi is classified as a low impact aerobic exercise comparable to walking that is used as a therapeutic exercise for people who are recovering from illness or injury, or for those who are beginning an exercise program.

There are new muscle activation techniques that provide maximum benefits in less time by utilizing a series of sequential movements designed to put the body in proper functional alignment, establishing increased strength and flexibility of the spine, better neuro-kinetic flow, lymphatic function, and an increased metabolic rate. In addition, you can utilize these muscle activation techniques while you are at work, shopping, walking, driving or doing everyday household chores – consequently, reducing the amount of time you need to spend exercising each day. Contact our wellness center for more information.

Nutritional Tips for Exercise

Utilize the following nutritional tips to optimize your exercise regimen.

1. Before you exercise, if you are hungry, you may need to eat a super snack to prevent cell dehydration and muscle damage.

2. After you exercise, replenish the body with the nutrients of a super meal to provide the necessary raw materials for the muscles and other body parts and to replenish the glycogen stores. Carbohydrates after an intense exercise session actually help to shuttle glucose into the muscle cells and accelerate the healing process to reduce most of the muscle soreness. If the exercise included intense weight-resistance training, ensure you include a quality protein supplement (e.g. an amino acid blend) to help repair and rebuild broken down muscle tissue and build new lean muscle tissue. And, don't forget to drink at least 16 ounces of filtered water before your meal.

3. Eat a super dinner meal of "live" enzyme-rich foods, especially raw vegetables, chlorophyll-rich wheat/barley grasses, dark fruits, and raw juices to provide all the enzymes and B vitamins, which are essential for food metabolizing and energy production. Also, eat beans or some whole grains to provide a sustained release of energy.

4. Based on your exercise regimen and health needs, utilize one or more of the following nutrients:
    - Acetyl-L-Carnitine (ALC): helps to reduce the buildup of lactic acid, which contributes to sore muscles after exercising.
    - CoQ10: supports the production of energy in the cells.
    - Ginseng: contains compounds called ginsenosides, which boost stamina, energy, and fight fatigue by sparing glycogen while utilizing fatty acids as energy.
    - L-carnitine (in liquid form): enables fat metabolism (and weight loss) – by transporting fat to the mitochondria of each cell to be burned as fuel – but, only when the body is *exercising*, using the heart and skeletal muscles, where 95% of the carnitine resides.
    - Vitamin B-Complex: provides the nutrients that break down carbohydrates, protein, and fat to provide energy to the cells.

Chapter 11. Blood Glucose Testing/ Doctor Visits

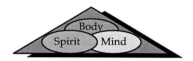

Blood Glucose Testing

Because of the major advances of medical science and technology, blood glucose testing is a very important tool for diabetics to track the progress of their blood glucose levels. Blood glucose (BG) testing is the **most powerful diagnostic tool** that a diabetic has to determine the state of their health on a daily basis. Next to nutrition and exercise, it is the most important key to effectively control the disease. And, for Type 2 diabetics, it has the power to *reverse* the disease – once effective nutritional, exercise and spiritual programs have been implemented. Unfortunately, most diabetics either do not test their blood glucose on a frequent-enough basis or do not understand the appropriate corrective actions to take based on their test results. Consequently, most diabetics can never get to a point where they can *proactively* control their blood glucose level and their diabetes.

By increasing your blood glucose testing, you can more readily determine the potential cause and effect relationships between your high glucose readings and the events that may be driving those high readings, e.g. meals, drugs, exercise, stress, illness, emotional state, menstrual cycle start (for women). Keep in mind that there will be times when your glucose levels will be high for no apparent reason, but, the more you test, the more infrequent will be those types of occurrences. Blood glucose testing is probably the most misunderstood and least-performed activity of the eight "living" elements for managing and controlling diabetes, so do not overlook this critical activity.

Blood Glucose Tests & Normal Ranges

The fasting blood glucose test is performed by pricking your finger and placing a drop of blood on a test strip. This drop of blood is analyzed by your blood glucose meter and translated into a number that is displayed in the window of your glucose meter. This number indicates your blood glucose level at that particular moment and is based on what you ate and did during the past few hours since your last meal. The following is the set of normal ranges for blood glucose levels.

Fasting glucose level before meals: 80 to 120 mg/dl
Optimum Range: 80 to 100 mg/dl
Optimum Running Average: less than 100 mg/dl

Postprandial glucose level (2 hours after meals): 90 to 130 mg/dl
Optimum Range: 80 to 110 mg/dl
Optimum Running Average: less than 105 mg/dl

Note: To convert mg/dl to mmol/l, divide the number by 18. Refer to the following table to compare readings in mg/dl vs. mmol/l.

Hemoglobin A1C Testing

Another important blood glucose test is the Hemoglobin A1C test. This test measures the percentage of glucose in the blood for the past two to three months and provides a more reliable measure of your blood glucose control during that time frame. Because A1C values are directly proportional to the concentration of glucose in the blood over this time period, they are not subject to the wide fluctuations of the day-to-day fasting blood glucose tests. The test is also known by several other names, including such variations as glycated hemoglobin test, glycosylated hemoglobin test and HbA1C test.

You will know whether your blood glucose has been under control during the past two to three months, based on the hemoglobin A1C percentage. The hemoglobin A1C normal range of 4.4% to 5.5% correlates to the blood glucose monitor normal range of 80 mg/dl to 120 mg/dl.

Refer to the following table, which correlates the hemoglobin A1C percentages and blood glucose meter readings.

HbA1C (%)	4	4.4	5	5.5	6	7	8	9	10	11
BG (mg/dl)	65	80	100	120	135	170	205	240	275	310
BG (mmol/l)	3.6	4.4	5.5	6.6	7.5	9.4	11.4	13.3	15.3	17.2

Figure 9. Hemoglobin A1C & Blood Glucose Readings

The hemoglobin A1C number indicates if your treatment strategy is working, making the A1C test one of the most effective tools in diabetes care. If your A1C is higher than desired, you and your health care team can adjust your strategy to help you better control your diabetes and prevent the onset of complications. If you can lower your A1C percentage, you will dramatically improve your chances of controlling the disease and preventing complications.

Your red blood cells contain hemoglobin, a protein that carries oxygen from your lungs to all the cells in your body. When a red blood cell first forms, it has no glucose attached to it. But with diabetes, you have too much glucose in your bloodstream. That extra glucose enters the red blood cells and attaches (glycates) to molecules of hemoglobin. The more glucose in your blood, the more hemoglobin that gets glycated. The A1C test measures the percentage of that glycated hemoglobin, offering a snapshot of your average blood glucose control for the past few months.

The hemoglobin A1C test helps to confirm the validity of your daily blood glucose self-testing. Some people, especially young children, may not perform their self-tests correctly. If you mistakenly think your blood glucose has been well controlled but your A1C is high, it could mean there's a problem with your self-testing routine. On the other hand, if the A1C reading is within the normal range but your average fasting blood glucose level is high, the A1C reading may be wrong, depending on your health state. Be careful not to draw any significant conclusions from the A1C test if it does not align with your fasting average blood glucose readings. You may want to retest the A1C and/or increase your fasting blood glucose tests to resolve any potential differences.

Because the normal range for glycated hemoglobin values varies among laboratories, ensure that you understand what numbers represent the normal range for your test. Your healthcare professionals will take that variation into account when they interpret the results of your A1C test.

You may also be able to check your A1C level at home with an over-the-counter test approved by the Food and Drug Administration. For this test, you draw a large drop of blood from your finger, mix it with a special solution, place it in the A1C monitor and receive results in several minutes. Talk to your doctor about using a home test if that's your preference.

Your A1C testing schedule may vary depending on your individual situation and how your diabetes changes over time. In general, have the A1C test two to four times a year. Here is the schedule recommended by the American Diabetes Association:
- First test your A1C when you are initially diagnosed with diabetes or when you start your initial treatment.
- Test every 6 months if you have Type 2 diabetes and you don't use insulin, and your blood glucose is well-controlled with diet and exercise or oral medications.
- Test every 3 months if you have Type 1 diabetes or you have Type 2 diabetes and use insulin.
- Test every 3 months if you change treatment, such as starting a new medication, or if your blood glucose is not well controlled.

However, as previously mentioned, if your A1C tests and blood glucose tests conflict with each other, you may want to have your A1C tested more frequently. Usually, the more you test your blood glucose at home, the more unlikely that you will have any major conflicts with any lab tests.

Objectives of Blood Glucose Testing

The key objectives of blood glucose (BG) testing include the following:
- Determine how well your BG levels are being controlled between meals.
- Determine how well your BG levels are being controlled *after* meals.
- Determine your cells' level of insulin resistance.
- Determine what actions to take, to better control your BG levels, reduce your insulin resistance and eventually eliminate your insulin resistance.
- Determine what actions to take to reduce and then eliminate the need for the diabetic drugs.
- Determine what actions to take to reverse the disease.
- Provide invaluable data/information to your doctor so that he/she can better help you make the right decisions to better control your BG levels.

Tip: Purchase a notebook of some kind to record your daily activities, including when/what you eat, your BG readings, medications/dosages, other health data, activities, appointments, events, etc. If you are comfortable with computer-based tools, then, you may want to consider purchasing a blood glucose monitor that provides a robust set of test data that can be transported to a computer (spreadsheet) for further analysis or to a tool that can provide corrective actions.

Blood Glucose Testing Techniques

Proper blood glucose testing requires practice and patience. The following are some guidelines and tips that will help to ensure that your readings are accurate.
- Purchase a glucose meter that aligns with your health needs, personal preferences and fits within your financial pocketbook. (Refer to the next section for details).
- Read the instructions that explain how to use your glucose meter. But, don't try to use the meter for the first time on your own – let the nurse or diabetes educator walk you through the steps.

- Then, demonstrate those same steps to the nurse/diabetes educator so that he/she can correct anything that you may be doing wrong.
- Set aside a quiet, isolated place to test your blood glucose and record the readings.
- Always wash your hands before testing. Ensure your fingers are dry. If you use alcohol, ensure the alcohol has dried before puncturing your skin.
- Use a clean lancet to prick your finger (or forearm).
- Ensure the drop of blood covers the test strip fully. Be careful not to touch the test strip to prevent any contamination. While waiting for the reading, dab the puncture with a cotton swab of alcohol and throw it away.
- Record the number that is displayed in the glucose meter window into your logbook as soon as it is displayed. If you don't like the number because it is high, don't despair. Keep in mind that this is normal and part of the journey to better health.

  Author's Personal Note: I believe that I learned more and healed faster because of the high readings. But, I must admit that I felt very anxious and nervous during my early testing. As I became more knowledgeable, I actually looked forward to the readings.
- Ensure that you store the test strips, lancets and meter in a cool, dry place.
- Recalibrate your glucose meter per the instructions, especially when you purchase a new set of test strips. This is to ensure the accuracy of the readings. If the readings seem to be off for some unknown reason, check the test strips for damage, expiration date and check the meter, e.g. for cleaning, a new battery. If you can afford it, use a second meter to compare your readings.
- Bring your meter to your doctor's office to perform the test and compare the number with the doctor's number. Keep in mind that your test readings are usually 10 to 15% lower than the readings at the doctor's office primarily because most home glucose meters measure whole blood, which consists of several ingredients including plasma fluid; whereas, your doctor measures only the plasma portion of the whole blood which is more concentrated. Also, your readings will be less accurate due to human error.

- While at the doctor's office, demonstrate to the nurse how you test your blood glucose so that he/she can identify any corrections that you need to make.
- Review what the blood glucose readings mean with your doctor to compare your understanding with his/her understanding. Reach agreement on any corrective actions to improve your blood glucose control.

Glucose Meters

Obtain a glucose meter system that aligns with your health needs, personal preferences and fits within your financial pocketbook. The following is a list of criteria to consider when purchasing a meter.

- Insurance: Ensure that you find out how much your insurance company or Medicare will pay before buying a glucose meter. If you buy from a website, ensure that the glucose meter supply site will work directly with your insurance company or Medicare on the processing, paperwork, and payment for the glucose meter. Many times, you won't need to pay for the glucose meter up front and will only be responsible for the co-pay and/or deductible.
- Price: Most meters cost between $40 and $100, depending on the feature set, but don't make price your only criterion for choosing a glucose meter. In some cases, you can get a free meter, because the company makes its money on the test strips.
- Features:
  o Some meters provide alternate test sites (e.g. arm, thigh) that require less blood and are almost pain-free because the arm/thigh are not as sensitive as your finger, e.g. Prodigy, One Touch, TheraSense (FreeStyle Flash). This is very important, especially if you plan to increase your testing. Because the readings at alternate sites may vary due to the actual glucose concentration being different, you should not switch sites in the same week.
  o Some meters contain built-in strips with discs or cartridges to make it easier to handle test strips, e.g. Accu-Check, Bayer.
  o Some meters provide (English/Spanish) voice for people with vision issues, e.g. Prodigy.

o   Most meters provide enough memory to store at least the latest 100 readings, with date and time, plus a running average of the last 14 to 30 days.

o   If vision is a concern, some meters are designed with bigger, easier to read displays; and, others include audible controls.

o   Some meters provide data processing and additional testing data such as a running average and trend reports, which can be downloaded into a computer.

o   Other more sophisticated meters allow you to record insulin doses, carbohydrates eaten and exercise performed; and can even provide suggestions, based on your glucose readings.

Author's Personal Note: My daughter bought my first glucose meter (Accu-Check) while I was in the hospital. I bought a second meter (TheraSense Freestyle) because it allowed me to more easily test my glucose several times a day by using my arm instead of my fingers.

When to Test & What to Do

The following are some guidelines to utilize when testing your blood glucose (BG) level. Keep in mind that the more you test, the more data you can capture, and the easier it will be for you (and your doctor) to draw conclusions and take corrective actions that will control your blood glucose level and improve your health. Unfortunately, many diabetics try to draw conclusions and take corrective actions from one or two tests a day. When this fails, they become discouraged and stop testing all together; or, they continue to test but they don't take any corrective actions with their nutrition and exercise.

1. Measure and record your BG several times a day, at the same times.
   a. Measure your BG at the following times each day: before breakfast; two hours after breakfast; before lunch; before dinner; two hours after dinner; before bedtime.
   b. For additional data, measure your BG at one or more of the following times each day: two hours after lunch; before snacks, two hours after snacks; after stressful events; before and after exercise; before driving your car (especially if your average glucose level is too high or low).

    c. Measure your BG at least 3 to 4 times a day if your objective is to manage and control your BG level from meal to meal; and, take corrective actions based on those readings.

    d. Measure your BG at least 5 to 7 times a day if your objective is to *reverse* the disease because you will need more data to evaluate the proper actions to take. If finances are an issue, then, spread your BG measurements throughout the week to ensure you get a good sample of fasting and post-meal readings. After 2 to 3 months, you will have enough data and will be able to decrease the number of daily BG tests.

    e. If your BG average is greater than **126** mg/dl, and/or your Hb A1C is greater than **5.5%**, then increase the number of blood glucose tests to help analyze what's causing your blood glucose level to be outside the normal range.

2. Review and analyze your BG readings before you take your medication to determine if you need to change your dosage. Also, review your readings in conjunction with your food log and other events at the end of each day, week, or month depending on your current health and health goals. Determine the specific corrective actions that you plan to take by modifying one or more of the following variables if your blood glucose level is too high (outside the normal range).

    a. **Nutrition** (Amount, Type of food, Frequency)
- Reduce eating the "dead" processed foods.
- Increase eating the "live" super foods to help the body repair the trillions of defective (insulin-resistant) cells.
- Increase the number of meals for the day, but ensure the meals are evenly spaced throughout the day.
- Decrease the total number of calories of the previous meal for those BG readings that are the highest.
- Ensure there is a balance of carbohydrates, proteins, and fats with each meal.

b. **Nutritional supplement** (Amount, Type, Frequency)
- Begin drinking 2 to 3 cups of raw vegetables juices daily, e.g. Brussel sprouts, string beans, carrots, parsley. Mix in 1 tbsp. of wheat grass or flaxseed for fiber, protein, and EFAs.
- Add one or more nutritional supplements, depending on health needs, e.g. natural multivitamin/mineral, wholefood supplement, Omega-3 EFAs, CoQ10, alpha lipoic acid, chromium, biotin. Stop taking any synthetic vitamins!
- Add a quality herbal supplement, e.g. gymnema sylvestre, bitter melon, organic cinnamon cassia bark extract.
- Add a food-based supplement to your juice, e.g. flaxseed, super greens (spirulina, chlorella, barley grass), glyconutrients.

c. **Exercise** (Frequency, Duration, Intensity)
- Increase the number of times that you exercise during the week.
- Add anaerobic (weight/resistance) exercise to your exercise program.
- Increase the amount of time of each exercise session.
- Decrease the intensity of the exercise, especially if you are constantly out-of-breath.

d. **Cleansing/Detoxification** (Frequency)
- Increase the number of times that you cleanse/detoxify the body, especially if you have not noticed an increase in your energy level and an improvement in your bowel regularity.
- Review the quality of the herbal products and the cleansing/detox process with an experienced herbalist, naturopathic doctor, or other healthcare professional. Ensure that you are not using synthetic supplements.
- Add or increase juicing with raw vegetables and grasses.

e. **Testing** (Frequency, Timing)
- Increase the number of BG tests to better understand the cause and effect relationships.
- Re-evaluate your records to ensure your corrective actions align with your readings. If you are not certain, review this chapter and discuss with your doctor and other diabetic experts.

- Change the timing of your blood glucose testing, e.g. test after the meal to better understand your body's level of insulin resistance.
- Work with your doctor to determine whether you need any additional medical diagnostic tests if your health is not improving.

f. **Medication** (Dosage, Frequency)
   (Obtain your doctor's approval before making any drug changes)
   - Work with your doctor to get weaned off as many drugs as possible to reduce the number of side effects and the toxic load on your liver, kidneys and other organs – which all work to prevent the body from healing.
   - Ensure you are taking the right dosage of each drug. Ensure the proper amount of insulin is in the syringe.
   - Change the timing of your drug dosage relative to your meal.
   - Increase/decrease your drug dosage before the meal.
     Note: Be careful – increasing your drug dosage will gradually increase your body's dependency on the drugs.
   - Increase/decrease the number of times that you take your drugs each day.
   - Decrease your drug dosage if you are experiencing hypo-glycemic (low blood sugar) episodes.
   - Switch to a new drug or a new combination of the drugs you're taking.
   - *Note:* The following types of drugs may increase your blood glucose level: ACE inhibitors, antibiotics, antidepressants, diuretics, steroids, and cancer drugs.

3. In general, if you optimize your nutrition, exercise, and testing regimens, you should see an improvement with your fasting BG readings within two to three weeks. You should see an improvement with your post-meal BG readings within another two to four weeks, depending on your health state and drug therapy.

4. Review the proposed corrective actions to your nutrition and exercise with your doctor before you make any changes.

Doctor Appointments & Annual Scheduling

You should ensure that you set up the necessary doctor appointments during the calendar year as specified by your doctor (Primary Care Physician). If possible, try to schedule your appointments during the same time period each year. The following is a list of the key doctor visits that you should complete during the year.

Visit	Purpose	Frequency
Primary Care Physician/ Endocrinologist	Check blood glucose, hemoglobin A1C, kidney tests, nerves (foot exam)	Every 3 to 6 months
Primary Care Physician	Physical exam; Other tests: blood pressure, cholesterol, kidneys, liver	Annual
Ophthalmologist	Eye tests for retinopathy, cataracts, glaucoma	Every 6 months or annual
Wellness coach; Dietitian/Nutritionist	Wellness planning; Nutritional planning, etc.	As required
Dentist	Cleaning of teeth and gums, dental examinations	Cleaning: every 3 mos. Exams: annual
Podiatrist	Examination of feet for nerve damage	Every 3 to 6 months or as required

Figure 10. Schedule of Doctor Visits

You should visit your primary care physician and/or endocrinologist on a regular basis to review your progress, your blood glucose readings, corrective actions, and other notes – at least until you have your blood glucose level under control. Depending on your health needs and your health goals, you should get a complete physical and set of blood work every 6 to 12 months to identify any trends that may be getting overlooked, especially if you're not making any significant improvements.

Concerning your feet, you should always clean and inspect them daily. Record any abnormalities to discuss with your physician at your next visit. Keep your feet clean and moist; and wear cotton socks for better absorbency. Concerning your teeth/gums, you should always check them for any bleeding that doesn't stop, and, notify your dentist and primary care physician immediately. Gum disease can increase internal inflammation and increase the risk of cardiovascular disease.

Depending on your health needs and your health goals, other members of your diabetes care team may include one or more of the following: cardiologist, neurologist, nephrologist, physiotherapist, naturopathic doctor, or psychiatrist. Other members may include a wellness coach, diabetes educator, pharmacist, community health nurse, or social worker.

Doctor Appointments
One of the best ways to manage your diabetes is to develop an effective working partnership with your doctor. Your doctor's role in this partnership is to provide medical advice, offer treatment options and recommend resources. Your role is to monitor your symptoms and blood glucose readings, report them accurately and do what you can to manage your disease on a day-to-day basis.

Doctor appointments are very important, but most people come ill-prepared to take full advantage of the time with their doctor. Then, they complain about the doctor not taking enough time with them. Or, they don't ask the doctor any pertinent questions; or, they don't bother to take any notes and forget what the doctor told them. The doctor could spend more time with them, but they must first take full advantage of the time that they have with their doctor. Then, they will be pleasantly surprised how well their doctor responds when they take a more active role in their health.

The following is a set of guidelines to help improve the effectiveness of your appointments and the relationship with your doctor. If you are unable to establish a better partnership with your doctor, let him/her know your concerns. If there is no improvement, or you have a concern with taking drugs, consider talking with a doctor in the field of alternative medicine, e.g. a naturopathic doctor (www.naturopathic.org); or, work with a diabetes wellness coach who has a medical background.

General Planning

1. Take responsibility for your own health. This may include making necessary lifestyle changes, eating healthy foods, getting enough exercise, maintaining a healthy weight, stop smoking, stop drinking alcohol, and stop using recreational drugs.

2. Ensure that you understand and are completely comfortable with the doctor's diagnosis of your health, your diabetes, and any other disease/ailment that you may have at this time. A proper diagnosis will enable you to focus on the proper actions that need to be performed to improve your health. An improper diagnosis will lead to incorrect actions, frustration, doubt, and eventually hopelessness. Ensure that you have obtained all the necessary medical diagnostic tests that will provide a correct diagnosis.

   Key Point: Ensure that the treatment is being designed to repair your body, specifically, the defective sick cells in your body – not just to treat the symptoms of high blood glucose levels.

3. Post the phone numbers for your primary care physician, endocrinologist and other healthcare professionals by your telephone, along with a list of your current medications, other medical conditions and allergies. Call the doctor right away if you experience a sudden change or your symptoms get worse.

4. If possible, have doctor appointments and the applicable tests performed at regular intervals to prevent confusion and complications. If you have not had a specific test within the recommended interval, ask your doctor about it.

5. Your family doctor will manage most of your diabetes care, but you may be referred to other medical specialists when necessary. For instance, you may be referred to an ophthalmologist for a dilated eye exam or a podiatrist for foot care. You may be referred to an endocrinologist if managing your diabetes is particularly difficult. Your family doctor and other medical specialists work together as a team. Don't hesitate to ask for a referral if you think it is necessary.

6. Work with your doctor to set reasonable goals for your blood glucose levels, A1C, blood pressure, cholesterol, and homocysteine (if applicable).

7. If you need to find a new doctor or you need information about your doctor or local hospital, go to one of the following websites:
    *   Contact information for your state's board of medical examiners (address, phone numbers, website):
        www.fsmb.org/members.htm
    *   Information about the rating and performance of doctors, hospitals, and nursing homes:
        www.healthgrades.com
    *   Government and nonprofit health and human services information, with links to 1,500 health-related organizations:
        www.healthfinder.gov

Doctor Appointments

1. During the appointment, become an active participant in your health planning. Communicate your health goals and concerns at all times. If you show interest, your doctor will be more inclined to provide more help and information. But, if you don't show a vested interest, why should your doctor?
2. Be honest about whether you're following recommendations about diet, lifestyle and taking medications. Your doctor can usually tell when you're not telling the truth. Also, your doctor can suggest strategies to help you get on track.
3. Start with your major concern first. Waiting until the end of an appointment to discuss an important problem may mean it won't get proper attention.
4. Be specific about your symptoms and pay attention to details. Things that don't seem important to you may be important to your doctor. The American Society of Internal Medicine has concluded that 75 percent of correct diagnosis depends solely on what you tell your doctor.
5. Speak up but be respectful. Make sure from the outset that your doctor knows you have questions and concerns and expect to be listened to. Don't be afraid to be an active and assertive patient. If you don't understand a word, idea or direction, ask your doctor to explain.

6. Ask specific questions. You can't make good health-care decisions if you can't understand the information provided or aren't given enough information. If a question is crucial, ask politely but firmly for an answer before you leave. At a minimum, you should ask your doctor the following questions:
    *   What is my **diagnosis** or what is my current state of health based on my physical exam, blood work and other health information?
        Note! If you have multiple diseases/ailments, ensure that your doctor has taken that into account concerning your diagnosis. For example, a person with high blood pressure and high triglycerides should be evaluated for root causes that are common to both ailments instead of being given separate drugs for each ailment.
    *   What are the **root cause(s)** of my current diseased health state? (It is very important to understand what is causing your health problem!)
    *   What specific **corrective actions** do I need to take to improve my health through natural means (without drugs/medications)?
        Note: If you decide to take drugs, ask your doctor how long you have to take them and what are the long term effects of the drugs.
    *   What is my **prognosis**? In other words, what is the doctor's projection of your future health state given his knowledge, expertise and the corrective actions you plan to take or have been taking?
7. Request additional tests if your doctor is puzzled with your health state. For example mineral tests, hormone tests and hair analysis tests (although controversial) can be invaluable in many cases involving fatigue, chronic pain, cognitive/memory, emotions, hyperactivity, violent behavior, learning disabilities, attention deficit disorder, high blood pressure, cardiovascular disease, osteoporosis, arthritis, neurological disorders, weakened immunity, hypoglycemia, diabetes, weak finger nails, and unhealthy skin and hair.
8. Ask your doctor to be honest with you about what you can expect to happen over the next few weeks, months and years.

9. Ask your doctor to tell you the three most important things you can do to manage your health condition.
10. Work with your doctor to develop an effective treatment plan. There may be times when you just don't think you can do what your doctor advises. Don't walk out in frustration and ignore it all. Work with your doctor to find an alternative that is acceptable to both of you.
11. Bring all your medications including over-the-counter drugs, vitamins and other supplements to your next appointment. To avoid drug interactions and over-medication, make sure that your doctor knows about every drug, vitamin and other supplement that you are taking.
12. Before you leave the office, know what you should do when you get home. It's difficult to recall everything a doctor tells you, especially if you're nervous or worried. Ask your doctor to write down the important points. Know who to call, and when to call, if you run into any problems. Obtain a copy of your blood test results.
13. Understand how well you are progressing and what actions to take, based on your doctor's diagnosis.
14. If this isn't working to your satisfaction, don't sit around and complain about your doctor. In most cases it's not your doctor's fault, so make sure that you are doing everything in your power to improve your health. Discuss your concerns honestly with your doctor. If you are doing your part, and the relationship with your doctor has not improved, or your health is not improving, then, find a new doctor.

Blood Glucose Testing Analysis

Unless you are someone who likes to work with numbers, then, recording and collecting data several times a day may seem like a drag. But, once you begin to realize that these numbers can actually help you get better, you will find the time to record and collect the data. These technologies and tools can truly be a Godsend. In order to analyze the data, you will need some graph paper to plot each data point. If you have computer skills, you can use an application like Microsoft Excel to plot a graph of your glucose readings. Some of the glucose meters have the capability for you to download the data to your computer. Once you plot the graph, you can review and analyze your data so that you can make any corrective actions to improve your blood glucose control.

So, how can a graph help you? The following line graph (Figure 11) is a subset of my blood glucose readings over a 7-day period during my recovery. This diagram shows my morning, midday and evening before-meal readings from Monday to Sunday. It shows how my readings were very inconsistent, up and down throughout each day during the entire week. But, I didn't really understand why I was so inconsistent. According to everything I had read about diabetes, if you are taking insulin and your blood glucose readings remain high it may be necessary to increase the insulin dosage to help lower and stabilize the readings. That seemed to make sense, but I was afraid that if I increased my insulin dosage, my body would become dependent on the extra insulin.

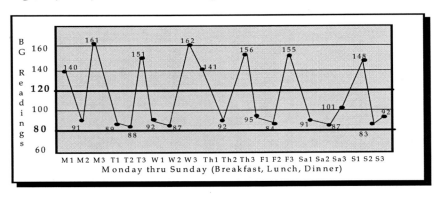

Figure 11. Line Graph of Blood Glucose Readings

However, as an engineer I knew that how data is sorted and categorized is very important to interpreting the data properly. So, I decided to sort the data and group the readings into 3 categories: Morning, Midday and Evening. Eureka! As you can see from the following bar graph, the Midday readings were the most consistent – in fact, every Midday reading was within the normal range. The Evening readings were the most inconsistent – in fact, every reading was outside the normal range. The Morning readings were the most puzzling – some readings were within the normal range and others were outside the range.

CHAPTER 11

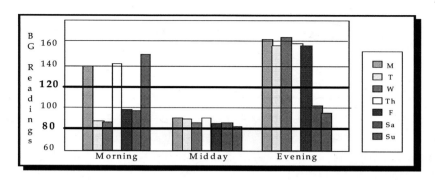

Figure 12. Bar Graph of Blood Glucose Readings & Meals

So, what did I conclude from this data? After reviewing my daily food log, I determined that I needed to do a better job with my meals and snacks during the middle of the day because that was driving my high glucose readings in the evening (before dinner). Also, I determined that my evening snack was too glycemic, driving my glucose readings higher the next morning. So, I changed my snack by reducing the carbohydrates and adding some quality fat (with a handful of walnuts/almonds) and a glass of filtered water. Within two weeks, I had my morning and evening readings under control. My morning average went from 114 to 102 and my evening average went from 140 to 105 within 2 weeks.

Although this is a simplistic example, you can see that by sorting the data differently, it may uncover an inconsistency in your blood glucose readings that may have something to do with your daily habits or other regularly scheduled events in your life. For example, I found out a couple weeks later that some of my high readings were connected to my exercise regimen that was too intense, causing my liver to release glycogen driving my glucose level as high as 270 mg/dl. Once I changed my regimen to one of moderate intensity, the high readings subsided.

Constant testing, recording the data, and analyzing the data are not activities that most people will enjoy. However, there are glucose meters on the market now that will do this analysis for you and provide corrective actions. For me though, God blessed me with the "perfect disease". Why? Because diabetes is the only disease where you (the patient) do your own blood testing, collect your own test data, analyze your test data, and take actions based on that analysis. And, what do engineers do for a living? We perform testing, collect test data, analyze the test data, and take corrective actions based on that analysis.

Recordkeeping/Analysis

As blood glucose testing is the most powerful diagnostic tool, recordkeeping (and its analysis) is the **next most powerful diagnostic tool** because it pulls together all the information that you've been recording and collecting throughout the day. The following information will prove to be invaluable to you and your doctor:
- Content of each meal/snack, including beverages
- Nutritional supplements (with dosages)
- Number of "live" super foods eaten at each meal
- Number of "dead" processed foods eaten at each meal
- Number of (approximate) calories of each meal
- Percentages of carbohydrates, proteins, fats, and liquids of each meal (optional)
- Fasting and post-meal blood glucose readings
- Drugs/dosages, indicate if the dosage is being increased or decreased
- Exercise type, duration and intensity level
- Sleep/relaxation time (number of hours)
- Feelings, e.g. how you feel after exercise, after a meal, especially after taking any drug/medication, when you awake. Pay attention when you are feeling tired, fatigued, low emotionally or overly energetic.
- Events during the day, including doctor appointments, work, shopping, and other travels
- Medical tests, physical exam results; the doctor's diagnosis, prognosis
- Weight, blood pressure, cholesterol (record these weekly/monthly if you have the appropriate test equipment in your home)

However, many diabetics do not take the time to record their daily events because they are unaware of its power and value to making corrective actions that will improve the quality of their lives. Most diabetics either over-respond to the last high reading to try to over-correct the problem, or become frustrated and give up trying to correct the problem.

Unfortunately, some diabetics believe that it doesn't really matter even when they believe that they did everything correctly. Recordkeeping also allows you to review when you had good readings and what you did for that to happen so that you can repeat your successes.

Analysis Tips

The following are some of the key points that you must keep in mind when reviewing your blood glucose (BG) readings and trying to analyze the data to determine what corrective actions to take:

- If the majority of your **BG readings are outside the normal range**, more than likely you are still consuming too many "dead" foods with refined sugar and flour; or, your body is still full of too many toxins, acid waste and parasites. Once you have eliminated food as a factor, perform a cleansing/detoxification to remove the toxins and other wastes that accumulate from high glucose levels. Then, review your exercise program – you may need to increase your exercise to burn the extra glucose in the blood. Also, increase your sleep, rest and relaxation times to help reduce any stress levels. Also, review with your doctor the diabetic drugs and other drugs you are taking for any possible side effects that could drive your glucose level up.

- If your **BG readings are high in the morning**, this is known as the "dawn effect", which is usually due to improper blood glucose and insulin management. Causes can include last night's dinner meal, last night's snack, the previous exercise session, or improper drug therapy, e.g. the amount of insulin before last night's dinner being too low, or the timing of the insulin dosage may be too early.

- If your **BG readings are inconsistently up and down**, this indicates that you are probably eating right some of the time and not eating right the other times. This inconsistent eating drives your pancreas to release too much insulin and too little glucagon, causing a vicious cycle that can only be corrected with the proper balance of "live" foods from meal to meal.
  - o Review and analyze the foods you were eating for the meal previous to the high glucose reading. Make any necessary corrective actions.

o   Inconsistent up and down readings could also be triggered by celebratory events, travel, work, or other stressful events, so you should review your daily log to see what's been going on during the past couple weeks that may be affecting your stress hormones and causing your glucose levels to rise. But, an important point to remember is that when you are eating and exercising properly, the body has the proper raw materials to handle stress without negatively affecting your health.

o   Also, take a look at ways to leverage your spiritual health to help you, especially when dealing with stressful events.

- In order to **stabilize your BG readings** and improve your running BG average, try to string together as many super meals and super snacks as reasonably possible – so that your body can build up some momentum in the healing process.

- Once your BG readings start to come down, you should review the foods that are giving you such a positive response; and, try to integrate them more into your nutritional profile (eating plan) throughout the week. For example, when I had such a positive response from eating Brussel sprouts, I began eating them for lunch, dinner, snack, and even breakfast until I got tired of them. And, then, because I didn't want to regress and lose all the progress I had made, I replaced the Brussel sprouts with another similar green vegetable, broccoli; and, then, I replaced the broccoli with spinach. Now, that was probably overkill, but I believe it helped to accelerate my body's ability to heal itself. Later, I learned how to prepare these vegetables differently (e.g. roast, stir fry) to vary their taste.

- If your BG readings have been steady in the normal range and all of sudden you have a high reading, check the content of the previous meal – more than likely, you ate some extra carbohydrates or you had a larger-sized meal.

- Check your running blood glucose average to ensure that your average glucose reading is decreasing over time. If your average reading is not decreasing, then, you need to review your nutritional profile and your exercise program. More than likely, you are still consuming too many "dead" foods with refined sugar and flour; or, not exercising consistently to burn off the glucose.

- If your post-meal BG average is still outside the normal range, this indicates your body still has some insulin resistance. Review your nutrition and exercise programs to look for ways to optimize one or both. Once you have optimized your meal and exercise programs, consider adding a nutritional supplement such as the herb gymnema sylvestre to help get you over this last hurdle.
- Check to ensure your fasting glucose level is consistently within a tighter range of 80 to 110 mg/dl, with a standard deviation of less than 15 mg/dl.

  Note: The standard deviation indicates a **stability of your blood glucose levels**, indicating that your readings are not too high and not too low, with a concentrated (tight) "Bell-curve" distribution. This is an **overlooked point** that most diabetics are not aware -- that you can have a good average reading, but it may be misleading if you have high readings that are offset by low readings!
- If you are unable to correlate a high BG reading to a previous meal, then, review the following culprits: change in drug therapy, change in drug dosage, not enough exercise, too much intense exercise, a highly stressful event, a cold or infection.
- Also, you must be very patient – it took a lot of years of abuse to your body before it succumbed to being diabetic. Consequently, it is unrealistic to expect the body to turn it all around in just a few weeks.
- Do not get upset over one or two high readings if your running average is moving in the right direction (towards the normal range). Getting upset or worrying will only cause your glucose level to rise.

The Dawn Effect

High blood glucose readings in the morning, known as the **"dawn effect"**, are the end result of a combination of natural biochemical and hormonal changes that occur during the sleep cycle. Some time between 3:00 a.m. and 8:00 a.m., your body starts to increase the amounts of counter-regulatory hormones (e.g. growth hormone, cortisol). These hormones work against insulin's action to lower your blood glucose level. The increased release of these counter-regulatory hormones, at a time when bedtime insulin is wearing out, results in an increase in your blood glucose level in the morning (at "dawn").

Another cause of high blood glucose readings in the morning is known as the **Somogyi effect**, named after the doctor who discovered this phenomenon.   The cause of this condition, also called "rebound hyperglycemia" is more "man-made" (a result of poor diabetes management). Your blood glucose level may drop too low in the middle of the night, so your body counters by releasing hormones to raise your blood glucose level. This could happen if you took too much insulin earlier or if you did not have enough of a bedtime snack. As a result, your doctor may require that you change the time that you take your long-acting insulin, the amount of insulin or the type of insulin. In my case, once I adjusted my dinner meal and bedtime snack, the high glucose readings in the morning subsided.

Stressful situations may also trigger the release of hormones such as cortisol, epinephrine, and norepinephrine, which can lead to the loss of lean muscle tissue and the increase of fat in the abdomen area, which can lead to an increase in insulin resistance and more insulin production.

These are just a few examples of the many scenarios that can occur during your journey. This is why it is so important that you test your blood glucose as frequently as possible and record any events that are occurring at that time. Because the more data and other information you record, the easier it will be to determine what to do or not to do. Next to not eating or exercising properly, **not testing your blood glucose is probably the biggest mistake that you can make to prevent your recovery from this disease.**

Contact our wellness center if you need help with understanding your blood glucose readings and what specific actions you should be taking..

Lab Work/Blood Tests

The following is a list of the major types of lab work/blood tests that your doctor may perform to help determine your current state of health (diagnosis) and your future state of health (prognosis).

Note: The symbol < means "less than"; and the symbol > means "greater than".

Blood Glucose measures the amount of glucose (sugar) in the blood after fasting. The **Hemoglobin A1C** test measures the percentage of glucose in the blood during the past 2 to 3 months. Glucose is regulated by insulin, glucagon, liver enzymes and thyroid/adrenal hormones. It is elevated by diabetes, liver disease, obesity, pancreatitis, steroids, blood pressure drugs, stress, or diet. Low levels may be indicative of liver disease, overproduction of insulin, hypothyroidism, or alcoholism.

- Range for Fasting Blood Glucose: 80 to 120 mg/dl
  Optimum value: < 100 mg/dl
- Range for Hemoglobin A1C: 4.2% to 5.5%;
  Optimum value: < 5.0%

Blood Pressure measures the pressure (force per unit area) exerted by the blood on the walls of the blood vessels. The first number is the systolic pressure, which measures the force at which the heart contracts. The second number is the diastolic pressure, which measures the pressure when the heart is at rest (between beats). High blood pressure is an indication that one or more of the body's systems is not functioning properly, causing the heart muscle to work harder to push the blood throughout the body.

- Systolic (first number): < 120 mm Hg
- Diastolic (second number): < 80 mm Hg

In addition, measuring the blood pressure in other parts of the body such as the ankle, leg or toe can help to diagnose other problems that may go undetected. For example, according to recent research from Sweden, measuring toe blood pressure can be an effective screening method to identify diabetics with lower extremity arterial disease. Unlike the routine arm blood pressures where diastolic and systolic pressure are measured, extremity blood pressures measure only systolic pressure.

Blood Cholesterol measures the amount of lipids (fat) in the blood. Cholesterol is a critical fat that is a structural component of cell membrane and plasma lipoproteins, and is important in the synthesis of steroid hormones, glucocorticoids, and bile acids. Mostly synthesized in the liver, some is absorbed through the diet, especially one high in saturated fats. High density lipoproteins (HDL), which indicates more (dense) protein and less cholesterol, is desired as opposed to the low density lipoproteins (LDL), which indicates less protein and room for more cholesterol within the molecule. Elevated cholesterol levels have been seen in atherosclerosis, diabetes, hypothyroidism and pregnancy. Low levels are seen in depression, malnutrition, liver insufficiency, malignancies, anemia and infection.

Triglycerides, stored in adipose tissues as glycerol and fatty acids, are reconverted as triglycerides by the liver. Ninety percent of the dietary intake and ninety-five percent of the fat stored in tissues are triglycerides. Increased levels may be present in atherosclerosis, diabetes, hypothyroidism, liver disease, pancreatitis, myocardial infarction, metabolic disorders, and toxemia. Decreased levels may be present in chronic obstructive pulmonary disease, brain infarction, hyperthyroidism, malnutrition, and malabsorption.

LDL or Low density lipoprotein is the cholesterol remnants of the lipid transport vehicle VLDL (very-low density lipoproteins). A high level of LDL is an indication of a clogged liver, an unbalanced metabolic system, or possible arterial wall damage (atherosclerosis). Due to the expense of direct measurement of LDL, the Friedewald formula is used to calculate LDL:
LDL = Total Cholesterol - HDL Cholesterol - Triglycerides/5.
When triglyceride levels are greater than 400, this method is not accurate.

HDL or High density lipoprotein is the cholesterol carried by the alpha lipoproteins. A high level of HDL is an indication of a healthy metabolic system if there is no sign of liver disease or intoxication. HDL inhibits cellular uptake of LDL and serves as a carrier that removes cholesterol from the peripheral tissues and transports it back to the liver for catabolism and excretion.

The normal ranges for these cholesterol parameters are:
- Total Cholesterol (TC): < 200 mg/dl
- Low Density Lipoprotein (LDL): < 130 mg/dl
- High Density Lipoprotein (HDL): > 40 mg/dl
- Triglycerides: < 150 mg/dl
- TC/HDL Ratio: < 4:1; LDL/HDL Ratio: < 3:1

Note: The cholesterol ratios are better indicators of your health than the absolute numbers, which can be misleading, especially if you have a high HDL, which is an indicator of good health.

Body Mass Index (BMI) provides a measure of weight relative to height to use as a guideline to determine whether your weight is at a normal, overweight, or obese level.
- BMI Range: 20 to 25
- BMI greater than 25 indicates an overweight level
- BMI greater than 30 indicates an obese level
- BMI formula: (703 times Weight in pounds) divided by (Height in inches times Height in inches)

Note: Actually your ***waist size*** is a better measure and indicator of one's health state (excess belly fat). In general, if the waist size exceeds 40 inches (for a male), or 35 inches (for a female), this indicates a risk factor for developing diabetes and cardiovascular-related diseases.

Cardiac Risk and Inflammation Factors include homocysteine, lipoprotein (a), C-reactive protein (CRP), and fibrin. These factors are better indicators of cardiovascular disease and inflammation than your level of cholesterol. However, since your doctor may not order these tests until he/she has determined that you may be at risk for cardiovascular disease, you may need to request these tests, especially if you are not making any significant progress with your health.
- **Homocysteine** is a sulfur-containing amino acid that causes inflammation.
- **Lipoprotein (a)** is produced by the liver to repair arterial injuries due to a lack of Vitamin C to produce collagen for tissue repair.
- **C-Reactive Protein (CRP)** is a plasma protein produced by the liver in response to inflammation.
- **Fibrin** is an insoluble protein that is deposited around a wound in the form of a mesh to dry and harden, so that bleeding stops. Platelets, a type of cell found in blood, release the enzyme thrombin when they come into contact with damaged tissue, triggering the formation of the soluble protein, fibrinogen. Fibrinogen is then converted to fibrin as the final stage in blood clotting, which helps to repair damaged arterial walls.

The normal ranges for these cardiac risk/inflammation parameters are:
- Homocysteine: < 17 umol/L
- C-Reactive Protein (CRP): < 10 mg/L
- Lipoprotein (a): < 25 mg/dl
- Fibrin: 145-348 mg/dl

Note: In addition to CRP, interleukin-6 (IL-6) and tumor necrosis factor (TNF-α) may be inflammation markers for Type 2 diabetes that promote insulin resistance and damage to endothelial cells within the artery walls.

Cardiovascular Stress test should be performed to ensure your heart is providing adequate blood flow under stress conditions.

Waste Product tests include blood urea nitrogen (BUN), creatinine, and uric acid. They indicate the health of the kidneys. Blood Urea Nitrogen (BUN) is the end product of protein metabolism and its concentration is influenced by the rate of excretion. Creatinine is the waste product of muscle metabolism. Its level is a reflection of the bodies muscle mass. Uric acid is the end product of purine metabolism and is normally excreted through the urine. Bun/Creatinine Ratio is a good measurement of kidney and liver function.

Electrolytes/Minerals tests (e.g. potassium, sodium, magnesium, calcium) indicate the health of the kidneys, adrenal glands, parathyroid glands, and the acid/alkaline status of the blood. Do not overlook these tests as diabetics tend to have low levels of magnesium, potassium, zinc.

Urine tests can be performed to provide additional insight, especially concerning the health of the kidneys. Microalbumin (or the microalbumin/creatinine ratio) measures the amount of protein that is not removed by the kidneys and has leaked into the urine. When the damage is just beginning, only very small amounts of albumin escape into the urine, a condition known as microalbuminuria. In later stages of kidney disease, large amounts of protein leak into the urine (> 30g/dl), causing a condition called macroalbuminuria, also known as proteinuria. The ketone test measure the level of ketones, which are the by-product of the fat burning process that occurs in the absence of insulin.

Protein tests measure the amount and type of protein in the blood. Albumin is the major constituent of serum protein (usually over 50%). It is manufactured by the liver from the amino acids taken through the diet. It helps in osmotic pressure regulation, nutrient transport and waste removal.

Liver Enzyme tests measure specific liver enzyme levels to assess how well the liver and the body's systems are functioning and whether there has been any tissue damage; indicating injury to the cells of the muscles, liver, or heart.

Food Sensitivity Tests can help to identify foods/chemicals that may be the direct cause of your illness.

Other Tests include insulin, ferritin, TNF- α, IL-6, Blood pH, Complete Blood Count (CBC), Thyroid tests, Hormone tests, Bone Density, antioxidant score (biophotonic scanner), and Spirometry (lung) tests.

Excretory Factors are usually overlooked, but they can tell your doctor a lot about what you've been eating and how your body has been processing what you eat. Infrequent bowel movements (constipation) or indigestion is usually the first sign of problems in the gastrointestinal tract.
- Bowel movement frequency, texture, shape: 3-4 times per day (1 per meal), soft, peanut butter-like texture, slightly S-shaped
- Urination frequency, color: 4-6 times per day, yellow-straw in color

Critical Health Parameters & Ranges

There is a subset of the aforementioned blood and urine tests that are defined as the "critical health parameters". This is the minimum set of health parameters that your doctor will check to evaluate your health. Ideally, you should know these numbers as well as you know your name, because these numbers help to define how your health is progressing over a period of time. In my case, my critical health parameters were not outside their normal ranges but if I had been tracking them over a period of time, I would have noticed some trends, indicating potential health problems. As an engineer I should have known to do this . . .

The minimum set of critical health parameters includes the top five in the following list; and, depending on your health state, the bottom three may be important.
- Blood pressure
- Fasting blood glucose
- Hemoglobin A1C
- Blood cholesterol
- Body Mass Index (BMI) or waist size
- Microalbumin (urine test)
- Cardiac risk/inflammation factors (homocysteine, lipoprotein (a), C-reactive protein, fibrin)
- Excretory profile

Medical Technology Advancements

Medical technology continues to make major advances with new insulin delivery systems that may not require needle injections, e.g. through the skin, nasal passages, etc. There are new technologies that eliminate the need for pricking your finger several times a day such as continuous monitoring systems. Research with organ transplants is moving forward.

The current insulin delivery systems include the following:
- Insulin with needle/syringe: The needles are much thinner today, reducing the amount of pain involved with using needles.
- Insulin pen (with built-in syringe): Provides easier administering of insulin. The pen is the most popular insulin delivery device in Europe, far surpassing standard needles and syringes. Two types of pens are available: reusable and pre-filled. With reusable pens, patients insert an insulin cartridge, attach a needle, and dial in the dose before pressing a plunger to administer the injection. The pre-filled pens are easier to use – they contain a built-in insulin cartridge and are discarded when empty, but they may be more costly. Also, pens may not be a good choice for people who must take large insulin doses or mix different types of insulin.

CHAPTER 11

- Insulin jet injector: Uses a high-pressure jet of air to send a fine, needle-like stream of insulin through the skin. They deliver accurate doses that are more rapidly absorbed than subcutaneous injections and may be of particular benefit to patients who are phobic about needles. On the down side, they may be as painful as needles – about 1 out of every 10 injections really hurts. The devices are bulkier than syringes and still require the user to carry vials of insulin. Also, they must be cleaned every 2 to 3 weeks unless a disposable model is used.
- External insulin pump: Provides easier administering of insulin for diabetics who need insulin on a more consistent basis. It delivers a constant, measured amount of insulin (basal dose) throughout the day; then, before each meal, the diabetic presses a button on the pump to release a large amount at once (bolus dose). The diabetic adjusts the size and timing of these bolus doses according to when and how much food he/she plans to eat.

The Future of Insulin Injection Systems

Researchers are working on a number of other approaches to make daily insulin administration less difficult and more effective. These include forms of insulin that can be inhaled like asthma medication, taken orally, or administered via skin patches, eye drops, or time-release gels. One of the more promising techniques is the implantable insulin pump (IIP), which is surgically placed beneath the skin and operated by remote control. These pumps, which have been tested on a limited basis in clinical trials, have proven quite popular and superior to multiple daily injections at controlling blood glucose in several hundred patients who have tried them. A recent study has indicated an oral insulin spray formulation may offer a pain-free and more effective way of administering insulin to control blood glucose after a meal. Also under development, but may be a few years away, is an implantable continuous glucose sensor that constantly measures blood glucose. This device could be combined with an IIP to control the automatic release of insulin by the pump, thus mimicking the natural function of the pancreas and totally eliminating the need for patient-controlled injections.

Chapter 12. Drugs/Medications

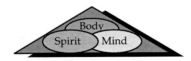

Drugs/Medications

According to the Center for Disease Control, close to 130 million Americans consume prescription drugs every month — more than any other country. In fact, over the past decade, the total number of prescriptions has increased by about two-thirds, to 3.5 billion a year. Practically every type of expert — doctors, public health officials, medical researchers — believes that Americans are overmedicated. We are willing to accept prescriptions for practically anything and demand them for conditions we think need medicating. If a condition has even the slightest potential to cause discomfort, there is a pill, patch, or prescription for it. And now, even TV commercials get you thinking about symptoms you may not have noticed before and suggest you ask your doctor for particular medications to combat them.

There are many life-saving drugs and medications that are invaluable to the quality of life such as antibiotics to help fight off serious bacterial infections. However, there are many other drugs and medications that, over a long period of time, interfere with the body's healing and immune systems, inhibiting the body from repairing, healing and protecting itself properly. Unfortunately, our dependency on these drugs in combination with bad eating habits and a sedentary lifestyle sentences the body to a slow, inevitable and sometimes painful death. However, if you are making the necessary lifestyle and nutritional changes, you should be working with your doctor to gradually wean yourself off the drugs. Unfortunately some people's health may have deteriorated to a level that prevents them from being able to totally live without any drugs.

If you are currently taking any prescription drugs, it is important that you continue to take them as prescribed by your doctor. But if you've been taking the drugs for more than three months or the drugs are causing side effects, you should notify your doctor about getting weaned off the drugs as soon as possible. Discuss the alternatives with your doctor and work out a safe weaning plan that does not put your health or life in jeopardy.

Limitations of Drugs/Medications

Although drugs provide life-saving benefits, they do have limitations, especially when they are taken over a long period of time for systemic degenerative conditions that can be addressed with proper nutrition and exercise, e.g. high blood pressure, high cholesterol, high blood glucose. Drugs that are taken for diabetes, pain relief or high blood cholesterol "fool" the body by altering the biochemical and hormonal functions within the body, leading to the artificial lowering of blood glucose, cholesterol, and the suppression of symptoms such as pain. Some diabetic drugs make the pancreas produce more insulin, which makes the diabetic fatter and can wear out the pancreas. Some of these drugs also prevent the liver from releasing stored glycogen to artificially keep the diabetic's glucose level lower. So instead of making the necessary nutrition, exercise and lifestyle changes, people depend on the drugs to do all the work in lowering their glucose level. Unfortunately, over a period of years, the oral medications lose their effectiveness because they never address the root causes of the diabetes – **excess insulin**, insulin resistance, nutritional deficiency, inflammation, oxidation, and toxicity. And, so the diabetic is eventually resigned to taking insulin injections.

Another example is the drugs that are taken for high blood pressure. Most people who start taking drugs to lower their blood pressure never get off the drugs. Why? Again, people refuse to make the nutrition, exercise and lifestyle changes and depend on the drugs to keep their blood pressure artificially lowered. Consequently, if they stopped taking the drugs, their blood pressure would start to rise again. Now, there is nothing wrong with depending on drugs – in the short term. It buys the patient time to make the changes to nutrition, exercise and lifestyle to help the body to heal itself and eventually wean it off the drugs with the assistance of their doctor.

Another example is the statin drugs used to lower cholesterol. These drugs have been very successful in lowering cholesterol. I should know since I used to take one of the statin drugs (Lipitor) for my high cholesterol. But, the biochemical pathway that allows the statin drug to inhibit the production of cholesterol also inhibits the liver from producing CoQ10, a very powerful and critical nutrient for the cells and the heart muscle. Also, there are some studies that show these drugs may cause a decrease in insulin sensitivity, a deterioration of the liver, neurological problems, severe muscle aches, and a condition called rhabdomyolysis, which is a deterioration of the muscles. Consequently, if you do take this drug, you should ensure that you are having your liver tested on a periodic basis. Also, if you are resigned to taking this drug, then, at least discuss with your doctor the benefits of taking a CoQ10 supplement to counteract some of the ill effects of the drug.

Drugs for these types of systemic degenerative conditions do not have the ability to heal the body; and, over a long period of time, they cause more harm than good to the health of the body. For example, the long-term uses of blood pressure and common pain-relieving drugs have been linked to heart attacks, liver failure, kidney failure, breast cancer and other systemic conditions. Only the body can heal itself — but it needs help from the individual to provide the body with the proper raw materials and nutrients to initiate the healing process.

For anyone who is taking any drugs for diabetes, high blood pressure, high cholesterol, or any other systemic disease/ailment, you should ask yourself the following question: Who do you think is smarter: God or man? God has provided superior nutrients in foods such as broccoli, Brussel sprouts, spinach, walnuts, olive oil, sesame seeds, wild salmon, barley, water, blackberries, blueberries, and other vegetables, fruits, fish, nuts and seeds. These food nutrients fight, reverse and prevent many diseases. On the other hand, man has developed processed foods such as French fries, mashed potatoes, tacos, macaroni, pasta, fried chicken, cakes, bottled juice, candy, and artificial sweeteners that cause diseases/ailments such as diabetes, heart disease, high blood pressure, high cholesterol, cancer, arthritis, osteoporosis, and Alzheimer's. And, to fight these diseases, man has developed various drugs to try to help us.

So, instead of looking to God's foods to help us improve our health, we look to man's drugs (for the "magic pill") to solve all our health problems. And the side effects of drugs, hospital/prescription errors (known as iatrogenic illness) account for more than 216,000 deaths a year, the number 3 cause of death in the United States!

Conflict of Interest?

Pharmaceutical companies have readily admitted that they routinely pay insurance companies to increase the use of their products and to be added to the recommended list of drugs. They admit that they give rewards and kickbacks to both pharmacists and doctors for switching patients from one brand of medication to a rival. And, they admit that they provide all sorts of gifts and gratuities to doctors, ranging from financial aid to educational programs to bags and writing pads, to encourage doctors to prescribe their brand of drugs.

If you are concerned with your doctor "pushing" drugs onto you, consider asking if he/she receives any financial gifts or benefits from the drug manufacturer. Such questions are uncomfortable, but ethical questions often are -- and they may be more uncomfortable for your doctor than for you. Otherwise, go to www.naturopathic.org to contact a naturopathic doctor who subscribes to the motto "Doctor do no harm."

Guidelines for Drugs/Medications

The following are only guidelines -- always defer to your doctor.
- Understand the purpose of the drug, how it's supposed to help your health and how it affects other aspects of your health (side affects), If the drug is not doing what it's supposed to do, notify your doctor immediately. Do not wait for your next doctor's appointment.
- Administer the drug properly per the directions from your doctor. If you are not certain, contact your doctor immediately.
- If you are taking insulin, make certain that you are extracting the right amount of insulin from the bottle. If possible, have a friend or partner verify for you. Also, unless otherwise specified, once an insulin bottle is opened, it is good for 28 days even if it's refrigerated. Unopened bottles of Lantus should be stored in the refrigerator.

- *Author's Tip:* In my case, because I was taking two different types of insulin with two different dosage amounts, I set up my needles for the week and kept each type of insulin in a separate (different color) basket that I stored in the refrigerator.
- Insulin pens that are not in use and are refrigerated are good until the expiration date. Insulin pens that are in use should not be refrigerated and are good for 10 to 28 days depending on the brand and type.
- Before drawing up your insulin or injecting with an insulin pen, check the bottle or cartridge for frosting on the inside of the glass and crystals or clumps in the insulin.
- Rapid-acting (Humalog, Novolog), short-acting (Regular) and long-acting (Lantus) insulins are clear. Pre-mixed, Lente, and long-acting (NPH, Ultra Lente) insulins are cloudy after rolling the bottle between your hands.
- If the drug is not helping to get your blood glucose within the normal range, discuss this with your doctor. After all, why take a drug and suffer through the side effects if it's not doing what it's supposed to do. Discuss with your doctor what you need to do to correct the problem. Also, discuss the effectiveness of the drug over time. In addition, discuss other alternatives before your doctor recommends putting you on a different drug.
- If appropriate, increase (or decrease) the drug dosage for your pending meal, based on the input from your doctor and other factors including your blood glucose average, and your pending meal size (number of carbohydrate calories, number of total calories, amount of fiber).
- Once your blood glucose is within the normal range, work with your doctor to develop a strategy and timeline to get weaned off the drugs by continual modification of your nutritional plan and exercise regimen. If the drug dosage is not decreasing over time, discuss the reasons why with your doctor and determine the actions you should be taking.
- *Note:* The following types of drugs may increase your blood glucose level: ACE inhibitors, antibiotics, antidepressants, diuretics, steroids, and cancer drugs.

Drug Weaning Process

Warning: If you agree that drugs are not the answer for you in the long term, then, work with your doctor to develop a drug weaning process that will enable you to slowly reduce your drug dosage and prevent **pancreatic beta cell dysfunction** and the **"insulin addiction trap"**. For Type 2 diabetics, long term use of most diabetic drugs overworks the pancreas, which can no longer meet the insulin demands of your cells. This leads to insulin injections, which signal the pancreas to reduce its production of insulin. With this reduction of insulin production by the pancreas, the insulin injections will be required for the rest of your life!

1.   Obtain a copy of a book such as the Physician's Desk Reference for detailed information about most drugs, or go to a website such as www.webmd.com.

2.   If you are taking more than one drug, work with your doctor to determine which specific drug to safely initiate the weaning process. If necessary, enlist the help of a natural health practitioner to assist you in the weaning process.

3.   Determine whether you need to obtain any measurement tools to allow you to closely monitor your progress, e.g. blood pressure monitor, blood cholesterol monitor, an additional blood glucose meter. Check your medical insurance for coverage.

4.   Establish a timeline (e.g. date) to initiate the weaning process for that specific drug.

5.   Identify a clear measurable goal that you need to achieve to begin the weaning process, e.g. The average blood glucose level is reduced 10 points over the previous week.
     Author's Personal Note: It was important that I could reduce my blood glucose level at least 10 mg/dl over the previous week before I would consider reducing my insulin dosage. It was also important that I had made specific changes to my nutrition (e.g. reduction of refined carbohydrates) -- to allow me to reduce my Humalog dosage.

6.   Identify the smallest reasonable increment that you can safely reduce your drug dosage. If this is not possible, discuss other alternatives with your doctor, e.g. using a pill cutter, taking a dosage every other time.

7. Use the measurement tool (e.g. glucose meter, blood pressure monitor) several times a day, ideally at the same times each day, to record and track your readings and progress.
8. Record any specific observations and events that may be occurring at that time, including how you feel.
9. At the beginning of each new week (or month), depending on your schedule and goals, review your readings, how you felt, and other notes with your doctor to decide whether to continue with decreasing your dosage.
10. Contact your doctor immediately if you notice that you don't feel well or you notice a trend in your readings going in the wrong direction.
11. Once you reach a zero dosage level, closely monitor your measurements/readings during the next several weeks to ensure there are no problems. In fact, to be on the safe side, you may even want to increase your measurements/readings – at least until your next medical exam/physical.
12. Initiate this process for the next drug that you and your doctor have agreed to wean you off.

Drugs for Diabetes

The following is a list of the major types of diabetic drugs.

Warning: Just because you don't feel any side effects of the drugs does not mean that your body is not being harmed!

Metformin, a biguanide, e.g. Glucophage (Metformin)
- Function: reduces insulin resistance in the liver and acts on the liver to reduce the release of stored glycogen.
- **Side Effects:** gastrointestinal problems, weight loss, diarrhea, decreased appetite, gas, lactic acidosis (buildup of lactic acid in the blood if kidneys are not functioning); blocks the absorption of folic acid from the intestines to raise blood levels of homocysteine, which leads to arterial plaque formation and heart disease.
- Caution: A large percentage of diabetics who take drugs such as Glucophage eventually end up with heart disease.

Sulfonylureas, Meglitinides, e.g. Amaryl, Glucotrol
- Function: acts on the pancreas to increase insulin secretion.
- **Side Effects:** weight gain, hypoglycemia, skin rash, headache, nausea.

Alpha-glucosidase Inhibitors, e.g. Acarbose (Precose)
- Function: slows absorption of carbohydrates from the intestines.
- **Side Effects:** diarrhea, gas, bloating, abdominal pain, headache, hypoglycemia.

Thiazolidinediones, e.g. Pioglitazone (Actos), Rosiglitazone (Avandia)
- Function: acts on muscles to enhance insulin sensitivity and glucose uptake.
- **Side Effects:** headaches, muscle aches, runny nose/sore throat, diarrhea, fluid retention, weight gain, fatigue, increased cholesterol levels; linked recently to heart attack and possibly death (Avandia).

Insulin, e.g. Humalog, Regular, NPH, Lente, Lantus
- Function: increases the amount of insulin in the bloodstream and reduces the blood glucose level (injected with a needle/syringe).
- **Side Effects:** weight gain (belly fat), heart disease, stroke, insulin addiction. Insulin acts as a (fat) storage-and-locking hormone, which leads to the body being in a catabolic (fat-building, muscle-burning) state; which, in turn, leads to weight (fat) gain. Insulin inhibits the breakdown of homocysteine, which causes inflammation, arterial plaque formation and heart disease. Insulin also causes a slower metabolism, higher cholesterol (lipid profile), fatigue, depression; vitamin/mineral loss; and bone (density) loss.
- Complications: long-term use increases fat cells, which require more insulin, increasing the dependency on the injections and ensuring a complete reliance on the insulin injections – creating **pancreatic beta cell dysfunction** and the **"insulin addiction trap"**.
- **Side effects (long term):** for Type 2 diabetics, leads to sustained obesity, heart disease, fatigue, and other weight-related complications. Long term use of insulin injections signals the pancreas to reduce its own production of insulin, creating a lifelong chemical dependency.

Combinations of Drugs, e.g. GlucoVance
Sulfonylureas & Metformin

- Function: combines a sulfonylurea (glyburide) and a biguanide (metformin) to trigger the pancreas to produce more insulin and inhibit the liver from releasing glucose.
- **Side Effects:** hypoglycemia, diarrhea, nausea/vomiting, abdominal pain, skin reaction, dark urine, increased sensitivity to sun. The most serious side effect is lactic acidosis. Because it may be life threatening, your health care provider will check your kidney and liver function to determine if you are at risk.

Thiazolidinediones & Metformin, e.g. Avandamet

- Function: combines a rosiglitazone (Avandia) and a biguanide (metformin) to target insulin resistance and inhibit the liver from releasing glucose.
- **Side Effects:** hypoglycemia, fluid retention or swelling, which could lead to heart failure and possibly death. The most serious side effect is lactic acidosis. Because it may be life threatening, your health care provider will check your kidney and liver function to determine if you are at risk.
- Signs of lactic acidosis: feeling very weak/tired, unusual muscle pain, unusual sleepiness, rapid breathing, nausea, vomiting, low body temperature, feeling dizzy or light-headed, a slow or uneven heartbeat.
- Signs of liver problems: nausea, vomiting, stomach pain, unexplained tiredness, loss of appetite, dark urine, yellowing of your skin or whites of your eyes.

Key Point: Most diabetic drugs focus on lowering your blood glucose, but do *not* address the **excess insulin**, which is depleting your body of vital nutrients, producing more fat, and preventing fat metabolism — leading to even more weight gain in the belly area. The body becomes dependent on the excess insulin to "push" the glucose into the cells, until the body requires insulin injections, creating beta cell dysfunction and the **"insulin addiction trap"** where the body requires insulin shots for life.

Drugs for Heart Disease

Because of the connection between diabetes and heart disease, the following list of drugs for heart disease, high blood pressure and high cholesterol is provided for your general knowledge. Also, listed are some, but not all, of the more common side effects associated with these drugs. Reference: www.americanheartassociation.org

Warning: Just because you don't feel any side effects of the drugs does not mean that your body is not being harmed!

ACE inhibitors:
- Function: reduces the activity of the angiotensin converting enzyme (ACE), which is responsible for causing the blood vessels to narrow. If the blood vessels are relaxed, your blood pressure is lowered and more oxygen-rich blood can reach your heart. They also lower the amount of salt and water in your body.
  Note: Angiotensin II antagonists act in a similar way to ACE inhibitors, but do not cause the persistent dry cough that ACE inhibitors can sometimes cause.
- **Side Effects:** a dry cough; headache, upset stomach, numbness or tingling in the hands or feet; an increase in blood glucose
- *Note:* Have regular blood tests to check the levels of salts in your blood and to test your kidney and liver function.
- *Note:* Natural ACE inhibitors include green tea, raw/aged garlic, hawthorn, olive leaf, taurine, proanthocyanidins, and ginkgo biloba.

Angiotensin II receptor blockers (ARBs):
- Function: acts in a similar way to ACE inhibitors, but does not cause the persistent dry cough that an ACE inhibitor can sometimes cause.
- **Side Effects:** diarrhea, stomach problems, muscle cramps, back/leg pain, dizziness, insomnia, nasal congestion, cough, sinus problems, upper respiratory infection, higher cholesterol level, kidney problems.

Anti-arrhythmic drugs:
- Function: controls the rhythm of the heart.
- **Side Effects:** may cause low blood sugar; dizziness, blurred vision.

Anticoagulants, e.g. Coumadin (Warfarin), Liquaemin (Heparin):
- Function: prevent fibrin from forming. Clots consist of platelets (small blood cells) clumped together, and a protein called fibrin.
- **Side Effects:** hemorrhaging, dermatitis, diarrhea.
- *Note:* Natural anticoagulants include: fish oil, raw/aged garlic, ginger, turmeric, Vitamin E.

Aspirin (and other anti-platelet drugs), e.g. Bayer Aspirin, Bufferin
- Function: reduces the stickiness of platelets, but may cause internal bleeding, weakening of artery walls. It is important that your blood pressure is normal before you start taking aspirin.
- **Side Effects:** bleeding, stomach pain, diarrhea.

Beta-blockers:
- Function: blocks the effects of adrenaline on your body's beta receptors, beta 1 and beta 2. This slows the nerve impulses that travel through the heart. As a result, your heart does not have to work as hard because it needs less blood and oxygen. Beta-blockers also block the impulses that can cause an arrhythmia. They are also effective in lowering raised blood pressure.
- **Side Effects:** drowsiness, fatigue, cold hands and feet, weakness, dizziness, dry mouth, eyes, and skin.
- *Note:* Beta 1 receptors are responsible for heart rate and the strength of your heartbeat. Beta 2 receptors are responsible for the function of your smooth muscles (muscles that control body functions that you do not have control over).

Calcium channel blockers (calcium antagonists):
- Function: slows the rate at which calcium passes into the heart muscle and into the vessel walls. This relaxes the vessels allowing blood to flow more easily through them, lowering blood pressure.
- **Side Effects:** feeling tired, flushing, swelling of the abdomen, ankles, or feet, heartburn
- *Caution:* There may be a danger of the heart rate becoming too slow when combining some channel blockers with beta-blockers.
- *Note:* Natural Calcium Channel Blockers include: magnesium.

Cholesterol-lowering (statin) drugs, e.g. Lipitor (Pfizer), Zocor (Merck), Pravachol (Bristol-Myers Squibb), Mevacor (Merck), Vytorin (Merck/ Schering-Plough Pharmaceuticals), Crestor (AstraZeneca)

- Function: lowers the total amount of cholesterol in the blood, particularly the LDL cholesterol, but does not lower triglycerides.
- **Side Effects:** nausea, diarrhea, constipation, neurological effects (e.g. memory loss), muscle aching, myopathy; inhibits CoQ10 production, an important nutrient for the heart and other muscles; increases liver enzyme levels, which may cause muscle pain and tenderness (statin myopathy). In severe cases, muscle cells can break down (rhabdomyolysis) and release a protein called myoglobin into the bloodstream causing myoglobinuria. Myoglobin can impair kidney function and lead to kidney failure.

Notes:

o People who take statins should have their liver function tested periodically because liver problems may develop.

o Certain drugs when taken with statins can increase the risk of rhabdomyolysis. These include gemfibrozil, erythromycin (Erythrocin), antifungal medications, nefazodone (Serzone), cyclosporine and niacin. If you take statins and have muscle aching or tenderness, consult with your doctor immediately.

o Avoid taking statins with grapefruit juice, which alters the body's metabolism of these drugs.

o Doctors generally recommend that people take statins late in the day because the body makes most of its cholesterol at night.

o One of the statin drugs Baycol was recalled because of deaths from rhabdomyolysis.

o Statin drugs have been the most popular and the most prescribed class of drugs in the U.S. for the past 15 years, with an annual revenue of more than $35 billion.

o To counteract the effects of the statin drugs that cause myopathy, Merck filed two US patents in 1989 recommending the use of Coenzyme Q10 with statins. But, to date, not one pharmaceutical company has developed a statin drug that contains this important nutrient – because they may not want to publicly acknowledge the danger associated with this drug.

Diuretics:
- Function: increases the output of water and sodium in the urine; causes an increased loss of potassium, which may lead your doctor to prescribe a potassium supplement; and, causes a loss of calcium, which may lead to osteopenia and osteoporosis (bone loss).
- **Side Effects:** increase in blood glucose. Too much potassium: irregular heartbeat; breathing problems; numbness or tingling in the hands. Too little potassium: fast or irregular heartbeat; weak pulse; nausea, vomiting; dry mouth; excessive thirst; muscle cramps or pain.
- *Note:* Natural diuretics include: dandelion, stinging nettle, lemons.

Nitrates:
- Function: relaxes the muscles in the walls of the veins and arteries (including the coronary arteries) and makes them wider. They are useful in relieving angina pain and in preventing "predictable'" attacks. e.g. glyceryl trinitrate (nitroglycerin) tablets.
- **Side Effects:** dizziness; headaches; flushing of your face and neck; upset stomach; low blood pressure; irregular heart rhythms.

Potassium channel activators:
- Function: relaxes the walls of the coronary arteries to improve blood flow (similar to nitrates).
- **Side Effects:** headache when you first take them, and flushing, indigestion or dizziness.

Thrombolytic drugs ("clot busters"):
- Function: is used only when there is an urgent need to dissolve a clot.
- **Side Effects:** may cause serious bleeding, so the doctor must be reasonably sure of the diagnosis and that the patient does not have a high risk of bleeding.

> **Warning:** Some drugs may be difficult to wean off, because the body develops a chemical dependency on the effects of the drug. If possible, try to delay any drug therapy until you have tried a nutritional/spiritual-based program. Otherwise, if you are concerned with the drug therapy, consider contacting a naturopathic doctor.

Chapter 13. Mind & Spirit

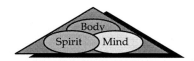

Body, Mind & Spirit

Man is a trinity that is comprised of the Body (Physical), the Mind (Mental), and the Spirit (Spiritual). The Body, Mind and Spirit work in harmony to make you the best that you can be in this life. If one of these three elements is "sick" or out of balance with the other two, then, your entire being will be sick.

Unfortunately, most of traditional medicine focuses on the Body by addressing and suppressing the symptoms and never fixing the underlying root cause of the unhealthy cells. Traditional medicine tends to overlook the importance of the Mind and the Spirit and its role in healing the Body. Man also tends to focus on the Body by taking drugs to relieve pain or by feeding his food cravings to satisfy hormonal hunger – both of which may be driven by emotions such as depression.

Consequently, there are psychological and psychosocial factors that may exert substantial influence on the biochemical control in diabetic patients. These factors have been shown to increase the risks of poor glycemic control, "brittle diabetes", and diabetic ketoacidosis. Depression has been identified as one negative influence of poor glycemic control among pediatric and adolescent patients. And, depression has been observed to affect family members of patients with Type 2 diabetes and influence family dynamics toward the condition.

As with any disease, after several years of fighting the good fight, you can become physically drained because your physical body has continued to weaken despite everything that you've done to fight the disease.

Consequently, you also become emotionally and spiritually drained; and, as a result, you lose hope and "give in" to the fact that the best you can do is to live with the disease – that you've done everything possible to fight the disease. This can be very disconcerting and difficult to overcome emotionally. Also, despite the support from your family and friends, you feel very alone and afraid at times. There are horror movies that can scare you, but I can truly tell you that there is nothing, absolutely nothing scarier than knowing that your doctor cannot help you and your time is limited. Only a strong belief in a power that is greater than yourself can give you the hope, the confidence and courage to fight for your life instead of giving in to the inevitable life of kidney failure/dialysis, amputation, and blindness.

Once you accept the fact that we live in a spiritual universe and that we are all spiritual beings, you will find yourself equipped with an instrument through which you can exert influence over your body and your blood glucose control. But, how do you go about tapping into your inner spirit and belief system? The following section will give you some ideas to get started. Anything and everything is possible if you have faith and you take responsibility of your health problems and follow up with the necessary actions; and, resist the negative influences that will discourage you from making yourself a healthier person.

How does food help or prevent us from getting to this inner spirit? There is no universal agreement about the relationship of food to the human body, mind or spirit. However, I believe that we can agree that "dead" food definitely harms the Body. And, since food can make us happy or console us when we're sad, we can make the case that food also harms the Mind and the Spirit. Food is an ever-present reminder that there is more to life than just filling stomachs. Our minds and spirits crave for more meaning.

Now, we can conclude that the inverse of those statements is true -- that the Body, Mind and Spirit affect the food we select to eat. If you have a positive mental attitude and truly believe that food can help you improve your health, then, it will because you will acquire the knowledge to make better food choices. The following section provides some guidelines that will help you to build and use your Mind and Spirit to improve the health of your Body.

So, how did we get here with all these convenience and fast foods and such poor health? When it comes to food, the irony is that just at the time nutritional scientists were identifying vitamins, minerals, and other nutrients that support life, technologists were perfecting the refining processes to separate the nutrients from the food or to reconstitute them in synthetic forms. Refined white flour, "enriched" cereal, homogenized milk, bottled juices, soda, high fructose corn syrup, margarine (partially hydrogenated oil), and fast foods are examples that are devastating our health today. All of this was motivated by profit for the seller and convenience for the buyer, as the age of boxed mixes and prepackaged foods brought new freedom in the kitchen and profits to food packaging industries and grocery stores. Unfortunately, that new freedom has come at a high price, which many people are ignoring, hoping that, maybe medical science will develop a magic pill in the near future. Medical science is very successful in handling trauma and emergency treatment, but not with their treatment of degenerative diseases such as heart disease, cancer and diabetes. Their treatment protocol for these diseases is drug therapy to *suppress* the symptoms instead of *fixing* the underlying root cause and get rid of the disease. If the drug therapy doesn't work or it stops working, the only other option is surgery.

Unfortunately, many people put their faith in these drugs that were created by man instead of the foods that were created by God. And, as long as we continue to believe that man is smarter than God, we will be trapped with poor health and our dependency on these man-made foods and drugs. So, become a *victor* of wellness, instead of a *victim* of disease.

Spiritual health allows you to focus on your inner faith and the belief that you must respect and protect what you put into your body to maintain a healthy balance with the mind and spirit. This supports Apostle Paul's requirement to glorify God in our body, as well as our spirit:

"Know ye not that your body is the temple of the Holy Ghost . . . therefore glorify God in your body, and in your spirit, which are God's." [1 Corinthians 6:19-20]

Discord between your Spirit and Mind usually leads to illogical behaviors and rationalizations. For example, as their reasoning for eating what they like even if it is bad for their health, I am amazed at the number of people who have told me "Well, you gotta die of something." This type of rationalization is due to a disconnect between that person's spirit and unconscious mind, leading to a negative effect on their body. It is also a disconnect between the spirit and conscious mind that is created as a defense mechanism when the person can't really explain why they're doing something that they know is harming their body. Research has shown that a diabetic who is not healthy emotionally will not respond positively to treatment, even though they may have the best care and medicine. Discord between the mind and body is a critical factor. Diabetics know that if they worry too much their blood sugar will go "sky high" and stay high until they stop worrying.

Be wary of systemic societal prejudices (e.g. sexism, racism), which may decrease your exposure to knowledge/education while increasing the anxiety and stress in your life. How you handle these problems and stress is very important. Do not neglect the problem. Acknowledge that stress can actually be helpful. For example, the stress that an athlete feels can actually help to improve their performance if they know how to channel the stress and nervous energy. Someone like a Magic Johnson or Michael Jordan handled stress well on and off the basketball court. But, you don't need to be Magic or Michael – just be yourself, embrace the challenge and don't neglect the problem.

Neglect is like an infection -- left unchecked it will spread throughout your entire being. When you neglect your health (by not eating right and not exercising), this may cause you to feel guilty and guilt leads to an erosion of your self-confidence. As your self-confidence diminishes, so does your activity level (of trying to get healthy). And as your activity level diminishes, your results inevitably decline. And as your results suffer, your attitude begins to weaken. And as your attitude begins the gradual shift from positive to negative, your self-confidence diminishes even more . . . and this downward spiral continues as your health suffers.

Review the next section and *God's Food for Thought* (page 385). Discuss options with your pastor or healthcare professional, and, if necessary, consider some type of relaxation therapy or other psychological support.

Mind & Spirit Practices

Review the following to help with your emotional and spiritual health.

Self
- Be selfish: Take care of Number One – You!
- You deserve the best – start treating yourself accordingly.
- Forgive others, but, more importantly forgive yourself.
- Love yourself – if you love yourself, you will take the time to prepare meals and find the time to exercise.
- Develop and maintain a positive attitude with life as well as an open mind to new ideas about health and nutrition. Don't hide behind the disease and look for sympathy from friends and relatives.
- Attitude is everything. Attitude is a choice. A person with a positive attitude will have a strong faith and belief in self, others, and in God. A person with a positive attitude will attract positive people and positive events.
- Identify a strong motive for getting healthy, e.g. financial, your children, family, quality of life, religious, disdain towards drugs, fear of a painful death. Ensure that your motive is strong enough to overcome the setbacks you're going to have during your journey.
- Change the way you think – *choose* to be healthy. More importantly, avoid your **food triggers**, e.g. driving past a fast food place, mall shopping, playing cards with friends.
- Become a *victor* of wellness, not a *victim* of disease and drugs.
- Be thankful, hopeful, cheerful, and prayerful. These attitudes produce the endorphins, which are merry hormones and happy chemicals that fight disease and promote a sense of well being.
- What you think you create. Therefore, change the talk-track in your head that tells you "dead" food is good for you because it taste good! Many of your favorite foods are poison to your body. Would you consume arsenic if it tastes good? These negative beliefs are powerful motivators that drive your fear and will actually cause you to repel getting healthy. Fear is driven by a lack of knowledge and a lot of misinformation from television and your doctors. Acquiring knowledge about nutrition and diabetes is very empowering and will set you free from the shackles of ignorance.
- State a daily self-affirmation to reinforce your positive attitude.

- You are not defined by being a diabetic. How you rise and face the adversity will define who you are.
- Be aware of societal "isms" that may affect your health.
- Embrace change and the adversity that you will face during your journey. Adversity will build your character or reveal it.
- "Listen to your inner voice, your true self: Get in touch with your true feelings, your calling, your purpose in life, your real passion – it's not what you want to do, it's what you want to be. It's what you were meant to be. Use your personality (the essence of who you are) and everything you've learned throughout your life to serve your soul and drive your true passion." [Oprah Winfrey]
- Share your knowledge, become an advocate in your community.

Faith & Spirit

- Strengthen your belief system: Trust in divine power. Recognize that a divine being, a guardian angel, is always with you. Believe in something that is a higher power – "more powerful than thee."
- Believe that God will help you, but don't sit around waiting for God – take action!
- Use your Spirit to make the Mind-Body connection and find your center. This will ensure that you maintain a positive attitude fueled by your internal motivation and drive to succeed no matter the odds.
- Walk with God for God is in you:
  o **G**iving: Learn to be a *giving* person by helping others, e.g. become a volunteer, join a support group. Say "thank you" with a smile to someone every day.
  o **O**bservant: Learn to be *observant* and aware of your surroundings and community, and, you will find ways to help yourself, your family and others. Learn something new every week. Increase your awareness by increasing your knowledge.
  o **D**iscipline: Use *discipline* to stop eating the addictive "dead" foods. Learn to use discipline to provide structure and guidelines for you and your family, especially your children. As a math tutor, I learned that children more than anything want discipline to help guide them and provide focus as they learn how to become productive adults.

- Connect to your inner spirit to change your state of mind and bring back the hope. You can't solve your problem (e.g. diabetes) with the same state of mind that created the problem in the first place.
- Change the way you look at things and things will change the way they look.
- No doctor, no herb, nor any medicine can cure you. It is the body that heals itself – with your help and with God's help.
- "Don't give up, don't ever give up." Jim Valvano, basketball coach
- You can neutralize your fears by making your faith bigger than your fear – by cultivating your faith. And, faith breeds more faith.
- Do not underestimate the power of the human spirit – as demonstrated by events such as the Tsunami and Hurricane Katrina.
- There is a fine line between denial and faith: Denial is believing you can't win the battle against the disease because of all the facts. Faith is believing that you *can* win the battle *despite* all of the facts.

Enjoyment
- Laugh! Laugh! Laugh! Laughter is a wonderful stress-reducer. Laughter relieves muscular tension providing a discharge of nervous excitement. It improves breathing, regulates the heartbeat and pumps endorphins (the body's natural painkillers) into the bloodstream. Smiling is also beneficial.
- Oprah, during one of her "After the Show" segments, said the following about passion and one's purpose in life: "Everybody has a calling, and your real job in life is to figure out what it is you're called to do; you use a job until you can figure out what the calling is . . . If you find your passion in life you will never get tired . . . because you're fueled by the passion and the energy . . . You know it's right when it feels right; you know it's right because it gives you your juice; you know it's right because you'd do it for nothing if you could . . . your passion is what gives your life purpose and meaning . . . listen to your inner voice . . . the Voice of God speaks through your heart, but you have to be still and very quiet to hear the Voice . . . don't look for God to speak to you like he did with Moses and the Burning Bush . . . he speaks to us everyday, if we just listen quietly . . ."

- "Try to do three things every day: laugh, cry and think. If you do, you will have had a full day." Jim Valvano, college basketball coach who was successful with increasing the visibility of cancer.
- Let go of the anger, jealousy, hopelessness, and envy in your life. These negative emotions trigger the release of stress hormones and weaken the immune system, making you more susceptible to disease.
- Forgive others, but don't expect anything in return.
- Participate in activities and with people that bring joy to your life.
- "Live each day with enthusiasm." [Rev. Joel Osteen]

How to Improve Rest & Relaxation

Relaxation is more than just sitting back, reading, or watching TV. It involves learning ways to calm and control your body and mind. Relaxation does not come easily, especially if you are ill. Some people find it difficult to relax. They feel they don't have time to practice it, or they don't believe it will help them. Others feel embarrassed or guilty for taking the time to relax. With practice, most people get some relief from relaxation.

There is no best way to learn how to relax. Everyone responds differently to different techniques. Try some of the following methods until you find one or two that work for you.
- Use deep breathing techniques, e.g. learn to breathe to slow down your heart rate by breathing in deeply, counting to 7 and breathing out, counting to 10; keep doing this until your heart rate slows down.
- Take a walk after dinner or during the day. If you live near a mall, walk around the mall with a friend a 3-4 times a week.
- Guided imagery uses your mind to focus on pleasant images. First, begin by breathing slowly and deeply. Think of yourself in a place where you feel comfortable, safe, and relaxed. This may be a favorite vacation spot, or a porch swing in your own backyard. Create all the details: the colors, sounds, smells, and how it feels. These images take your mind away from pain and focus it on something more pleasant. If necessary, obtain a couple of imagery video tapes.
- Prayer is very relaxing and comforting for some people. You may want to make a tape recording of a soothing inspirational message.

- Use prayer to talk to God, use meditation to listen to God.
- Biofeedback uses sensitive electrical equipment to help you to be more aware of your body's reaction to stress and pain, and to learn how to control your body's physical reactions. The equipment monitors your heart rate, blood pressure, skin temperature or muscle tension. These body signals are shown on a screen or gauge so you can see how your body is reacting. Biofeedback helps you learn how you feel when your muscles are tense or relaxed.
- Relaxation audio tapes help guide you through the relaxation process. These tapes provide directions for relaxation, so you don't have to concentrate on remembering the instructions.
- Use meditation to bring a sense of fullness and tranquility. Meditation increases self-discovery and awareness of the natural phenomena that is actually going on behind your own eyes.
- Hold the hand of a loved one to help him/her relieve their stress.
- Take a meditation, yoga or T'ai Chi class. They are two excellent ways to establish harmony between the Body, Mind and Spirit, get the physical activity you need, learn to relax, and prepare the Body and Mind to better handle the stress of daily life. Yoga is a physical way of life emphasizing the harmony of the body and mind, and a philosophical way of life that is based on Eastern metaphysical beliefs. T'ai Chi is an ancient Chinese art of exercise and self-defense with an emphasis on relaxation of tension, both physical and mental, which leads to developing internal strength. Through T'ai Chi practice, an individual can become a more willing participant in the process of change, understanding that it is inevitable anyway.

How to Improve Sleep

Sleep is even more important than rest and relaxation. The purpose of sleep is to allow the body to repair and rejuvenate itself. Sleep also reduces fatigue and stress. There are five distinct stages of sleep. Stages 1 and 2 are considered light sleeping which takes place the majority of the night. Stages 3 and 4 are deep sleeping or "delta sleep" and rest and restoration. Stage 5 is the dream state, which helps to clear the nervous system and generally involves rapid eye movement or REM.

Patterns of sleep generally look like this: light sleep - deep sleep - REM - light sleep - deep sleep - rest and restoration, with the first period of light sleep lasting about 45 minutes.

In general, babies need 16 hours of sleep a day, teenagers perform best with 10 to 11 hours, older college students need about eight hours, and people between 45 and 60 often report that seven hours is enough. If you consistently rely on your alarm clock to wake up every morning, then, more than likely you are not getting enough quality sleep. An easy way to determine if you're getting enough quality sleep is to turn off your alarm clock and see how long you sleep before you wake up naturally. Then, make the necessary adjustments by going to bed a little earlier, if necessary.

In addition to how much sleep you get, it's important what type of sleep you're getting. For instance, your memory, learning ability, and adaptability to change are all linked to Stage 5 REM sleep while your body's ability to restore and repair itself is largely dependent on Stage 4 sleep, which is also important for maintaining many other aspects of your physical health. Unfortunately, the amount of Stage 4 sleep declines as we age, when it would be nice if the body repaired itself more, not less. Many people, including some diabetics, have trouble sleeping (and especially in entering Stage 4 sleep) because they don't stay physically active.

Insomnia problems include: you can't get to sleep; you wake up in the middle of the night, and can't go back to sleep; and, waking up too early, between 3:00 and 5:00 a.m., and you can't get back to sleep. Common causes of insomnia include poor eating habits, too much caffeine, too much alcohol, too much tobacco, nutritional deficiencies, blood glucose imbalances, physical pain, improper breathing, anxiety, stress, and the lack of exercise. To improve the quality (and quantity) of your sleep:

- Establish a consistent a regular daily routine and bedtime ritual, e.g. the same meal times, the same bedtime, the same pre-bed activities.
- Keep your bedroom cool and well ventilated. Maintain a relaxing atmosphere in the bedroom.

- Do not eat (especially processed grain and sugar carbohydrates) less than 2 hours before going to bed. These foods raise your blood glucose and inhibit sleep. Later, when your blood glucose drops too low, you may wake up and not be able to go back to sleep.
- Reduce your caffeine intake and avoid it altogether four to six hours before bedtime. Reduce your intake of alcohol, tobacco, and other stimulants especially in the evenings.
- Eat a handful of walnuts or drink a glass of warm milk or a cup of chamomile or fennel tea to soothe your nervous system 15-20 minutes before going to bed.
- Take a hot bath 2 hours before bedtime -- it increases your core body temperature, and when it abruptly drops when you get out of the bath, it signals your body that you are ready for sleep.
- Ensure you have a quality firm bed that properly supports your body's frame and a quality pillow to properly support your neck.
- Try to sleep in complete darkness or as close as possible. When light hits the eyes, it disrupts the circadian rhythm of the pineal gland and the production of melatonin and serotonin.
  Note: The body operates on the 24-hour cycle (12 on, and 12 off), which is called "Circadian Rhythms". When it gets dark, the body clock stimulates the pineal gland, which produces melatonin to enable sleep. Bright light or sunshine shuts off melatonin production and inhibits sleep, causing insomnia.
- Sleep on your back – it's the best position for relaxing, and allows all your internal organs to rest properly. If you must sleep on your side, do it on your right side, not your left. Sleeping on the left side causes your lungs, stomach and liver to press against your heart. If possible, do not sleep on your stomach. It causes pressure on all your internal organs including your lungs, which results in shallow breathing. It can also cause a stiff neck and upper back problems.
- Try to avoid watching too much TV just before going to bed. TV is too stimulating to the brain and it will take longer to fall asleep.
- Listen to calm music, or read something spiritual to help to relax. Do not read anything stimulating, such as a mystery or suspense novel.
- If possible, avoid using a loud alarm clock, which can be very stressful on the body when it is awoken suddenly. If you are getting enough sleep, an alarm clock should not be necessary.

Causes of chronic insomnia associated with psychological problems can be deeply rooted in stress, anxiety or depression. Insomnia associated with medical problems can be caused by a variety of factors including: iron deficiency anemia, breathing disorders, kidney dysfunction, diabetes, and medication side effects.

Support Systems

There are several types of support groups to meet individual needs. Support groups may be led by a professional, such as a nurse, social worker, diabetes educator, psychologist or by other patients. These groups usually focus on providing key information and sharing their personal experiences, successes and failures, but they also provide hope and emotional support, so that members realize that they are not alone in their battle with diabetes. Because support groups can vary in approach, size and how often they meet, patients should find a group that they are comfortable with and that meets their individual needs.

Sharing your feelings and experiences with a group that's struggling with the same disease you have can be very empowering and relaxing. A support group can make living with diabetes or any disease a lot easier in the short term. The basic goal of a support group is to give you a way to share and learn about your disease. A group also helps you to feel understood, and can give you new ideas to help cope with problems. It can also help you feel good about yourself because you'll be helping others in the group.

Author's Personal Note: The American Diabetes Association (ADA), the ADA director and their local diabetic support were instrumental in my success. I personally found participating in a support group to be very relaxing, enjoyable and inspiring – you get to meet some real heroes. When I started facilitating a diabetic support group, I found it to be very invigorating and exciting because there was so much to learn and so much to share with people who were struggling with the same disease. However, be careful not to become lulled into accepting the disease and the drugs because most of the group will likely be in that situation.

Here are some tips that will help you to maximize your support system:

- Surround yourself with positive people that strengthen your hope.
- Join a local diabetic support group to learn how to help yourself and to help others. Join a diabetic support forum if you have a computer.
- Educate yourself about the science – this will prevent you from being misled by well-intentioned people in the support group or forum.
- Learn from others in the support group by being observant. This may sound a little crude, but you should observe what sick people do and do the opposite, that is don't do what sick people do.
- If you are married or have a significant other, share your diabetes management with them. Most diabetics have better glucose control, a better sex life and a better relationship when they openly communicate and share their diabetes management with their spouse or partner. For example, if your partner knows that you tend to get down or moody when you have a high or low glucose reading, then, they will realize that it wasn't something that they did and, as a result, they may be able to help to lift your spirits.
- Speak out and let other family members know that you're diabetic. Don't be embarrassed to share what is happening to you. For whatever reason, diseases like diabetes are not shared among family members. It's kept quiet, which only increases the probability that someone else in the family will become diabetic, primarily because of the silence and the poor eating habits being passed down to each new generation.
- Design your own support team of family members, relatives, church members, friends, and others.
- Be wary of those who may become jealous once you start to feel and look healthy. Reach out to help them but if they don't want to be helped, don't allow them to drag you down. You must let them go until they are ready.
- Join a community or church group of some kind to help others in your local community. Become a community advocate. This will take your mind off the disease and bring hope to others.
- If necessary, consider some form of counseling. Many diabetics become depressed when they are initially diagnosed or after fighting the disease unsuccessfully for several years. Some diabetics feel so

bad they cannot sleep or eat. In these cases, therapy or counseling may help. Some people are afraid to admit they need help. They believe that others will think they are crazy if they talk to a professional about their problems. But it's smart to get help when you need it, especially if you have the symptoms of depression, e.g. poor sleep, changes in appetite, crying, sad thoughts, self-pity.

Knowledge & Education

Knowledge can be very powerful. Educate yourself about nutritional science, the human body and disease. If you are sick and/or overweight, more than likely your current thinking about nutrition is seriously flawed. In order to think differently, you must educate yourself by acquiring knowledge from various reliable sources. Acquiring knowledge to educate yourself about diabetes brings back the hope and can be very empowering. The more you learn, the more you will see the real power of this book and other resources. Also, the more that you learn, the more confidence you will have in making the important decisions and taking actions that will improve your health. It is also scary because some of the knowledge that you acquire may conflict with your current knowledge base and belief system. For example, it took a while for me to believe that consuming more fat was going to improve my health! Once I realized that it was the type of fat that mattered, I was more comfortable with making the change. And, when my health actually improved, it gave me even more confidence to make more changes.

Consequently, be accountable and take responsibility for your health -- acquire the knowledge. Once you acquire the knowledge you will have the power to control your life. As someone once said, "With power comes great responsibility." *However*, that power is not realized unless you *take action* based upon that knowledge!.

God said: **"My people perish for lack of knowledge." Hosea 4:6**. Educate yourself about the science – take some educational classes to learn more about diabetes and other related diseases. If you educate yourself about the science, you will feel more hopeful about making the necessary changes. When you *know* better, you *do* better.

Author's Personal Note: At various diabetic support group meetings, I was amazed at the knowledge that people had about food and drugs. Now, if only they had *applied* that knowledge and had *taken action* based upon that knowledge, they would be healthier today . . .

There are many resources that you can use as a starting point to acquire additional health-related information and knowledge. But, keep in mind that information in websites and books may be out of date or conflict with information in this book and other reference documents, especially when it comes to drug therapy and nutritional supplements. Also, keep in mind that many websites are trying to sell you one of their products, so buyer beware. The important point here is that the more knowledge that you have, the more empowered you feel and the more confident you will feel in making important health-related decisions.

Note: To help increase your knowledge about health and wellness, different diseases, and drugs, contact our wellness center concerning our new diabetes education program, which is gradually becoming the standard in diabetes care.

Nutritional & Exercise Tips for the Mind & Spirit

The previous chapters of this book focused on the Body portion of the Body-Mind-Spirit trinity, with nutrition, exercise and testing being the keys to optimize the health of the Body. Similarly, nutrition and exercise can also help to optimize the health of your Mind and Spirit.

Utilize the following nutritional and exercise tips to optimize your Mind and Spirit:
1. Utilize fun exercises and hobbies to free your Mind, lift your Spirit and help cleanse your Body.
2. Review the following nutrients and their descriptions to identify the nutrients that can support the health state of your Mind and Spirit. Ideally, try to find a wholefood supplement that contains the nutrients that you are not obtaining from your super meals.
    Important Note: Ensure the supplements are certified as pure and free of toxins, pesticides, and other chemicals; and, do not conflict with your drug therapy.

- Ashwagandha: is known as "Winter Cherry"; and, has anti-inflammatory, anti-tumor, anti-stress, antioxidant, mind-boosting, immune-enhancing, and rejuvenating properties that improve the body's ability to maintain physical effort and helps the body adapt to various types of stress. It works as an adaptogen, promoting the body's ability to maintain homeostasis and resist stress; and, is especially beneficial in stress related disorders such as arthritis, hypertension, and diabetes.
- Cayenne: stimulates the flow of blood to the brain, and accelerates the delivery of other key nutrients to the brain such as gingko biloba.
- DMAE (dimethylaminoethanol): increases production of brain chemicals essential for short-term memory, concentration, and learning capacity. It is referred to as a "cholinergic" because it may increase levels of the neurotransmitter acetylcholine, one of the chemicals in the brain that enhances mental powers. DMAE is found in high concentrations in sardines and anchovies.
- Gingko biloba: contains the flavonoid compounds collectively known as "ginkgolides" that act specifically to dilate the smallest segment of the circulatory system, the micro-capillaries, which has a widespread affect on the body's organs, especially the brain. The flavonoids and organic acids in gingko biloba increase the oxygen content to the brain by improving the blood flow in the small cerebral capillaries to enhance memory, increase mental focus and clarity; and inhibit age related reduction in brain chemicals. Because ginkgo is a blood-thinning agent, check with your doctor, especially if you are taking Coumadin or aspirin.
- Ginseng: contains active compounds called ginsenosides, which boost stamina, energy, and fight fatigue by sparing glycogen while utilizing fatty acids as energy. It also contains flavonoids, a group of antioxidants common in plants that neutralize free radicals.
- Phosphatidyl serine (PS): assists in regulating membrane transfer of nutrients and neurotransmitters necessary for proper mental function. Therefore, it is essential for nerve cell function and the production and release of neurotransmitters. PS supports the integrity of nerve cell membranes and the formation of other

important phospholipids to improve the health of the brain and nervous system. PS has been shown in numerous studies to help support memory and overall cognitive function, positive mood, and concentration. It also helps support the body's natural response to certain forms of stress.

- L-Tyrosine: is an amino acid that relieves the stress that sometimes accompanies weight loss by boosting your brain's levels of mood-regulating neurotransmitters like dopamine. L-tyrosine can be converted by neurons in the brain to dopamine and norepinephrine (noradrenaline), hormones that are depleted by stress, overwork and certain drugs.
- L-Phenylalanine: is an essential amino acid that can be converted to L-tyrosine by a complex biochemical process, which takes place in the liver. It aids and accelerates the production of l-tyrosine for optimum protection against anxiety and tension.
- Rosemary: contains tannins, flavonoids, rosmarinic acid, and carnosic acid. Rosmarinic acid may relieve pain and have antioxidant and anti-inflammatory properties. Carnosic acid has antioxidant properties.

3. Utilize one or more of the following nutrients (within a wholefood supplement) to improve the health state of your Mind and Spirit by helping to provide quality rest and sleep:

- Melatonin: supports the body's natural sleep rhythm by helping it to relax and prepare for sleep, which is often difficult when dieting and exercising. It also helps you feel more alert and rested after a night's sleep. Melatonin is produced by the pineal gland, located in the center of the brain. It is a hormone that plays a vital role in aging, energy and sleep.
- Melatonin-rich foods: include oats, barley, ginger, tomatoes, cherries, bananas, cucumber, beets and rice. If you're not sleeping well, increase your intake of melatonin-rich foods before resorting to a supplement; or, eat foods that raise your melatonin production, such as spirulina seaweed, soy nuts, cottage cheese, chicken, pumpkin seeds, turkey, and dried watermelon seeds. In addition, perform the following:

- o   Always turn off the lights and TV when you turn in for the night. Sleeping with the lights on may inhibit your body's natural production of melatonin.
- o   If melatonin foods don't help, talk to your primary care physician or naturopathic doctor before starting a nightly regimen of melatonin supplements.
- Rhodiola: acts as an adaptogen that strengthens the body's resistance to the effects of physical stress and stress-related fatigue, while enhancing the body's stamina and work performance by promoting higher levels of ATP in the mitochondria. It also provides calming benefits and promotes feelings of well-being by influencing serotonin, norepinephrine, and endorphin levels.
- Valerian Root, Passionflower, Chamomile, Hops: help you wind down to experience a good night's sleep by decreasing sleep latency (the length of time it takes to get to sleep) and the number of nighttime awakenings; and, without interfering with rapid eye movement (REM) sleep. Also, these botanical extracts improve well being by decreasing nervousness and anxiety; and, do not cause side effects that are common with sedative drugs, including addiction and morning "hangovers".
- 5-HTP: supports serotonin production, which is associated with sound sleep, positive mood and appetite control. L-tryptophan is converted to 5-HTP, which is converted to serotonin in the brain. In addition to increasing serotonin levels, 5-HTP is also a precursor molecule to melatonin, which contains sleep-enhancing properties. This can help you to feel less fatigued, and have a better mood due to enabling a good night's sleep. Europeans have been taking 5-HTP for decades to treat insomnia and depression.

  Caution: Be aware that if you are taking other agents that increase serotonin levels (such as l-tryptophan or drugs like Prozac), you should consult your physician before adding another product to your regimen. Also, an impure l-tryptophan supplement was connected to thousands of cases of illness and more than 30 deaths in the 1980s.

Inspirational Quotes

The following are quotes from some well-known people (in alphabetical order) that I found to be very inspirational when I was tutoring high school students and at different times during my recovery. Hopefully, one or more of these quotes hits a special chord within you.

"To be a great champion, you must believe you are the best. If you're not, pretend you are." Muhammad Ali

"Courage may be the most important of all virtues, because without it one cannot practice any other virtue with consistency." Maya Angelou

"Someone once told me that God figured that I was a pretty good juggler. I could keep a lot of balls in the air at one time. So He said, Let's see if you can juggle another one." Arthur Ashe

"I don't know the key to success, but the key to failure is trying to please everybody." Bill Cosby

"You can't solve a problem with the same mind that created the problem. You must change the way you think." Dr. Wayne Dyer, author of *The Power of Intentions*

"He's the best physician who knows the worthlessness of most medicines." Benjamin Franklin

"I always tell my kids if you lay down, people will step over you. But if you keep scrambling, if you keep going, someone will always, always give you a hand. Always. But you gotta keep dancing, you gotta keep your feet moving." Morgan Freeman

"You must be the change you wish to see in the world." Ghandi

"When wealth is lost, nothing is lost; when health is lost, something is lost; when character is lost, all is lost." Billy Graham

"Let your food be your medicine, and let your medicine be your food." Hippocrates, the Father of Medicine

"When you face a crisis, you know who your true friends are." Earvin (Magic) Johnson

"My father and mother had two simple rules about truth and living a long life: Rule Number 1: Don't ever lie to me. Rule Number 2: Don't ever forget Rule Number 1." DeWayne McCulley

"You have to be twice as good to be good – don't fight it, figure out how to be that good and do it." Melcan McCulley (my father)

"Boy, you tell them doctors that there is a science (listen to me now), tell them there is a science that is bigger than medical science – that science, it's called *God's* science, and God's science can fix any disease." Minnie McCulley (my mother)

"The inferior physician treats the disease once it occurs. The mediocre physician prevents the disease from coming back. The superior physician *prevents* the disease from ever occurring." Old Chinese Proverb

"Know ye not that your body is the temple of the Holy Ghost . . . therefore glorify God in your body, and in your spirit, which are God's." Apostle Paul (1 Corinthians 6:19-20)

"There are no secrets to success. It is the result of preparation, hard work, and learning from failure." Colin Powell

"He causeth the grass to grow for cattle, and herbs for the use of man." Psalms 104:14

"A hero is an ordinary individual who finds the strength to persevere and endure in spite of overwhelming obstacles." Christopher Reeve

"The greatest discovery of any generation is that human beings can alter their lives by altering the attitudes of their minds." Albert Schweitzer

"The road to success is through commitment." Will Smith

"Cancer can take away all my physical abilities, it cannot touch my mind; it cannot touch my heart, and it cannot touch my soul. And those three things will carry on forever." Jim Valvano

"A sure way for one to lift himself up is by helping to lift someone else." Booker T. Washington

"What I've learned from God personally is that as soon as you get the lesson, it's over . . . that's what Grace is." Oprah Winfrey

"I don't believe in failure. It is not a failure if you learned during the process." Oprah Winfrey

"Ya gots to work with what you gots to work with." Stevie Wonder

"Do not let what you cannot do interfere with what you can do." John Wooden

Chapter 14. The 6 Stages of Diabetes Control & Reversal

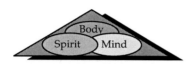

The 6 Stages

This diabetes wellness program will guide you from a state of no blood glucose control and sick cells to complete glucose control while reducing your cells' insulin resistance and inflammation to repair your sick cells — as you move from Stage 1 to Stage 6. However, it is your choice to stop at any stage if you are happy with your health at that point. Hopefully, you will progress through all the stages or as far as you possibly can in order to optimize your health. As you continue through each stage of this wellness program, your body will reduce its insulin resistance, oxidation, inflammation, and toxicity as it detoxifies and rebalances itself biochemically, hormonally, emotionally and spiritually. Your degree of success will depend strongly upon how much you really want to modify your behavior after several decades of poor eating habits and a sedentary lifestyle. It will be imperative that you develop and maintain a positive attitude because **behavior modification** is the most difficult challenge that you will face during this journey. Also, you must maintain an open mind to these new ideas about health and nutrition. After all, your current ideas about health and nutrition aren't working that well.

The previous chapters reviewed the eight "living" elements of diabetes control and reversal; and, now, it is time to put some structure around these eight elements. The following six stages provide a defined structure, a set of metrics, and a systematic approach for utilizing the eight "living" elements — in order to track, manage, control and reverse your diabetes. Being able to track and measure what stage you are in and knowing what you need to do to move forward will provide the necessary motivation to continue on your journey to better health.

If you find that you need structure and guidance in your planning, work with an experienced wellness coach that understands diabetes.

The six stages are as follows:
- Stage 1 No Blood Glucose (BG) Control
- Stage 2 BG Control with Drugs
- Stage 3 BG Control with Reduced Drugs
- Stage 4 BG Control without Drugs
- Stage 5 BG & HbA1C Control (without Drugs)
- Stage 6 BG & HbA1C Tighter Control (without Drugs)

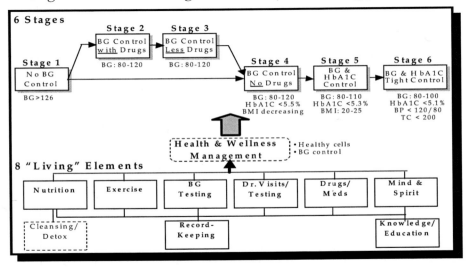

Figure 13. The Diabetes Control & Reversal Model

The six stages, depicted in the diagram above, are based upon the following targets/ranges to evaluate your blood glucose control and progress:
- Average fasting BG level: 80 to 120 mg/dl; Optimum: less than 100 mg/dl.
- Postprandial BG level: less than 130 mg/dl; Optimum: less than 120 mg/dl.
- Hemoglobin A1C of 4.2 to 5.5%; Optimum: less than 5.1%.

Timeline and Expectations

Because of the many factors that affect your blood glucose control, it is difficult to define the exact number of days/weeks that it will take to progress from Stage 1 to Stage 6. But, as you progress through each stage, you will obtain enough data to estimate how long it will take to reach the final stage. As depicted in the following chart, increasing the number of super meals, the frequency of exercise, and the amount of testing will decrease the recovery time, especially from Stage 1 to Stage 4. In general, it will take more time to get from Stage 1 to Stage 4 than from Stage 4 to Stage 6 because it will take more time for the body to repair the cells and reduce the insulin resistance/inflammation during the early stages. Once the body has started to heal, it accelerates the timeline for the remaining stages. Additional health problems (besides the diabetes) and any additional drugs you may be taking will increase the amount of recovery time, especially from Stage 1 to Stage 4.

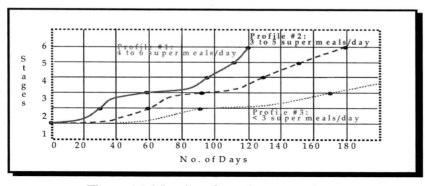

Figure 14. Timeline from Stage 1 to Stage 6.

As you progress through each stage of the wellness program, your body will repair and rebalance itself, while preventing further damage and complications. It is imperative that you wean your body off as many drugs as possible. How long it will take will vary from person to person, but the degree of your success will depend primarily upon your health state and drive to overcome the odds. Once you see how your body responds to the changes to nutrition, exercise, and testing, it will be easier to estimate your personal recovery timeline.

Stage 1 No BG Control

This is the stage where most diabetics usually find themselves in the beginning, with **excess insulin production** and an average fasting blood glucose (BG) level that is greater than 126 mg/dl or an oral glucose tolerance reading of at least 200 mg/dl.

The biggest challenge that you face at the beginning is the range of emotions from shock to denial, anger, and frustration. Once you face the reality that you have a *disease* of excess *insulin* (not a *sugar* problem), this becomes the first step to recovery. Remember – you cannot solve this health problem unless you accept the fact that you have a serious disease that needs your full attention. Whether you get your insulin/glucose under control and in the normal range is largely dependent on how you handle your emotions during this initial stage. The second biggest challenge is acquiring the motivation to change your behavior – changing human behavior is one of the most difficult challenges to overcome. As a result, some Type 2 diabetics *never get out of Stage 1* because they are unable to get their emotions under control or they are unable (or unwilling) to change their behavior. Consequently, they are unable to get their insulin/glucose under control with proper nutrition and exercise. Unfortunately, this leads them to try to fix the problem by taking diabetic drugs, but they still do not make the changes that need to be made to their nutrition, exercise, and testing. In the meantime, the disease continues to, slowly and without detection, cause deterioration of the small blood vessels that feed the kidneys, eyes, heart, feet, and brain. This deterioration is a microvascular disease and is part of an accelerated biological aging process. You may even feel good and look good on the outside, but inside your body is silently "rusting away".

Some diabetics are fortunate to get their blood glucose under control with minimal changes to nutrition, exercise and testing, but they usually relax thinking the disease has gone into remission. So, instead of making additional changes to nutrition, exercise, and testing to reduce the insulin and eradicate the disease, they underestimate the disease and end up regressing to a state of higher insulin/glucose levels within several years.

Other diabetics rely heavily on the drugs to temporarily control their blood glucose levels but not their *insulin* levels. Unfortunately, the excess insulin increases the toxic load within the body, requiring additional energy to get through the day. And as a result, these diabetics end up missing a major opportunity to actually eradicate the disease before it takes a stronghold in their bodies.

Caution: If your doctor has diagnosed you as "marginally diabetic" or "pre-diabetic", your doctor has noticed a high blood glucose reading in your most recent blood tests. You should heed this warning from your doctor who is trying to save you from a life of torment and serious health complications that diabetes brings with it. Instead, make the changes to your nutrition and exercise regimen to prevent the disease from progressing to a more serious state in your body. Specifically, read the information in Stages 1 and 4 to prevent yourself from progressing from pre-diabetes to full-blown diabetes.

Overall Planning

Planning will be the ultimate key to the success or failure of your journey. *If you fail to plan, then you are planning to fail.* It is also imperative that you get rid of the so-called "diet mentality" – this program is *not* a diet. Despite all the TV infomercials, books and marketing gimmicks, diets just don't work. The low-fat diets, the high carb diets, the high protein diets, and low cholesterol diets all failed and left us heavier, fatter and sicker people. Diets are too focused on restriction, deprivation, negativity, "falling off the wagon", and special foods. With this program you cannot "fall off the wagon" because you will include the foods and events that would cause you to fall off the wagon in the first place!

But you must first (temporarily) stop eating "dead" food just because it tastes good! Would you consume arsenic because it taste good? Identify your weaknesses (e.g. cravings for pasta, bread, sweets) and develop a strategy to include them as part of your overall plan. If you ignore them they will only come back to bite you in the future.

For example, eating rice, ice cream and drinking bottled juice were three areas that I had to address. I initially addressed these areas by adding kidney beans to my rice (for the extra fiber) and eventually moving to organic brown rice; adding blueberries and walnuts to my ice cream (to provide protein and fiber), and adding grounded flaxseed to my bottled juice. Almost any so-called "unhealthy" food can be turned into a "healthier" food either by adding something or switching to a healthier alternative. Refer to Figure 16 in the Appendix for a list of favorite foods and their more nutritious alternatives to help you through your transition.

Events such as picnics, holidays, birthdays, reunions, funerals, graduations, weddings, and other celebrations tend to be our downfall. Instead of dreading them or ignoring them, embrace them and develop your own strategy so that you will be successful and not feel "bad" after the celebration. Feeling "bad" or disappointed is counter-productive and causes the release of stress hormones, which is not healthy. During most celebrations, we are usually celebrating a happy (or sad) event. And, what do most people do when they are happy (or sad) and celebrating an event? They eat! Unfortunately, they usually eat too much of the wrong foods. So, how can you address this without putting a damper on all the fun or the event? There are so many creative ways to handle this – all you have to do is select one that fits you.

For example, if you ensure that you eat a fiber-rich super meal the night before and a vegetable-based super meal for the breakfast the following morning, this will prevent excess insulin production and provide you with the sustenance that will reduce your capacity to overeat a lot of the sweets and other goodies at the celebratory event. Although this strategy may not prevent you from eating the sweets and other goodies, it will definitely reduce the amount you consume, which should make you feel happy the next day. Also, if you ensure that your next meal at home is full of fiber and other "live" foods, this will help your body get rid of the waste from the sweets and other goodies instead of them sitting in your gut rotting away. And, if you perform a cleansing/ detoxification of the colon and liver, this will ensure that the waste and its toxic byproducts don't accumulate in the body.

By embracing these challenges instead of dreading them, you will be more successful and happier because you will realize that you cannot fail! No matter what happens, there is always a fallback plan of some kind to get you through any possible scenario – as long as you customize the plan to fit you. With this program, *there is no such thing as failure* – only opportunities to be even more successful than you had ever dreamed possible. Do not dread failure -- plan for it and be prepared to handle it.

Proactive planning, organization and consistency are the foundation of a solid diabetes wellness plan. Therefore, you should try to eat, exercise, and test at the same times every day. In order to acquire relevant and useful data to determine what changes to make, it is important that the data is being collected within some consistent boundaries. This also prevents the accidental introduction of other variables that may affect your data and corrective actions. Even with all of this planning and positive attitude, accept the fact that you *will* make mistakes. We all make mistakes, but it's how you respond once you make that mistake. As Oprah Winfrey once said: "All mistakes happen in our lives to teach us who we really are. . . and, how we respond to failure is what determines our real character."

Note: If you need help with your planning, contact our wellness center to obtain health coaching and a customized nutritional program.

Nutrition
During the first stage, you will be making the most significant changes relative to what you're currently eating and drinking. Unfortunately, many diabetics only make a few changes because they don't want to give up their "favorite foods", even though those are the very foods that are killing them one day at a time.

If you have multiple health issues, during the early stages, it may be critical to **stop eating wheat and other conventional grain-based foods** for breakfast -- because of the gluten protein and embedded chemicals. It may also be necessary to temporarily **stop eating fruit**, and replace it with vegetables. Once your body has cleansed, detoxified and begun to heal, you can gradually re-introduce some organic grains such as oat, barley, and quinoa, or gluten-free foods, during Stage 4 or Stage 5.

Do not try to make too many changes all at once unless your health is such that you need to make a lot of changes immediately. Of course, the *more* changes you make in Stage 1, the *faster* your body will begin to heal and be able to control its blood glucose level. I probably would not have made the major changes that I made if it hadn't been for my daughter and my mother. So, in my case, I was blessed to have a support system that accelerated the changes that needed to be made at the beginning.

Change your definition of food. Many of your favorite foods are your favorites because they taste good, but they're poison to your body. Would you consume arsenic if it taste good? Initiate the shift from eating "dead" processed, inflammatory foods to eating "live" anti-inflammatory foods (e.g. green, leafy and colorful raw land vegetables, sea vegetables; and, plant oils, nuts, and fish with the Omega-3 EFAs – to help repair the damaged cell membranes. Key vegetables include broccoli, Brussel sprouts, spinach, cauliflower, string beans, grasses, plankton, onions, and mushrooms. Avoid beets, carrots, eggplant, and winter squash temporarily due to their high carbohydrate levels. Eliminate as many **refined flour, starchy and sugary foods** as possible, since these are the major food groups that cause inflammation and the rise in **glucose** and **insulin** levels – especially bread, rice, pasta, wheat, potatoes, corn, soda, diet soda, pizza, bottled juices, sweets, fruits, and store-bought baked goods. Avoid foods that contain high fructose corn syrup, including some yogurts, cereals, applesauce, and ketchup. This will initiate the cleansing and detoxification process; and, will help to reduce the cravings, control your appetite, provide critical nutrients and bring the body chemistry into a better acid-alkaline balance, with more vitalized cells and energy and less acidity and inflammation. Increase fluids (filtered water, raw juices, green/white teas, vegetable broths) to increase hydration and elimination of acid waste and toxins, which deplete the energy from your cells.

Then, eliminate as many of the processed foods that contain **partially hydrogenated oil (trans fat)**. This artificial fat damages the insulin receptors and reduces the body's sensitivity to insulin leading to increased insulin resistance. Once you feel comfortable with those changes, gradually replace the **saturated fat** foods such as conventional animal meat and dairy products with leaner versions and more of the monounsaturated and Omega-3 polyunsaturated fats such as olive oil, macadamia nut oil, almonds, and fish, and saturated fats such as extra virgin coconut oil. These "good" fats will help the liver to metabolize the old fat and support the cardiovascular, nerve and immune systems.

If you have the time and patience, use a juicer to prepare fresh vegetable juices throughout the day to accelerate the body's healing and the removal of excess toxins, glucose, and waste. This will help repair your cells and tissues, and reduce the cravings for refined white flour products. Start juicing with several carrots and two cups of spinach leaves; and, slowly increase the amount of green vegetables while decreasing the amount of carrots. Add a tablespoon of wheat grass powder and ground flaxseed to provide some quality plant protein, fiber and Omega-3 fats to help control your appetite and absorb the fat-soluble nutrients. Use other vegetables such as Brussel sprouts, parsley, celery, cucumber, broccoli, and cabbage to provide some variety. Use half an apple to suppress the strong taste of the vegetables and satisfy your craving for sweets. If you don't have the time to juice, try something like low-sodium V-8 juice.

Because of the high sugar content, **avoid most fruits** except for lemons, limes, grapefruit, and tart cherries during the first four to six weeks. Once you have your blood glucose under better control, you can eat some fruits, especially apples, blackberries, blueberries, strawberries, and cherries – because of their fiber content, which helps to slow down their absorption. These "super" fruits provide antioxidant protection, help to cleanse your cells, and satisfy your cravings for sweets. However, be wary of tropical fruits that lack sufficient fiber and contain a lot of sugar, e.g. bananas, grapes, mango, oranges, pineapple, tangerine, watermelon. Your body can better handle these fruits in Stage 4.

To save time, prepare, cook, freeze and store foods on the weekend or when you have spare time during the week. Purchase portable nutritious snack foods, such as trail mixes or pulse food, for those times that you are in a hurry or you don't feel like preparing a healthy meal.

From a nutritional perspective, quality trail mixes and pulse food contain whole food ingredients such as vegetables, nuts, seeds, grains, legumes and fruit, which are free of additives and other chemicals. However, avoid roasted nuts, salt, and milk chocolate.

If you have high blood pressure, high homocysteine, high C-reactive protein, high cholesterol, or another health issue along with your diabetes, then, this indicates that your body has excess inflammation, toxins and acid waste. Therefore, perform an in-depth cleansing/ detoxification of your colon, liver, gall bladder, and kidneys, using quality herbal foods, glyconutrient foods, and wholefoods identified in Chapter 9. Depending on your health state, you may need to cleanse and detox every few weeks initially to reduce the inflammation and remove a lot of the excess chemicals, toxins, and acid waste. If you have never performed this type of procedure, discuss this with your doctor or other healthcare professional familiar with proper cleansing and detoxification. This in-depth cleansing and detoxification will accelerate the healing process and reduce your blood glucose level because the now healthy cells will be able to increase their uptake of glucose. In the meantime, increase the number of super meals/snacks to at least four a day to help the body perform its own cleansing and detoxification.

For those times that you consume an unhealthy meal (e.g. eating out at a fast food restaurant), don't worry about it excessively. In fact, you should expect this to happen instead of trying to avoid it. The key here is to know how to handle it and reduce the impact to your health. Do the best you can with your food selection at the restaurant (refer to the dining out guidelines in Chapter 7) and follow up your next meal with super foods.

Nutritional Supplementation
Use nutritional supplementation to close the gap between your new nutritional profile (of "live" super foods) and your nutrient needs based on your health state. Start with a wholefood or 100% natural, additive-free multivitamin/mineral supplement as a foundation. Although this will not help to lower your blood glucose level, it will ensure that your body is obtaining a minimum set of nutrients to complement your new super meal regimen. Other critical supplements to consider include CoQ10 (300 mg), alpha lipoic acid (500 mg), chromium (800 mcg), Vitamin C (500 mg), Vitamin E (500 IU), pharmaceutical-grade fish oil (1500 mg), l-

carnitine (1000 mg), and glyconutrients (1400 mg) – to help with energy, fat burning, antioxidation, immune system support, glucose control, and insulin sensitivity. If you are not obtaining at least 32 grams of fiber each day, add 2 tablespoons of freshly ground flaxseed to your beverage or salad at least twice a day; and, take a plant-based digestive enzyme supplement if you are eating primarily cooked vegetables.

Note: Refer to page 129, pages 139-144, or page 374 for a list of nutritional food-based supplements.

After several weeks of eating super meals, if you need help to lower your blood glucose level that final 10 points, perform a cleansing/detox or increase your exercise frequency. If you still need help, use one of the nutrients that help to increase insulin sensitivity, e.g. 150 to 200 mg of gymnema sylvestre before each meal. However, do not rely on these nutrients as a constant crutch to lower your insulin/glucose levels.

Exercise

Request a cardio stress test from your doctor before you start an exercise regimen. Start with a safe exercise regimen such as walking 20-30 minutes each day. Do not make the mistake that I made and try to make up for all the years of not exercising by overdoing the exercise. It is a long journey and the key here is consistency, not duration or intensity. Also, try to get 30 minutes of sunlight daily.

In two to three weeks, add 10-15 minutes of weight-resistance training on alternate days. This type of exercise eventually increases the uptake of glucose in the muscle cells, which is similar to what some of the diabetic drugs attempt to do.

Recordkeeping

During the first stage, you should use a daily record logbook of some kind to keep track of your meals, readings, drugs, exercise, activities, sleep patterns, how you feel, and appointments. This will be invaluable to you and your doctor, especially when you're trying to figure out why your readings are too high. Also, it will be invaluable because it will show what you did well when your blood glucose readings were in the normal range. It is important to record and track your progress as your health improves;

and, use that progress to motivate yourself to continue on your journey to better health.

Set aside specific times of the day (e.g. first thing in the morning, before meals, after meals, the end of the day) to update your record log. Use the weekend or other spare time to analyze the data to identify any corrective actions. If you implement any corrective actions, document them in your logbook along with the rationale for the corrective action.

Testing
Blood glucose testing is the *most powerful diagnostic tool* that you have to collect data and help you understand the cause and effect of how your body is performing and reacting to food, exercise, drugs and other events in your life. Ensure that you have completed a physical with your doctor so that you have a complete understanding of your health in all areas, not just your diabetes. For example, high homocysteine and C-reactive protein levels are indicators of increased "quiet" inflammation that will need to be addressed with cleansing and anti-inflammatory foods.

It is critical to increase your blood glucose testing (especially post-meal testing) to collect more data to help determine when and why your blood glucose levels are too high and too low. The post-meal test is very important because it is a strong indicator of your body's level of insulin resistance and inflammation. The data that you collect from the testing will be invaluable to help you and your doctor decide what corrective actions to take to get your blood glucose level back into the normal range. Please keep in mind that there will be times when your glucose levels will be high for no apparent reason, but, the more you test, the more infrequent will be those types of occurrences.

During the first stage, you will want to ensure the changes to your nutrition are working and your blood glucose level is moving in the right direction. If you have past records of your meals, your drugs, and your glucose readings, then, you will have a good base of information to compare when you begin eating the "live" super foods. You will be pleasantly surprised at how quickly your body will respond to the eating of the "live" super foods. This will give you the motivation to continue to make the necessary changes.

BG Testing Analysis

Because we all respond differently to foods, you must increase your blood glucose (BG) testing to collect more data and help determine the specific foods that keep your glucose level high, especially after meals. Also, you will be able to determine most cause-and-effect relationships with food, exercise, drugs, and other events including stress. With more data, you can perform a better analysis of what is really happening so that you can make the appropriate corrective actions to improve your future blood glucose levels.

Author's Personal Note: The following are some of the mistakes I made during the first stage (and proceeding stages). Keep in mind that although we are all different, and, we biochemically respond differently to foods and other stimuli, these mistakes may give you some insight into your specific situation. Hopefully, it will give you some confidence because despite all the mistakes I made, I was *still* able to get my glucose under control and eventually reverse the disease in less than four months. Ironically, it was these mistakes that provided me with the most invaluable knowledge that I was able to use to improve my future blood glucose levels, and reduce my insulin resistance and inflammation.

- When I had high BG readings in the morning, I was able to trace this back to 3 primary reasons: large dinner meals, a high sugar-based snack before bed, and an intense exercise session after dinner. When I had other high readings, I determined that I had taken the wrong amount (too little) of insulin.

- When I had low BG readings during the mid-morning, this was primarily due to: not eating breakfast; eating too small of a breakfast; an imbalanced breakfast of too much grain (cereal) and sugar; and, injecting too much insulin a couple of times.

- When I had high BG readings in the afternoon, this was due to: eating lunch at a fast food restaurant; vending machine food that didn't have much fiber; drinking too much apple juice or other bottled beverage; forgetting to take my insulin shot; having a snack of just some fruit.

- When my post-meal BG readings were still high, my body's cells still had a high level of insulin resistance, due to: eating too large of a meal; and, eating too much rice that my body was unable to process. Perform a thorough cleansing/detox, increase your intake of green foods to reduce the insulin resistance and get enough sleep.
- When I had high BG readings in the evening, this was due to: eating out; eating a large meal; eating too much macaroni and cheese; eating too much garlic bread; drinking too much bottled juices; and, not taking enough insulin.

Author's Personal Note: I was fortunate that my mistakes led me through a successful journey without setting me back in any significant way.

Check to ensure your average fasting glucose levels are consistently within a tighter range, with a standard deviation of less than 11 mg/dl. The standard deviation denotes a stability of your blood glucose readings, indicating that your readings are not too high and not too low, with a concentrated (tight) "Bell-curve" distribution. This is an overlooked point that most diabetics are not aware that you can have a good average reading, but it may be misleading if you have high readings that are offset by low readings. For example, the average for the readings of 80 and 120 and the readings of 90 and 110 is the same (100), but the deviation for the first two readings is 20 while the deviation for the second set of readings is 10. Consequently, the second set of readings indicates more stability and is a better indication of tighter glucose control.

Other Medical Testing
Ensure the following preventive measures are being taken:
- Foot care: filament test and proper bathing – to prevent ulcers and amputation.
- Eye care: early screening for retinopathy – to prevent blindness.
- Kidney care: early screening for protein in the urine and high blood pressure – to prevent kidney failure.
- Cardiovascular care: cardio stress test; tests for high blood pressure, inflammation markers (e.g. homocysteine, lipoprotein(a), C-reactive protein) – to prevent a heart attack or stroke.

Drugs/Medication
Hopefully, you are taking this disease seriously enough so that you don't have to take any diabetic drugs. If you have to take diabetic drugs during the first stage (as I did), you should be following your doctor's orders, but working with him/her to eventually wean off the drugs.

Mind & Spirit
This is the time to be selfish – remember to take care of Number 1 – You! Develop and maintain a positive attitude with life as well as an open mind to new ideas about health and nutrition. Focus on what you need to do to *be* healthy, not the reasons why you *cannot* be healthy. What you focus on will be what defines you and your journey – so focus on the positive, not the negative. Establish relationships with positive people full of hope, and healthy people who have either beat their diabetes or are controlling it with nutrition and exercise.

Look for what you love about your family members and friends instead of what's wrong with them. Acknowledge these positive perspectives to each of them individually and together. Keep in mind that discord with family members and friends can create stress. Also, starting out on this new journey may threaten some relationships that are founded on co-dependency. Some of their resistance to your changes may be due to their concern that they may lose your friendship. Assure them that that is not the case. But also assure them that you will not allow them to deter you from your new journey. Try to find a partner or friend who will work with you and support you on your journey.

Review Chapter 13 for ways to relax and sleep to improve the health of your Mind and Spirit; and, leverage your Mind and Spirit to improve the health of your Body. Many diabetics do not obtain enough *quality* rest or sleep, which doesn't give their bodies a chance to heal during the night. Do not hesitate to use meditation, prayer or a relaxation technique to help you sleep better and build your Spirit to provide strength and stability to your emotions (Mind) and your physical health (Body). Read a daily passage from the Bible or a similar book. Review the inspirational quotes in Chapter 13 to define your own inspirational quote -- to repeat and reaffirm yourself every day, e.g. "I am somebody."; "Don't give up, don't every give up."; "I will defeat this disease, it will not defeat me."

During this stage, you should be setting up your support system – with positive-minded people, including a wellness coach. Find a local support group by contacting your church, the American Diabetes Association (ADA) or other local agency. Look for an Internet diabetic forum or go to the following ADA website: www.diabetes.org/communityprograms-and-localevents.jsp and select "Community Programs & Events" to find local diabetic support groups in your community.

Education

Diabetes is your enemy. During the first stage, it is very important to increase your knowledge about your enemy, diabetes. Otherwise, without that knowledge, your enemy will defeat you. In order to defeat your enemy, you must develop a "war mentality" and learn everything you can about your enemy. Try to obtain as much information as possible from the web, the library and your doctor. Also, buy a book about natural healing, health and nutrition. Attend local health fairs and take a class about heart disease, stroke or diabetes. Knowledge will empower you.

During the first stage, it is also very important to increase your knowledge about food and drugs. It is very important to learn how to read food labels and know what to look for when buying any food. Some of the key ingredients to be wary of include: partially hydrogenated oil, high fructose corn syrup, refined sugar, artificial sweeteners, processed flour, enriched flour, low fiber. Be wary of such words as low fat, low cholesterol, low carb, no sugar, no fat, fortified, enriched, artificial, or any word that you don't understand.

It will take some time to educate yourself about purchasing the right foods. Initially it will be difficult to stop purchasing the "dead" processed foods. But, it will come easier when you start to feel the benefits of eating properly. Then, you will actually enjoy grocery shopping – because you will truly know what you're doing; and, you will know in your heart and soul that this is right for you and for your family. Personally, I used to dislike grocery shopping, but now I really enjoy it.

Knowledge about diabetes will set you free and empower you to make the changes to improve your health. Ignorance of this disease will create fear and make you uncertain of what to do and will sentence you to a state of poor health. You must also increase your knowledge about nutrition, vitamins and specific wholefood and superfood nutrients associated with cardiovascular health, diabetes and blood glucose control, e.g. Brussel sprouts, stringbeans, fiber, plant protein, flaxseeds, pulse food, sea vegetables, glyconutrients, cinnamon bark extract, gymnema sylvestre, bitter melon, fish oil, alpha lipoic acid, CoQ10, chromium, l-carnitine, and carnosine. This will allow you to spend your money wisely when buying food and nutritional supplements. This will also allow you to identify alternative solutions to your high blood pressure, high cholesterol, or other diabetes-related ailment. Refer to the wellness protocols in Chapter 15 and the clinical studies listed in the Appendix for additional information about nutrition and various nutritional supplements that have been studied and used successfully to fight diabetes and other related diseases.

Stage 2 BG Control with Drugs

This is the stage where most diabetics transition to when they are unable to control their blood glucose level with nutrition and exercise and they need drug therapy to help lower their glucose level. Type 1 diabetics automatically transition to this stage because they need insulin to control their blood glucose level.

During this stage you and your doctor are trying to use drugs to force your blood glucose level lower and eventually bring it within the normal range. If your average glucose level is above 200 mg/dl, your doctor will probably prescribe drug therapy to get the glucose level below 200 as a first step. Once successful with that, then, your doctor will work with you to try to get your glucose level below 120 mg/dl, by making changes to your nutrition and exercise. If unsuccessful, your doctor may propose an increase or a change in your drug therapy to affect a lowering of the blood glucose level.

Hopefully this will buy some time for you to make the necessary changes to your nutrition and exercise. However, it appears that many diabetics rely heavily on the drugs and do not make the necessary changes to their nutrition and exercise.

Warning: The biggest mistake that diabetics make during this stage is the total reliance on the drugs to bring and keep their blood glucose level within the normal range. The drugs are usually effective initially in forcing the blood glucose lower, but eventually the drugs lose their effectiveness. In addition, the drugs do very little to help the body repair itself and reduce its dependency on the drugs. Consequently, the disease continues to quietly deteriorate the body internally, increasing the diabetic's reliance on more drugs.

Nutrition
Because you are now using drugs to force your body to lower your blood glucose level, you should be making more significant changes to what you're currently eating and drinking by increasing your consumption of the 5 "live" super foods and decreasing your consumption of the 5 "dead" processed foods, especially the refined flour and sugar products that stimulate the glucose spikes and the excess insulin production.

Warning: Because your drug dosage may be too strong once you start eating the "live" super foods, be wary of potential low blood sugar episodes – ask your doctor to reduce your drug dosage.

And, now that you are using drugs to try to lower your blood glucose level, it becomes even more important to perform periodic cleansing and detoxification because the drugs add to your body's toxic load and inhibit your body from repairing and healing itself. Cleansing/detoxification will help your body to more effectively remove the excess toxins, acid waste and other chemicals from the drugs and to ensure optimum absorption and utilization of the nutrients you are now consuming from the "live" super foods. Add nutritional supplements (from page 120 or page 374).

Exercise
More than likely you were not exercising enough in Stage 1, so start an exercise regimen and gradually increase your frequency (number of times per week). Then, increase your duration (number of minutes per exercise session) to burn more glucose and prevent its conversion to fat. It is the consistency and duration that will eventually lead to your body burning fat – especially when you exercise daily and reach the 30-minute duration level.

If you have not started any type of weight-resistance exercise, then, start with something simple such as carrying a three-pound weight in each hand while you walk. Weight-resistance exercise will increase the uptake of glucose in the muscle cells and is similar to what some of the diabetic drugs are trying to do. As a result, this will eventually allow you to reduce the amount of diabetic drugs that you're taking. Exercise also helps to stimulate the lymphatic and gastrointestinal systems, helping the body to remove accumulated toxins and other waste.

Testing/Recordkeeping/Analysis
During this stage, you need to increase your blood glucose testing to collect more data – to help you and your doctor to determine what corrective actions to take to get your blood glucose under control and *prevent* your body from becoming *dependent* on the drugs.

If you are not making significant progress, you may want to have your doctor conduct additional testing, especially of your cardiac risk/inflammation factors (e.g. homocysteine), which may be preventing your cells from getting healthy because of the high level of inflammation in your body. If these factors are high, go to the appropriate wellness protocol section in Chapter 15 for natural solutions to reduce their levels.

Drugs/Medication
During this stage, continue to follow your doctor's orders concerning any drugs you're taking. Continue to keep detailed records of your drug usage and results. Contact your doctor if you are no longer able to maintain your blood glucose control with the drugs. It doesn't make sense to take a drug if it isn't working properly.

Mind & Spirit

Continue to improve the health of your Mind and Spirit by learning how to relax, sleep better and find time for yourself. You will eventually notice an increase in a positive attitude and motivation. If not, use your Spirit to improve your Mind-Body connection and find your center.

Leverage the people in your support group to help you and you help them. If the support group isn't working because it's controlled by negative people, find a new support group or go to your church pastor and set up your own group. Begin to use more of your support system to provide motivation and also to help others. You will find that helping others will motivate you even more.

Education

During this stage, you need to acquire more knowledge about nutrition and diabetes. As previously mentioned, knowledge about this disease will set you free and empower you to make the changes to improve your health. You must also learn about the drugs you're taking so that you fully understand their drawbacks and dangerous side effects.

If you choose to adopt the mentality that there is a war going on inside your body, then, diabetes is the enemy that is waging that war within your body. And, knowledge about the enemy is self-empowering because it drives your actions to help your body fight and defeat the enemy. One way is to envision grocery shopping as the way to obtain the "weapons and ammunition" (the super foods) to fight the "enemy" (diabetes).

Stage 3 BG Control with Reduced Drugs

This is probably the most difficult stage to reach once you and the doctor have chosen to use drug therapy to lower your blood glucose level. It becomes a more difficult battle because your body has to deal with the disease *and* the drugs, which bring along their own toxins and side effects and impedance to the body's healing process. But, it is not impossible for the body to overcome this, as I am living proof of that. I was able to methodically reduce my insulin dosage over a period of three months from more than 60 units a day to less than 5 units a day – until I reached 0 units and my glucose level remained within the normal range.

This will be an important stage for you and the doctor to achieve because your body chemistry will now be able to control its glucose level and keep it within the normal range with a lesser dependence on the drugs. With the proper medical guidance, some Type 1s may reach this stage.

You should be noticing an increase in your energy level and a decrease in your weight (fat) by now. At a minimum, you should be noticing that your clothes are starting to fit more loosely. If not, you will need to optimize your nutrition and exercise regimens.

> **Warning:** If you are able to reach this stage, do not return to your old eating habits because you believe the disease is under control. The disease is partially under control, but your body is still dependent on the drugs! If you return to your old eating habits, your blood glucose levels will increase, causing you to increase your drugs to the previous dosage level; and, you will regress to Stage 2.

During this stage, you should be settling into your nutritional program. At this point, your "super" meals should be dominated by the "live" super foods. If you have not noticed a decrease in cravings by now, perform a periodic cleansing and detoxification to remove the excess acid waste, chemicals, and toxins from the drugs and to ensure optimum absorption of the nutrients from the food. Add one or more nutritional food-based supplements (refer to the list on page 120 or page 374).

Continue to gradually increase your exercise frequency and duration. You should be noticing an increase in energy and a feeling of exhilaration after exercise. Use weight-resistance exercise to train your body to increase its uptake of glucose into the cells and reduce the need to use the diabetic drugs to perform the same function.

Continue with your blood glucose testing, cause-and-effect analysis, use your inner spirit, acquire more knowledge, and implement any corrective actions to your nutrition and exercise regimens.

Stage 4 BG Control without Drugs

Congratulations! This is the first significant sign that your body is healing and winning the war in its fight with diabetes because your body is able to control your blood glucose level and keep it within the normal range *without* any assistance from any diabetic drugs. At this stage your blood glucose level and hemoglobin A1C are both in the normal range because you took the disease seriously enough to make the necessary changes.

The following is a list of other signs that may have occurred so far:
- A loss of body fat, a lower Body Mass Index (BMI), a smaller waist size, looser-fitted clothing
- A noticeable increase in energy level, stamina/endurance
- Steady, average glucose readings of 100 mg/dl with less than 15 mg/dl deviation
- Steady, average post-meal glucose readings of 110 mg/dl or less
- Some improvements in blood cholesterol, blood pressure
- An increase in muscle tone (if you've been performing any weight/resistance training on a consistent basis)
- An increase in well-being, positive attitude

You may have heard of diabetics who were able to get their blood glucose under control with diet and exercise – this is the stage that they were in. Unfortunately, the biggest mistake that these diabetics make is that they relax and as the years pass, the disease progresses ever so slowly and silently until one day they are shocked to find that they have full-blown diabetes. So, if you are able to reach this stage, you are truly blessed – so don't slip up now! The disease is not gone! It is only "under control" at this point. If you return to your old eating habits, your blood glucose levels will return to their previous high levels. And, you will find that it will be even more difficult to lower your blood glucose level.

During this stage, make slight modifications with your nutritional plan to address other health issues, e.g. high blood pressure, high cholesterol. At this point, look for creative ways to improve your nutritional plan with other "live" foods and nutritional food-based supplements.

Refer to Chapter 15 for wellness protocols and specific actions that you can take for high blood pressure, high cholesterol, and other health conditions.

Now that you have your blood glucose under control, you can eat more fruits and use your blender to prepare fresh fruit juices, which help to cleanse your cells and contain fiber to slow down their absorption and reduce your body's craving for sweets. Some of these fruits include apples, blackberries, blueberries, strawberries, and cherries. Although your body can handle some sweet fruits, be wary of tropical fruits and use them sparingly, e.g. bananas, pineapple, watermelon.

If your average post-meal fasting glucose levels are not consistently within a tighter range, this indicates your body's cells still have some insulin resistance. Perform a thorough cleansing/detox, or increase your intake of green foods. Also, add one or more nutritional supplements.

During this stage, continue with your exercise regimen, recordkeeping, cause-and-effect analysis, use your inner spirit, acquire more knowledge, and make any changes to your nutrition and exercise regimens.

Medical Testing
During this stage, you should be discussing alternatives with your doctor for the (non-diabetic) medications that you may be taking. Now that you have reached Stage 4, you've completed the toughest part of the journey, Although it is tempting to stop at Stage 4, hopefully, this information will motivate you to transition to Stage 5.

Stage 5 BG & HbA1C Control

This stage and the next stage indicate that your average blood glucose level is consistently within a tighter range, meal to meal, day to day, without any medication; and the hemoglobin A1C percentage is less than 5.3%. In addition, the critical health parameters of other related ailments are moving towards their normal ranges, e.g. cholesterol, blood pressure, body mass index, minerals, enzymes.

During this stage, continue with your nutritional program, exercise regimen, blood glucose testing, recordkeeping, use your inner spirit, acquire more knowledge, and make any minor changes to your nutrition and exercise regimens. Use supplements to help maintain your health. Because your body is now back in balance biochemically and hormonally, you can eat some "dead" foods once in a while, but don't over do it. You should continue to increase your knowledge and obtain more information about nutrition, supplements and other diseases. This information will motivate you to want to transition to Stage 6.

Stage 6 BG & HbA1C Tighter Control

Congratulations! You will have reached this final stage if:
- Your hemoglobin A1C percentage is less than 5.1% and your fasting and post-meal glucose levels are consistently less than 100 mg/dl, with a standard deviation of less than 11 mg/dl.
- You were able to eat some "dead" foods without negatively affecting your post-meal average glucose level and your hemoglobin A1C.
- You have not taken any diabetic medication since Stage 3.
- Your other critical health parameters for cholesterol, blood pressure, body mass index, minerals, etc. are all within their normal ranges.

During this stage, continue with your nutritional program of "live" foods, but you can eat some "dead" foods, but don't overdo it. Also, you can reduce the number of daily meals, but do not significantly increase the size of the other meals. Utilize wholefood supplements as part of your nutritional maintenance program to maintain a high nutritional level. Continue with your exercise program and increase/decrease the duration or intensity, depending on your health goals.

Reduce your blood glucose testing, but do not stop testing completely. Make certain that you are getting a good sample of different readings during the week, especially post-meal tests. You should continue to have your hemoglobin A1C tested to be fully certain that your health has not regressed. Once all your blood tests (for cholesterol, blood pressure, etc.) are in the normal range, you will have fully reversed and eradicated the disease and other ailments from your body.

Have a party and celebrate! This is a major accomplishment! You can finally enjoy parties, picnics, weddings, holidays, and other celebrations without being frantic and overly concerned about the food. However, you should continue to rely upon your inner Spirit – it is probably the single most important factor that got you through this journey.

Take the time to share your testimony with others. Become an advocate within your church or community – you have first-hand knowledge, experience and insight that others will be seeking. Don't forget to acknowledge those who helped you along the way. They deserve your gratitude and recognition, as much as anyone.

Review your logbook and other notes. You will uncover some interesting information about your journey, especially during the tough times when it didn't appear you were going to get better. This new insight will be invaluable to you becoming an advocate and helping others who don't believe there is a way out. You are now one of the blessed ones, you are now one of the true believers who made it, despite all the odds. Now, it is your responsibility to help others and spread the new ministry that God has given you.

Increase your knowledge – not to help you, but to help others. Talk to experts in the fields of nutrition, supplements, exercise, spirit, disease, drugs, and other areas in which you may have some interest. Reread this book – there are concepts that you will grasp better now that the pressure is off and you can relax. For up-to-date information about diabetes and nutritional supplements, contact the author at:
Email: Engineer@DeathToDiabetes.com
Website: www.DeathToDiabetes.com
Business address: 940 Holt Rd. #190   Webster, NY 14580-9101

Document your journey, based on your journal and personal experiences. Have a loved one review your document and provide his/her feedback. This document will become your personal testimony. You will be pleasantly surprised how much you have learned and how far you have come on your journey. And, this will help to fuel your life and the lives of those around you. May God continue to bless you on your journey.

Chapter 15. Diabetic Complications

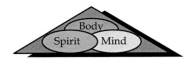

Diabetic Complications

There are several long-term microvascular and macrovascular complications that develop if your diabetes is not managed properly and your blood glucose is not maintained within the normal range. They are kidney disease, eye disease, nerve disease, and heart disease. Other health complications that can occur before or after you become diabetic include: high blood pressure; high inflammation (high homocysteine, C-reactive protein, cholesterol, fibrinogen); fatigue; and, frequent infections (especially gum disease). The first section of this chapter describes these diabetic complications, including how they develop and how they are medically diagnosed. The second section provides a set of wellness protocols that prevent, control, or reverse the effects of these complications. Each wellness protocol identifies and describes a list of specific (*food*-based) nutrients that are listed in alphabetical order.

> **KEY MESSAGE:** If you control your blood glucose level and hemoglobin A1C within their normal ranges, you will not develop these long-term complications because of your diabetes. Otherwise, at least 4 out of every 5 diabetics will develop one or more of these complications.

> **WARNING!** Although the nutritional supplements listed in this chapter can be beneficial to your health, some of them may conflict with your current drug therapy. Consequently, *always* review your nutritional supplementation strategy with your doctor to prevent any life-threatening health complications.

Kidney Disease (Nephropathy)

Diabetic nephropathy occurs when there is too much inflammation and glucose in the bloodstream, clogging the small capillaries that feed into the kidneys. In addition, there is an excess amount of acid waste in the blood that further clogs these small capillaries. The accumulation of calcium (due to the extra insulin) and acid waste in the kidneys causes the formation of kidney stones and ultimately causes kidney cells to die. Because kidney cells cannot be regenerated or repaired, the remaining cells have to work that much harder to filter substances from the blood. To help with the filtering process, the heart increases the flow of blood plasma to the kidneys, which in turn elevates blood pressure. As the kidney cells continue to die, the risk of kidney failure increases dramatically. This eventually leads to one or both of the kidneys losing their ability to function properly, characterized by high protein levels in the urine. Alcohol, tobacco, conventional animal meat, and many of the other "dead" processed foods accelerate the deterioration of the kidneys.

Each kidney is comprised of more than a million units called nephrons. Each nephron has a tuft of blood vessels called a glomerulus. The glomerulus filters blood and forms urine, which drains down into collecting ducts to the ureter. The earliest detectable change in the course of diabetic nephropathy is a thickening in the glomerulus. At this stage, the kidney may start allowing more albumin (protein) than normal in the urine, and this can be detected by sensitive tests for albumin. This stage is called "microalbuminuria" (micro refers to the small amounts of albumin). As diabetic nephropathy progresses, increasing numbers of glomeruli are destroyed. This increases the amounts of albumin being excreted in the urine, and may be detected by ordinary urinalysis techniques. At this stage, a kidney biopsy clearly shows diabetic nephropathy.

Protein may appear in the urine for five to ten years before other symptoms develop. High blood pressure often accompanies diabetic nephropathy. Over time, the kidney's ability to function starts to decline.

Diabetic nephropathy may eventually lead to chronic kidney failure. The disorder continues to progress toward end-stage kidney disease, usually within two to six years after the appearance of high protein in the urine (proteinuria).

Diabetic nephropathy is the most common cause of chronic kidney failure and end-stage kidney disease in the United States. People with both Type 1 and Type 2 diabetes are at risk. The risk is higher if blood glucose levels are poorly controlled. However, once nephropathy develops, the greatest rate of progression is seen in patients with high blood pressure.

Diabetic nephropathy is generally accompanied by other diabetic complications including high blood pressure, retinopathy, and vascular (blood vessel) changes, although these may not be obvious during the early stages of nephropathy. Nephropathy may be present for many years before high protein in the urine or chronic kidney failure develops.

Diagnosis & Tests
The first laboratory abnormality is a positive microalbuminuria test, which implies that you are very likely to develop diabetic nephropathy. Most often, the diagnosis is suspected when a routine urinalysis of a person with diabetes shows too much protein in the urine (proteinuria). The urinalysis may also show glucose in the urine, especially if blood glucose is poorly controlled.

There may or may not be signs of other diabetic complications. High blood pressure may be present or develop rapidly and may be difficult to control. Serum creatinine and BUN (blood urea nitrogen) may increase as kidney damage progresses. If there is any doubt in the diagnosis, a kidney biopsy may be performed to confirm the diagnosis and to study the extent of the disease.

Foods and nutrients such as filtered water, celery, cucumbers, lemons, limes, and cranberries nourish, protect and cleanse the kidneys and the bladder. Refer to the wellness protocol section in this chapter for more details.

Eye Disease (Retinopathy)

After the kidneys, the eyes are usually the second major organ that is damaged by the effects of diabetes. The signs of damage to the eyes include blurry vision, spots, and loss of vision, which can lead to blindness if the macula is damaged and there is a loss of blood supply to the retina.

The retina is a nerve layer at the back of the eye that senses light and helps send images to the brain, similar to film in a camera. Diabetic retinopathy is caused by damage to blood vessels of the retina, leading to the loss of vision and even blindness. In the initial stages (called non-proliferative diabetic retinopathy), the arteries in the retina become weakened and leak fluid or blood, forming small, dot-like hemorrhages. This can blur or distort the images that the retina sends to the brain leading to blurred vision, called "background retinopathy".

In the next stage (proliferative retinopathy), circulation problems cause areas of the retina to become oxygen-deprived or ischemic. New, fragile blood vessels develop in the retina and branch out into the vitreous humor in the middle of the eye as the circulatory system attempts to maintain adequate oxygen levels within the retina. This is called neovascularization. Unfortunately, these blood vessels are fragile and hemorrhage easily, causing blood to leak into the retina and vitreous. This creates spots or floaters, causing a decrease in vision and scarring. In the later stages of the disease, continued abnormal blood vessel growth and scar tissue cause serious problems such as retinal detachment and glaucoma.

The likelihood and severity of retinopathy increase with the duration of diabetes and is likely to be worse if blood glucose is poorly controlled. Almost all people who have had diabetes for more than 30 years will show signs of diabetic retinopathy, as it is the *leading cause of blindness* in working-age Americans.

Diagnosis & Tests

The diagnosis of diabetic retinopathy is made following a detailed examination of the retina with an ophthalmoscope. Ophthalmoscopy is an examination of the back part of the eyeball (fundus), which includes the retina, optic disc, choroid, and blood vessels. Ophthalmoscopy is performed as part of a routine physical or complete eye examination to detect and evaluate symptoms of retinal detachment and eye diseases such as glaucoma and cataracts. Most patients with diabetic retinopathy are referred to vitreo-retinal surgeons who specialize in treating this disease.

Cataracts & Glaucoma

Diabetics are twice as likely to develop eye diseases such as cataract and glaucoma. A cataract is a clouding or opaque area that develops over the lens of the eye, and thickens, preventing light rays from passing through the lens and focusing on the retina. You may have a cataract if you need a stronger light for reading or sewing, but, no matter how bright the light, your vision seems dim; or, the glare of a car's headlights makes it difficult to see.

The primary causes of cataracts include glycosylation and oxidation -- due to the accumulated exposure to ultraviolet sunlight, tobacco, or diabetes with uncontrolled glucose levels that damage the proteins in the eye lens. Consequently, one of the key strategies to either slow down or even prevent the formation of a cataract is to reduce the amount of glycosylation and oxidation – by wearing sunglasses and eating foods and supplements that contain antioxidants, e.g. spinach, red grapes, carrots, bilberry, beta carotene, Vitamin C, l-carnosine. Studies continue to show that people with cataracts tend to have low serum levels of beta carotene and Vitamin C. These nutrients will not cure cataracts, but they will prevent further damage. Even after someone has had cataract surgery, he/she will still need to consider antioxidant nutrients, otherwise, the new lens will become cloudy from the same oxidative process.

Glaucoma is an increase in fluid pressure inside the eye that leads to optic nerve damage and loss of vision. Glaucoma is called the "sneak thief" of sight because it has no obvious signs at first – it is painless and has no effect on vision. By the time you notice that your vision has deteriorated, glaucoma has done its damage. Consequently, **annual exams are a must, especially if glaucoma runs in your family.**

A normal eye is filled with fluid, which drains through tissue between the iris and the cornea. With glaucoma, the draining of the fluid slows down or stops completely as the eyes' "drainage pipes" become backed up like a clogged drain. The backup of the fluid builds intraocular pressure throughout the eye, damaging blood vessels that feed the retina and optic nerve. Without the proper nutrients, the optic nerve begins to die, and so does your vision.

It is important to note that many people with glaucoma don't realize there is a loss of vision because they don't actually "see" dark areas – there are no visible "walls" of the so-called "tunnel". People with peripheral vision loss just have a narrower visual field. People with normal vision see images of their surroundings and have a naturally limited range of vision. They do not "see" darkness all around them. People with glaucoma don't "see" darkness either – they just see less of their surroundings. This is why annual eye exams are so important – they can catch the glaucoma before irreparable damage is done.

Once your doctor diagnoses glaucoma, eye drop medication will be necessary to reduce the eye pressure and prevent any further loss of vision. High doses of supplements such as natural Vitamin C with bioflavonoids (1000 to 2000 mg) and bilberry/eyebright (350 to 500 mg) may help to draw fluid out of the eye, but this has not been completely verified with any well-controlled clinical studies. Refer to the wellness protocol section in this chapter for more details.

Nerve Disease (Neuropathy)

About 15 million Americans suffer from neuropathy, a nerve problem that can damage the nervous system and cause unrelenting aches and pains. In particular, 60% of diabetics develop peripheral neuropathy when their blood glucose reaches and remains at dangerous levels for several years. When blood glucose levels rise too high and remain too high, the glucose molecule attaches itself to cells permanently and is eventually converted to a poison sugar called sorbitol that destroys nerve cells (nerve death). The signs of nerve damage include tingling, burning, and the loss of feeling (touch) in the feet, which lead to a high incidence of foot infections, foot ulcers, and amputations. If motor or autonomic nerves are damaged, this can lead to the loss of muscle control, bladder control, and bowel control. Eventually, after many years of poor blood glucose control and deterioration of the nervous system, the cells in the brain may also become damaged.

Peripheral Neuropathy

The peripheral nerves that go to the arms, hands, legs, and feet are responsible for relaying information from the central nervous system (brain and spinal cord) to muscles and other organs. Peripheral nerves also relay information back to the spinal cord and brain from the skin, joints, and other organs. High blood glucose levels create trace chemicals that damage the blood vessels that bring oxygen to some nerves and cause oxidative stress to nerve cells, and the degeneration of nerve fibers and the myelin sheath covering on the nerves. In addition, the high glucose and insulin levels can cause calcium and other minerals to leech from the synaptic junctions. Synaptic junctions can only retain a limited amount of glucose, insulin, and electrolytes; therefore, when glucose or excess insulin enters, something else must be released. Since there is usually a plentiful supply of calcium and potassium from food, as well as a plentiful supply of oxygen from the lungs, these elements are generally the first to be discharged. However, once the nerve cell becomes shorter, it remains in that condition until it is over stimulated.

The calcium ion pump is responsible for the propagation of the nerve impulse along the myelin sheath. As a result, each time the synaptic junctions and nerve cells lose calcium, they conduct fewer impulses. A similar process is facilitated by the electric fields of tiny electrical charges, which are keyed to potassium levels. Atrophy occurs when any body part is used with less and less frequency. Similarly, when the electrical signals are not propagating correctly and the body assumes that the nerve is no longer necessary and, to conserve energy, further reduces support for that nerve cell. In turn the nerve cell shrinks in order to function due to a reduced input of fuel and oxygen while still keeping itself viable until the nerve ceases to function. Consequently untreated diabetes, hypoglycemia or poor glucose control could cause wide variations in the blood calcium, potassium, sugar, insulin, and oxygen levels thereby resulting in oxygen deprivation and loss of nerve integrity. Damaged nerves stop sending messages or send messages too slowly or at the wrong times. This leads to neuropathic symptoms such as tingling or numbness in the feet.

As a result, damage to these peripheral nerves can make the arms, hands, legs, or feet feel numb. Also, you might not be able to feel pain, heat, or cold when you should. You may feel shooting pains, burning or tingling like "pins and needles". These feelings are often worse at night and make it difficult to sleep. Most of the time these feelings are on both sides of your body, like in both of your feet, but they can be on just one side. Some of the other symptoms of peripheral neuropathy include prickly or burning pains, tightness of the skin, hypersensitivity to touch, impaired coordination, balance problems, difficulty climbing stairs or difficulty getting up from a sitting position, urinary urgency, erectile dysfunction, acid reflux and lightheadedness. The numbness that typically accompanies neuropathy can be particularly problematic because minor injuries may go unnoticed, turning into health problems that are not minor at all.

Peripheral nerve damage can change the shape of your feet because foot muscles get weak and the tendons in the foot get shorter. In some cases, failure of nerves controlling blood vessels, intestinal function, and other organs results in abnormal blood pressure, digestion, and loss of other basic involuntary processes. Peripheral neuropathy may involve damage to a single nerve or nerve group (mononeuropathy) or may affect multiple nerves (polyneuropathy).

Damage to Autonomic Nervous System & Brain

After a period of years, diabetes can damage the nerves of the autonomic nervous system, and eventually, even affect the nerve cells of the brain. Damage to the autonomic nervous system causes one or more of the following:

- Difficulty in feeling the symptoms of hypoglycemia (low blood sugar).

- Nausea, vomiting, constipation, or diarrhea due to damage to the autonomic nerves that go to the stomach, intestines, and other parts of the digestive system, making food pass through the digestive system too slowly or too quickly.
- Erectile dysfunction or impotence due to the damage to the autonomic nerves going to the man's penis nerves.
- Prevention of a woman's vagina from getting wet when she wants to have sex or having less feeling around her vagina.
- A faster beating of the heart or the heart beating at different speeds.
- Difficulty in knowing when to go to the bathroom due to damage to the autonomic nerves that go to the bladder. The damage can also make it hard to feel when your bladder is empty. Both problems can cause you to hold urine for too long, which can lead to bladder infections.
- Slow movement of your blood to keep your blood pressure steady when you change position due to damage to the autonomic nerves going to the blood vessels that keep your blood pressure steady. When you go from lying down to standing up or when you exercise a lot, the sudden changes in blood pressure can make you dizzy.
- Double vision due to damage to the autonomic nerves going to the cranial nerves that control the eye muscles. Damage to these nerves usually happens in one eye. This problem happens all of a sudden and usually lasts for a short time.
- A side of the face hangs lower or sags due to damage to the autonomic nerves going to the cranial nerves that control the sides of the face. Damage to these nerves usually happens on only one side of the face. This nerve damage causes that side of the face to hang lower or sag. Usually the lower eyelid and lips sag. This problem, which is called Bell's palsy, happens all of a sudden and tends to correct itself most of the time.

Diagnosis & Tests
The diagnosis of diabetic neuropathy is made on the basis of symptoms and a physical exam. During the exam, the doctor may check blood pressure and heart rate, muscle strength, reflexes, and sensitivity to position, vibration, temperature, or a light touch.

The doctor may also perform other tests to help determine the type and extent of nerve damage including a foot exam, nerve conduction test, electromyography test, sensory testing, heart rate variability check, ultrasound, and a nerve or skin biopsy.

A comprehensive *foot exam* assesses skin, circulation, and sensation. The test can be done during a routine office visit. To assess protective sensation or feeling in the foot, a nylon monofilament (similar to a bristle on a hairbrush) attached to a wand is used to touch the foot. Those who cannot sense pressure from the monofilament have lost protective sensation and are at risk for developing foot sores that may not heal properly. Other tests include checking reflexes and assessing vibration perception, which is more sensitive than touch pressure.

A *nerve conduction test* checks the transmission of electrical current through a nerve. With this test, an image of the nerve conducting an electrical signal is projected onto a screen. Nerve impulses that seem slower or weaker than usual indicate possible damage. This test allows the doctor to assess the condition of all the nerves in the arms and legs.

An *electromyography (EMG) test* shows how well muscles respond to electrical signals transmitted by nearby nerves. The electrical activity of the muscle is displayed on a screen. A response that is slower or weaker than usual suggests damage to the nerve or muscle. This test is often done at the same time as nerve conduction tests.

An *ultrasound test* uses sound waves to produce an image of internal organs. An ultrasound of the bladder and other parts of the urinary tract, for example, can show how these organs preserve a normal structure and whether the bladder empties completely after urination.

Brain Damage

Current research indicates a connection between diabetes and Alzheimer's disease. Since diabetes damages the nerves of the peripheral and autonomic nervous systems, it would follow that, eventually, it would affect the nerve cells of the brain itself.

The average human brain, which weighs about 3 pounds, is comprised of billions of neurons (brain cells), water, and phospholipids, namely arachidonic acid and docosahexaenoic acid. The brain produces electrical signals, which, together with chemical reactions, lets the parts of the body communicate. Although the brain is only 2% of the body's weight, it uses 20% of the oxygen supply, more than 50% of the glucose, and gets 20% of the blood flow. Blood vessels (arteries, capillaries, veins) supply the brain with oxygen and nourishment, and take away waste. More subtly, the blood-brain barrier protects the brain from chemical intrusion from the rest of the body. Blood flowing into the brain is filtered so that many harmful chemicals cannot enter the brain.

When a part of the brain (e.g. brain cells, blood vessels, neuro-transmitters) becomes damaged due to a combination of consistently high blood glucose levels and other factors, after a period of years, a diabetic may develop Alzheimer's or some other brain-related ailment. These other factors may include exposure to aluminum (e.g. sodas, aluminum utensils) and other chemicals and toxins that have gradually built up in the body, and some accumulating in the brain. This can lead to a formation of a sticky plaque that inhibits the transmission of brain signals. This decrease in signal transmission causes atrophy and death of the brain cells, which leads to further decreased signal transmission, and decreased neural transmission, which leads to further deterioration of the brain's function. This decrease in brain function may be exhibited in many ways, including a significant increase in memory loss, e.g. confusion, forgetfulness, or a major change in behavioral and personality such as unprovoked anger or loss of social skills.

Note: Neurotransmitters are small molecules whose function is to transmit nerve signals (impulses) from one nerve cell to another. Neurotransmitters are chemical messengers that neurons use to tell other neurons that they have received an impulse. There are many different neurotransmitters - some trigger the receiving neuron to send an impulse and some stop it from doing so. Neurotransmitters include: acetylcholine, serotonin, histamine, glutamate, gamma aminobutyric acid glycine, aspartate, histamine, norepinephrine, epinephrine (adrenalin), endorphins, dopamine, adenosine triphosphate (ATP), and nitric oxide.

Because of the amount of time that it may take for the brain to begin deterioration, the diabetic will experience problems with one or more of the other organs long before a disease like Alzheimer's settles in. Consequently, there is time to nourish, protect, and exercise the brain to prevent these types of complications. Refer to the wellness protocol section in this chapter for more details.

Cardiovascular (Heart) Disease

The circulatory system, which consists of the heart, arteries, veins, capillaries, and blood, is responsible for delivering oxygen and other nutrients to cells throughout the body. The heart's pumping action forces oxygenated blood from the lungs to reach millions of cells throughout the body via arteries and capillaries. After the cells have been nourished, blood returns to the heart through the venous system and is then re-oxygenated in the lungs.

A muscle-vein system, often referred to as the "second heart", is a system of muscles, veins, and valves in the calf and foot that work together to push deoxygenated blood back up to the heart and lungs. The second heart vein valves act as trapdoors that open and close with each muscle contraction to prevent the backflow of blood.

The major types of vascular disease that affect the circulatory system are cardiovascular disease, which affects the heart (and, is sometimes referred to as heart disease); cerebrovascular disease, which affects the brain; and, peripheral vascular disease, which affects the legs. If blood flow is blocked in one of these areas, it may cause a heart attack, a stroke, or a cramping pain in the leg muscles on exertion (intermittent claudication). When second heart vein valves in the legs become defective or weak, blood can pool in veins causing varicose veins, spider veins, and swelling.

A **heart attack** (or myocardial infarction) occurs when a blockage develops in one of the arteries supplying blood to the heart. A **stroke** occurs when the blockage develops in one of the arteries supplying blood to the brain. A leg cramping occurs when the leg muscles are not being supplied with enough blood for the physical effort demanded. In the case of a heart attack or a stroke, a lack of blood stops the heart or brain from working so it shuts down and the body collapses. In the case of leg cramping, a condition called normal inadequate leg circulation (NIC) can develop when leg valves do not close completely, resulting in feelings of heaviness, a sensation of tension (chiefly located in the calves), restless legs, and edema (swelling). The ropy, swollen knots known as varicose veins occur when the incompetent valves cause blood to pool in the larger leg veins, forcing them to bulge against the skin surface. This slowing of the blood transit time triggers the clotting response causing pockets to form, trapping blood and resulting in minor clots and inflammation. This condition, called phlebitis, can become life threatening if the clot breaks free and travels to the heart, brain, or lungs.

Heart disease is the number one killer disease in most countries including the United States, where over a million people die each year, one death every 33 seconds. More than 60 million Americans have some form of cardiovascular disease, 50 million have high blood pressure, 12.6 million have coronary heart disease, 1.2 million have heart attacks, and 4.6 million have suffered a stroke. Coronary heart disease and atherosclerosis are the two major degenerative forms of heart disease that account for most of the deaths.

For most people who don't have diabetes, heart disease speaks loud and clear. Inadequate blood flow to the heart muscle causes a variety of signs and symptoms, such as chest pain or pressure, pounding heartbeat, shortness of breath, jaw or arm pain, and sweating. They know something's wrong and are more likely to seek help. In people with diabetes, heart disease often doesn't offer such clues. That type of heart disease is called silent ischemia. The lack of symptoms may give you a false sense of good health. And that may prevent you from seeking medical care or treatment until noticeable and more serious complications have occurred. You may have had a heart attack and not even know it.

Unfortunately, most people with diabetes believe that amputation and blindness are their biggest threats. They aren't aware that they are at an increased risk of heart attack and stroke. **In fact, two out of every three diabetics die from a heart attack or a stroke.** According to a recent study conducted by the Yale University School of Medicine, more than one fifth of patients with Type 2 diabetes have decreased blood flow to the heart, but no symptoms to suggest there is a problem. Known as myocardial ischemia, this serious condition occurs when the heart does not receive enough blood to meet its metabolic needs, usually due to inflammation and plaque build-up in the coronary arteries. When no symptoms are present, this is usually due to "silent" inflammation. As a result, the risk of sudden death from a heart attack, even though there is no history of heart disease, is as high as the risk in people without diabetes who have had a heart attack. That's why diabetes is called a heart disease equivalent: Having diabetes is like having survived a heart attack.

Symptoms of Cardiovascular (Heart) Disease
Symptoms of cardiovascular (heart) disease vary according to the type of heart disease, and they vary from person to person. The following is a list of some of the early signs or symptoms of heart disease/stroke: shortness of breath; shortness of breath after exercise; pain or tightness in the chest (angina); swelling (edema) in the legs and feet; pain in one of the legs, usually in the lower leg, with swelling and discoloration; pain in the legs with walking (claudication); heart palpitation, arrhythmia; cold feet and/or cold hands; high C-reactive protein level; high homocysteine level; slurred speech, memory loss, muscle weakness, numbness. But, you may not exhibit any of these signs. If you do exhibit any of these signs, you should contact your doctor for a physical or check up – to avoid one of the major symptoms of heart disease: sudden death from high stress.
Note: The 64-slice CT scanner can provide detailed images of the heart and arteries for an easier, non-invasive diagnosis.

According to the Mayo Clinic: "Diabetes damages your cardiovascular system, putting you at increased risk of a sudden heart attack or stroke." Your risks are higher because of the damage that diabetes can cause to your major arteries, including the blood vessels that supply blood to your heart and brain. Another grave complication is gangrene, due to poor circulation, which usually leads to nerve damage and amputation.

WARNING: If you believe that you are having a heart attack, sit down, call 911, chew an aspirin tablet (if you're not allergic), take deep breaths to inhale extra oxygen, and cough every few seconds to keep your heart beating at a reasonable rate.

When the circulatory system is working properly, it delivers blood throughout the body, utilizing and providing specific nutrients to all the organs, tissues, and cells of the body. These key nutrients include CoQ10, l-carnitine, Vitamin C, Vitamin E, Omega-3 EFAs, magnesium, folate, and arginine. But, when there is a chronic deficiency of these or other nutrients, the circulatory system starts to struggle and does not work as effectively. Over time, components of the circulatory system such as the blood vessels may become inflamed and damaged. This puts additional stress on other components of the circulatory system such as the heart, which can lead to a *sudden* stroke or heart attack. However, a consistent exercise program and a well-designed nutritional program that addresses these specific nutritional deficiencies can be very beneficial in preventing and reversing heart disease and other circulatory issues without the need for drugs. Refer to the wellness protocol section in this chapter for more details.

High Blood Pressure

High blood pressure, or hypertension, is usually one of the first signs that the cardiovascular system is lacking key nutrients and is under serious stress and deterioration. This is due to the heart's extra force required to push the blood through the arteries eventually causing damage to the inner lining of the arteries. This, in turn, causes inflammation and leaves the arteries susceptible to the buildup of fatty plaque that can narrow or block the arteries and reduce blood flow to the body's organs. When untreated, high blood pressure can lead to kidney damage, heart failure, stroke, and loss of vision from damage to the retina.

Unfortunately, high blood pressure is a "silent" *symptom* that goes undetected until another problem arises that triggers the need for a physical exam, e.g. blurry vision, constant headaches, heart arrhythmia, kidney problems. The key organs that are involved with high blood pressure include the heart, kidneys, arteries, and the neural and hormonal systems. **The combination of high blood pressure, obesity and diabetes is particularly stressful on the kidneys.**

High blood pressure is generally defined as a level exceeding 140/90 mm Hg on multiple occasions. The systolic blood pressure, which is the first number, represents the pressure in the arteries as the heart contracts and pumps blood throughout the circulatory system. The diastolic pressure, which is the second number, represents the pressure in the arteries as the heart relaxes after the contraction.

An elevation of the systolic or diastolic blood pressure increases the risk of developing heart (cardiac) disease, kidney (renal) disease, hardening of the arteries (arteriosclerosis), glaucoma (eye damage), and stroke (brain damage). Usually a high systolic number indicates problems with the cardiovascular system and the liver, while a high diastolic number indicates problems with the kidneys and the liver. These complications of high blood pressure are often referred to as end-organ damage because damage to these organs is the end result of chronic (long duration) high blood pressure. Accordingly, the diagnosis of high blood pressure in an individual is important so that efforts can be made to normalize the blood pressure and, thereby, prevent the complications.

For some people, high blood pressure may be defined at a level lower than 140/90 mm Hg. For example, in certain situations, such as in patients with long duration (chronic) kidney diseases that spill protein into the urine (proteinuria), the blood pressure is ideally kept at 125/75, or even lower. The purpose of reducing the blood pressure to this level in these patients is to slow the progression of kidney damage. Patients with diabetes may likewise benefit from blood pressure that is maintained at a level lower than 140/90. In addition, African-Americans, who have an increased risk for developing the complications of high blood pressure, may decrease this risk by reducing their diastolic blood pressure to 80 mm Hg or less.

> **Important:** Not only can kidney disease cause high blood pressure, but high blood pressure can cause kidney disease. Therefore, all patients with high blood pressure should be evaluated for the presence of kidney disease so that they can be treated appropriately.

Diagnosis

The diagnosis of high blood pressure is more than reading the numbers off the monitor. It may take several months of doctor visits, monitoring and testing, including an electrocardiogram to prevent a false reading. The diagnosis starts with measuring your blood pressure using a mercury manometer and a properly fitted arm cuff, with your elbow at the same level as your heart, not below it. There is usually a small difference between the left and right side. Ideal systolic-diastolic pressure values are under 120/80. Values over 180/110 are a definite concern. If the difference between the systolic and diastolic pressure exceeds 60, advanced atherosclerosis may be present. Values greater than 140/90 are a concern if you have other risk factors such as being overweight. You may require further testing, which may involve wearing a small automatic measuring device and recorder for 24 hours. To prevent a false diagnosis, have your blood pressure checked while sitting, standing and lying down – if readings skyrocket when you change position, this may indicate a problem with the adrenal glands. All this information is collected and analyzed by your doctor for a proper diagnosis.

Primary Root Causes

In order to understand the best ways to treat high blood pressure (without drugs), it is very important to understand the primary root causes which cause the heart muscle to work harder to push the blood throughout the body. They include: an increase in the volume of blood and fluids, e.g. fluid retention due to cell dehydration; a decrease in the diameter of the artery walls; a decrease in the elasticity of the arteries; an increase in blood viscosity (thick blood); a clogged liver; a clogging of the smaller capillaries in the kidneys; reduced nitric oxide; a constriction of the arteries due to an increase in cortisol levels; a defective heart muscle or heart valve; and, poor filtering of the blood by the kidneys.

When the heart tries to "push" thick, sticky blood through the blood vessels, it's similar to forcing ketchup out of a bottle. You have to pound the bottom of the bottle to provide enough force to get the ketchup out of the bottle. This is analogous to the pounding that the heart has to perform to generate enough force to push the thick blood throughout the body. And, this extra pounding can cause headaches and blurry vision while creating more pressure that causes injuries to the linings of the arterial walls. These wall injuries cause inflammatory and repair responses that lead to the production of various proteins and extra cholesterol to form plaque to repair the injured walls. The arterial walls become thickened (arteriosclerosis); and, if there is high homocysteine, this can lead to the formation of more plaque and blood clots (atherosclerosis).

As you can see, there are many causes of high blood pressure. In order to determine which ones are causing your high blood pressure, it is critical to have your doctor perform all the necessary blood tests and other diagnostic tests that may help to better diagnose the root cause(s) of your high blood pressure, including testing for inflammation markers such as homocysteine, C-reactive protein, lipoprotein(a), and fibrin.

When the circulatory system is working properly, it delivers water and blood throughout the body, providing nutrients to all the cells and tissues of the body. Specifically, the blood provides key nutrients to the millions of artery wall cells, which are responsible for the availability of "relaxing factors" that decrease vascular wall tension and keep the blood pressure in the normal range. These key nutrients include Omega-3 EFAs, CoQ10, water, Vitamin C, Vitamin E, magnesium, folate, and arginine. But, when there is a chronic deficiency of these nutrients, blood viscosity can increase, the artery walls can become damaged leading to plaque formation, or the artery walls can spasm and become thickened, leading to an increase in blood pressure. Consequently, a consistent exercise regimen, stress reduction, and a nutritional program that addresses specific nutrient deficiencies can be beneficial in preventing high blood pressure. Refer to the wellness protocol section in this chapter for more details.

Cardiac Risk & Inflammation Factors

Homocysteine, lipoprotein (a), cholesterol, and C-reactive protein are all cardiovascular risk factors and inflammation markers – some actually *cause* cardiovascular disease, others are just *indicators* or the result of cardiovascular disease. This is important because if you do not address the factors that actually cause the disease, then, you cannot get rid of the disease. You end up controlling the symptoms and indicators, but the disease is still in the body doing more harm as time progresses.

Homocysteine (discovered by Dr. Kilmer McCully, 1969) is a toxic amino acid that is produced normally as a byproduct of protein synthesis when protein foods are metabolized; and, is converted to another amino acid, methionine, unless it's blocked due to high insulin levels or low consumption of vegetables and beans. Poor nutrition (consisting of too much animal meat and not enough vegetables and beans containing folic acid, Vitamins B6 and B12) impairs the metabolism and breakdown of homocysteine. Refined sugar, flour, processed foods and a sedentary lifestyle lead to high insulin and homocysteine levels, which combine with LDL cholesterol to promote oxidation. This irritates and cuts the blood vessels causing inflammation, fatty plaque formation and gradually, as the plaque accumulates in the arterial walls, leads to atherosclerosis. Elevated homocysteine may also make blood more likely to clot, raising fibrinogen levels and increasing the stickiness of blood platelets, which may precipitate a heart attack or a stroke. Elevated homocysteine may reduce brain function, increasing memory loss and triggering the development of Alzheimer's. In addition, high homocysteine accelerates telomere ("genetic clock") shortening of vascular lining cells and impairs endothelial nitric oxide production, preventing blood vessels from relaxing and restricting blood flow to tissues.

To prevent high homocysteine levels, there are three principal pathways through which the body breaks down homocysteine. The first of these pathways uses Vitamin B6 (pyridoxine) and zinc to convert homocysteine to the beneficial sulfur amino acid cysteine. The cysteine may then be used to synthesize glutathione, one of the body's most powerful antioxidants. The second pathway requires folic acid and vitamin B12 and converts homocysteine to the beneficial and lipotropic amino acid methionine. The third and most potent pathway uses a nutrient (from beets) known as trimethylglycine, or TMG, to break down homocysteine and produce methionine and boost the generation of SAMe, or S-adenosyl-methionine, which can help with our mood (depression).

In addition to heart disease, high homocysteine levels may also be a risk factor for the development of other conditions, including osteoporosis, inflammatory bowel disease (Crohn's disease and ulcerative colitis), death from diabetes, miscarriage, other complications of pregnancy, and hypothyroidism.

Lipoprotein (a) is a protein with sticky, adhesive properties that is produced by the liver to repair the endothelium of the artery walls when there is insufficient Vitamin C to produce the collagen and elastin to repair the walls of the (damaged) blood vessels. In addition, the liver produces fibrinogen to develop fibrin, which is deposited in the form of a mesh; and, dries and hardens so that any bleeding stops. Lipoprotein (a) bonds with fibrin to complete the repair of the damaged walls.

Triglycerides, which are produced by the liver to provide a major source of energy to the body tissues, are chains of high-energy fatty acids that circulate in the bloodstream and provide much of the energy needed for cells to function. Triglycerides are also the chemical form of most fats in the food we eat. The liver takes up dietary cholesterol and triglycerides from the bloodstream and packages the cholesterol and triglycerides, along with special proteins, into tiny spheres called lipoproteins. The lipoproteins are released into the circulation, and are delivered to the cells of the body. When the body needs energy, the cells release the triglycerides, which are burned as fuel to meet our energy needs. If we eat too many refined sugar foods and do not exercise, the high insulin level triggers the liver to produce more Very Low Density Lipoproteins (VLDL), which is a main carrier of triglyceride. And, the excess triglycerides will build up in the blood and be stored in the body as adipose (fat) tissue. Consequently, many diabetics who have a high total cholesterol, may have high triglycerides, since the same foods that cause the blood glucose level to rise are the same foods that cause triglycerides to rise. A high triglyceride level is also a risk factor for stroke.

If you have a high cholesterol level because of high triglycerides, then, a statin drug like Lipitor will *not* help because the drug is not designed to reduce the triglycerides. This is why it is important that you get a *complete* lipid profile, a blood test that will provide a reading for each of the cholesterol components: total cholesterol (TC), low density lipoprotein (LDL), high density lipoprotein (HDL), lipoprotein(a), and triglycerides (TG). Refer to Chapter 11 for more details about blood tests.

Cholesterol, a waxy, fatty substance, 80% of which is produced by the liver and the cells, is a very important nutrient that is used to build cell membranes and hormones. It is packaged in a fat-protein package called a lipoprotein so that it can be transported throughout the body. There are four types of fat-protein lipoproteins: chylomicrons, very low density lipoproteins (VLDL), low density lipoproteins (LDL), and high density lipoproteins (HDL). Lipoproteins are differentiated by how much triglyceride they contain such that the more triglyceride that is in these particles, the less dense they are and the more they "float". Chylomicron contains the most triglyceride, followed by VLDL, LDL, and HDL.

If one's total cholesterol level is too high, this may be an indication that the body has constant high insulin levels (hyperinsulinemia) triggering the liver to produce more triglycerides and cholesterol; or, that the liver is clogged with too much fat and cannot effectively filter the cholesterol out of the blood; or, that the cardiovascular system may be in a repair mode due to damaged blood vessel walls. Conventional medicine's use of statin drugs has proven to effectively lower the cholesterol level by inhibiting the liver's production of the enzyme HMG-CoA reductase. But, this lowers CoQ10 levels predisposing the patient to muscle deterioration (rhabdomyolysis) and heart disease, the very condition that these drugs are intended to prevent! In addition extra cholesterol continues to be produced until the root cause of why the liver is producing the extra cholesterol is addressed (e.g. high insulin levels, damage to the artery walls, a clogged liver, insufficient nutrients).

High levels of LDL ("bad") cholesterol result because of interference with the body's utilization of cholesterol due to the suppression of thyroid function and the lack of sunlight. Suppression of thyroid function is caused by trans fats (partially hydrogenated oil in processed foods, margarine, shortening) and clear vegetable oils (corn, soybean). Under normal conditions, sunlight converts the cholesterol on the skin to hormone precursors, including Vitamin D. Then, cholesterol in the bloodstream migrates to the surface of the skin, to replace the cholesterol that was converted. But, if you do not obtain at least one hour's worth of sunlight every day, this process of producing Vitamin D (to fight cancer) and naturally lowering your cholesterol does not occur.

A sedentary lifestyle and a poor nutritional profile of excess refined carbohydrates, insufficient soluble fiber, and excess saturated fat may also contribute to higher cholesterol levels. In addition, if the LDL particles are small-sized and dense, recent studies have shown that these particles become trapped in the inner lining of the artery walls, and, after being attacked by the immune cells, are highly inflammatory and toxic to the lining of the arterial walls. Consequently, someone with a normal cholesterol level could have a high cardiovascular risk or a sudden heart attack if the LDL particles are small and dense.

C-reactive protein (CRP) is a reactant released by the body in response to acute injury, infection, fever, or other inflammatory stimuli, indicating a heightened state of inflammation in the body. CRP measures inflammation, part of the immune reaction that protects you from infection when you injure yourself. It causes redness, pain and swelling, and can damage the inner lining of arteries, and break off clots from arteries to block the flow of blood triggering strokes and heart attacks.

C-reactive protein levels fluctuate from day to day, and levels increase with aging, high blood pressure, alcohol use, smoking, low levels of physical activity, chronic fatigue, coffee consumption, elevated triglycerides, insulin resistance or diabetes, taking estrogen, eating a high protein diet, suffering sleep disturbances, or depression.

Note: In addition to CRP, possible inflammation markers for Type 2 diabetes include tumor necrosis factor (TNF) and interleudin-6 (IL-6).

Fibrinogen is a protein that plays a critical role in normal and abnormal clot formation, a mechanism referred to as coagulation. An interaction between clotting factors and naturally-occurring anticoagulants normally results in healthy levels of fibrinogen and normal coagulation. If fibrinogen levels increase above normal, however, a blood clot becomes a threat; if fibrinogen levels decrease below normal, a hemorrhage can result.

Excess fibrinogen is produced by the liver due to inflammation, high homocysteine levels, and an immune response that releases a specific cytokine (interleukin-620) into the bloodstream. Platelets release the enzyme thrombin when they come into contact with damaged tissue, triggering the release of this cytokine, which leads to the formation of the soluble protein, fibrinogen. Fibrinogen is then converted to fibrin, an insoluble protein that is deposited around a wound in the form of a mesh to dry and harden, so that bleeding stops as the final stage in blood clotting. In addition, fibrinogen increases the viscosity of the blood, making it thicker and slow moving.

> **Key point:** High C-reactive protein, high homocysteine and small, dense LDL particles are indicators of high inflammation, and may be reasons why more than 60% of heart attack victims actually have normal cholesterol levels.

As a result of the high inflammation, the blood vessels become damaged and the body goes into a repair mode that is indicated by high levels of these specific cardiovascular risk factors and inflammation markers. In order to reduce these levels of internal inflammation and reverse its effects, utilize a consistent exercise program and a nutritional program that includes fiber-rich anti-inflammatory foods and Omega-3 fatty acids such as broccoli, spinach, beans, blueberries, avocados, flaxseed, and wild salmon. In addition, utilize other wellness principles such as cleansing/detoxification and spiritual health. Refer to the wellness protocol section in this chapter for more details.

Wellness Protocol for Diabetes & Its Complications (General)

Use the following set of procedures as a guideline to control, prevent, or reverse your diabetes and its other health-related issues.

Education, Doctor Visits & Planning

1. Educate yourself about diabetes and its complications especially since it requires less effort to prevent the complications than to treat them.
2. Maintain a tight blood glucose level of 80 to 100 mg/dl and a blood pressure level of less than 120/80 mm Hg to prevent problems with the kidneys, eyes, nerves and heart.
3. Visit your doctor and healthcare team on a periodic basis to obtain up-to-date test results for your kidneys, eyes, nerves, and heart.
4. Develop an overall "get well" plan and a set of health goals, based on your physical exam, blood tests, and your doctor's diagnosis. Track your progress and make any necessary changes to your nutrition, exercise, and test regimens to achieve your health goals.
5. Contact our wellness center if you need help with your planning.

Nutrition: Food, Beverage & Supplements

1. Eat bright-colored raw vegetables, dark fruits, legumes and super foods for the antioxidants, vitamins, minerals and fiber to control your glucose and nourish/protect the kidneys, eyes, nerves and heart.
2. Eat avocado and fish such as wild salmon, sardines and tuna at least three times a week to obtain the Omega-3 oils that will reduce inflammation. The Omega-3 oils lubricate the blood vessel walls; provide anti-inflammatory properties to the kidneys, eyes, nerves, and heart; and, help the body absorb the fat-soluble nutrients (e.g. beta carotene, chlorophyll, lutein) in the vegetables. Use borage oil and extra virgin olive oil, which contains oleic acid to increase the absorption of the Omega-3s and keep your cells supple.
3. Drink raw vegetable juices 2-3 times daily to provide the necessary carotenoids and Vitamin C to protect the kidneys, eyes, nerves, and heart. For example, juice 6 carrots, 2 handfuls of spinach, a handful of parsley, 1 tablespoon of freshly ground flaxseed, two endive leaves, 8 ounces wheat/barley grass and 12 ounces of filtered water.

4. Take a daily *food*-based multivitamin/mineral supplement(s) that provides the following nutrients to control your blood glucose and nourish/ protect your kidneys, eyes, nerves, and heart:

400-750 mg **Alpha Lipoic Acid**	1200 mg liquid **L-Carnitine**
300-500 mg **CoQ10**	400-600 mg **L-Carnosine**
400 mcg **Chromium** 2 times daily	600 mg **N-Acetyl Cysteine**
200-300 mg **Borage Oil (GLA)**	1750 mg **Omega-3 Fish Oil**
2-4 tbsp. **Flaxseed**	500-750 mg **Vitamin C**
100 mg **Gymnema Sylvestre** 3 times	400-500 IU **Vitamin E**

5. Depending on your health needs, add one or more of the following nutrition-rich foods to close your nutritional gap: aloe vera, pulse food, royal jelly, grasses, plankton, chlorella, spirulina, kelp.

Nutrition: Cleansing & Detoxification

1. Perform periodic cleansing and detoxification of the colon, kidneys, liver and gall bladder to remove excess glucose, toxins, and waste.
2. To help the body to perform cleansing and detoxification, drink filtered water and eat fiber-rich foods, including bright-colored vegetables, fruits, organic whole grains and super foods such as sea plankton, grasses, chlorella, spirulina, pulse foods, and royal jelly.
3. Work with your doctor to get weaned off as many prescription drugs as possible to reduce the body's toxic load.

Exercise, Mind & Spirit

1. Implement a consistent exercise program of aerobics and weight-resistance training to lower blood glucose level, improve motor skills, remove toxins from the body, and reduce stress.
2. Address any negative emotional issues (e.g. anger, resentment, jealousy, envy), which create hormonal imbalances such as high cortisol levels, putting a strain on the cardiovascular and immune systems. Forgive others, but don't forget to forgive yourself.
3. Perform mental exercises or learn a new hobby or skill to increase brain activity, e.g. scrabble, crossword puzzle, pottery class.
4. Learn how to relax and use your spiritual health to improve the health of your body and mind.
5. Get 6-8 hours of quality sleep and 30 minutes of sunlight daily (or 2 tbsp. cod liver oil or 1000 IU Vitamin D).

Wellness Protocol for Kidney Disease

Utilize the following specific steps as a guideline to help slow down or prevent kidney disease.

1. Visit your doctor on a periodic basis to ensure your kidneys are functioning properly and no protein is leaking into your urine. If protein has started to leak into your kidneys, discuss alternatives with your doctor and begin implementing the following steps.

2. Eat alkaline-forming foods such as lemons, limes, cranberry; cabbage, cauliflower, grasses, kohlrabi, spinach, summer squash, kale, mustard greens, turnip greens; and raw juices (cucumber; parsley, dandelion, spinach, carrots) to nourish the kidneys and reduce inflammation. Drink 5 to 7 cups of filtered water each day to help cleanse the kidneys and bladder and address any cell dehydration issues.

3. Reduce/eliminate the consumption of the "dead" refined carbohydrates to lower the production of insulin, which causes extra calcium to be excreted into the urine and become a binding agent for the formation of kidney stones. Reduce/eliminate consumption of animal meat, which contains too much uric acid such that when the body metabolizes the protein, it produces sulfuric and phosphoric acids. And, these acids must be neutralized by ammonia and alkaline minerals before they can be discharged safely by the kidneys.

4. Reduce/eliminate the drinking of beverages such as soda, coffee, and beer because they contain dehydrating agents such as sugar, caffeine, and alcohol. Your body becomes more starved for water as you drink more of these beverages. This forces the body to draw water from your cells to cleanse the toxins found in these beverages. This puts a strain on your kidneys and may raise your blood pressure.

5. Reduce/eliminate the consumption of tobacco, over-the-counter drugs, and, if possible, prescription drugs. All drugs have to be detoxified by the kidneys, especially the nonsteroidal anti-inflammatory drugs (NSAIDs) and other painkillers, which have been shown to cause kidney failure and death.

6. Take a *food*-based nutritional supplement that provides two or more of the following nutrients to complement your super meal program, close any nutritional gaps and support your kidney health.
   - Apple cider vinegar, apple juice (organic): contain mallic acid, which dissolves calcium stones in your kidneys.
   - Blueberries: contain ellagic acid and tannins that help prevent urinary tract infections.
   - Cranberry extract: contains flavonoids that provide antioxidant protection and cleansing nutrients to the kidneys. Cranberry extract inhibits microorganisms from adhering to the mucosal cells lining the urinary tract and bladder, making it a less hospitable environment for the proliferation of E. coli and other infection-causing bacteria. Avoid bottled cranberry juice because it contains too much sugar.
   - Ginger: encourages the removal of toxins (as a diuretic) through increased kidney filtration and (as a diaphoretic) through the skin.
   - Juniper berries: contain a volatile oil, terpinen-4, that acts as a kidney irritant to stimulate increased kidney filtration and urine output, and for relief from symptoms of gout and kidney stones. Caution: Pregnant women and people suffering from kidney ailments are cautioned to avoid eating juniper berries.
   - Parsley: contains flavonoids (e.g. apiol, myristicin) that stimulate urination and provide relief when urination is painful and incomplete due to an enlarged prostate. It provides diuretic effect to address stones or gravel in the urinary tracts, and is effective for upset stomachs by stimulating digestive enzymes.
   - Uva ursi: contains a glycoside called arbutin that is responsible for its diuretic action, and is used to treat chronic inflammation of the bladder or kidneys, bladder infections, kidney stones, or incontinence. It helps to dissolve calculi in the kidneys, and may help to control the sugar levels in diabetics.
   - Water (filtered), raw juices: dilute the toxins in your urine stored in your bladder, and increase urine flow to reduce the exposure time of the toxins in your bladder, preventing bladder infections.

Wellness Protocol for Eye Disease

Utilize the following specific steps as a guideline to help slow down, reverse or prevent eye disease.

1. Eat lutein-rich and antioxidant-rich green, leafy vegetables and bright-colored vegetables, and dark-colored fruits such as spinach, broccoli, kale, collard greens, carrots, zucchini, blueberries and egg yolks, which also contain zeaxanthin. These carotenoids and antioxidants nourish and protect the eye tissues from oxidation and degeneration. Blueberries contain anthocyanins, which are the bioflavonoids responsible for the deep purple-blue color. Other sources of anthocyanins include red grapes, cherries, pomegranates, and red cabbage. Red vegetables and fruits (e.g. tomatoes, red peppers) contain lycopene, another carotenoid that provides antioxidant protection to combat free radicals in the eye.

2. Reduce/eliminate the consumption of the "dead" processed foods such as margarine and potato chips, which contain partially hydrogenated oil (trans fat). Trans fat appears to contribute to macular degeneration and may interfere with the Omega-3 fats.

3. Schedule regular eye examinations with an ophthalmologist at least once a year to detect any early signs of eye disease, such as small problems in the blood vessels of the retina.

4. Wear sunglasses that filter UVA, UVB and blue light to reduce the oxidative damage to the retina.

5. Take a *food*-based nutritional supplement that provides two or more of the following nutrients to complement your super meal program, close any nutritional gaps and support your eye health.
   - Acetyl-L-Carnitine (ALC): is one of the nutrients that can fuel the mitochondria in cells, including the photoreceptor cells in the retina. ALC may be able to cross the brain-retinal barrier to assist in cellular energy production in the retinal lining.
   - Astaxanthin: is the carotenoid responsible for the pink color of salmon and crustacean shells. Testing has shown its ability to cross the brain-retinal barrier to reduce oxidation in the eye tissues.

- Bilberry: contains anthocyanocides, which speed up the regeneration of rhodopsin (a purple pigment in the rods) to help the retina to improve adaptation to light and dark, improving night vision. Bilberry and other dark berries nourish the small capillaries that feed the retina to help treat diabetic retinopathy, macular degeneration, glaucoma, and cataracts.

- Eyebright: enhances circulation of blood vessels in the eyes to optimize the delivery of nutrients to every part of the eye including the eyelids. It is especially useful for eyestrain, eye inflammations, conjunctivitis, and other eye infections. Eyebright has anti-inflammatory, astringent properties that draw out secretions and discharges; and, can greatly relieve runny, sore, itchy eyes due to colds or allergies.

- Fish oil: from wild salmon, sardines, other cold-water fish, and krill contains the Omega-3 EFA docosahexaenoic acid (DHA), which is the fat found in the retina's photoreceptor cells; and, is protective against macular degeneration.

- Ginkgo biloba: maintains and increases the flow of blood to the tiny capillaries of the eye, and helps maintain the elasticity and flexibility of the eye's blood vessels.

- Grapeseed extract: is a concentration of the oligomeric proanthocyanidins (OPCs) found in grape seeds and skins. It provides nutrient support to strengthen the walls of small capillaries to prevent capillary leakage in the eyes, legs and skin reducing fluid retention. It also provides antioxidant protection to safeguard the integrity of the retina and cornea of the eye.
  Note: Grapeseed extract works synergistically with resveratrol.

- L-carnosine: is a di-peptide (composed of the amino acids alanine and histidine) that is found in relatively high concentrations in several body tissues, most notably in skeletal muscle, heart muscle, nerve tissue and brain. Carnosine concentrates in the lens of the eye to slow down or prevent glycation and cataracts. A form of l-carnosine, in the form of eye drops, may prevent cataracts, according to recent research by Russian scientists.

- Lutein, Zeaxanthin: are the colorful pigments in green, leafy and bright-colored vegetables and give the yellow color to corn and egg yolks. These carotenoids can be found in the macula, a tiny yellow dot in the center of the retina that lets you see fine details and helps you distinguish people's faces. They are the only two carotenoids present in the lens of the eye that help maintain proper lens density and play a role against free radical stress in the cortex of the lens. They act as "sunglasses" by absorbing the harmful UVA, UVB and blue light, helping to maintain the photoreceptors and lining of the retina. Recent research shows that zeaxanthin is the more powerful antioxidant that protects the macula from the free radical oxidative damage caused by sunlight. Food sources: spinach, broccoli, greens, zucchini, eggs.
- N-Acetyl Cysteine (NAC): helps to neutralize toxins by increasing glutathione, the principle antioxidant of the eye's lens that protects it against oxidation. NAC helps the lens to register images clearly, and may help prevent retinopathy.
- Pine bark extract: contains pycnogenol and is similar in composition to grape seed extract as it provides a similar benefit in strengthening blood vessels.
- Quercetin: is a plant pigment (found in onions) that helps to maintain lens transparency by keeping out unwanted deposits of calcium and sodium. It also provides protection against cataracts in diabetics by blocking an enzyme inhibiting the accumulation of sorbitol, a type of blood sugar. Ultraviolet (UV) rays, particularly the burning UVB rays, damage proteins in the lens of the eye, causing them to clump together in a whitish cloud.
- Resveratrol: is a polyphenol found in the skins of red grapes that acts as an antioxidant to protect the eyes from oxidative damage.
- Selenium: acts as an antioxidant that helps to flush out toxic heavy metals from the eye tissues. Food sources: fish, grains, eggs, garlic, chicken.
- Zinc: supports the immune system; and, provides oxidative protection of the retina, which has a high concentration of zinc, more than any other organ. Food sources: meat, legumes, nuts.

Wellness Protocols for Nerve & Brain Diseases

If major nerve damage has not occurred, utilize the following steps as a guide to slow down, reverse or prevent nerve and brain-related diseases.

1. Taking care of your feet is very important. The nerves of the feet are the longest in the body and are often affected by neuropathy. Utilize the following guidelines for proper foot care.

   - Look at your feet every morning and every evening to check for cuts, sores, blisters, redness, calluses, or other problems.
   - Wash your feet in warm water every day. Do not soak your feet. Dry your feet well, especially between your toes. Rub lotion on your feet, but do not put lotion between your toes
   - If your skin is dry, especially the heel of your foot, use a salt scrub to carefully remove the dead skin. (Thanks, Cynthia!).
   - Cut your toenails once a week or when needed. Cut toenails when they are soft from washing. Cut them to the shape of the toe and not too short. File the edges with an emery board.
   - Always wear shoes or slippers to protect your feet from injuries.
   - Always wear socks or stockings to avoid blisters. Wear thick, soft socks. Do not wear socks or knee-high stockings that are too tight below your knee.
   - Wear shoes that fit well. Shop for shoes at the end of the day when your feet are bigger.
   - If you have neuropathy, talk to your doctor about orthotics to improve circulation and relieve pressure.
   - Check the temperature of bath water with your hand or arm before getting in the tub.
   - Do not cross your legs when sitting.
   - Make sure your doctor checks your feet at each checkup and performs the filament test by lightly rubbing a feathery filament across the bottom of your feet - to check for a loss of touch sensation. If you do not feel the filament, it is imperative that you use your eyes to check your feet every morning and night.
   - *Note:* If your feet do not sweat at all, this may indicate a loss of sweating and eventually a loss of touch sensation. Unfortunately,

this may eventually lead to foot ulcers. Notify your podiatrist and endocrinologist.

- Use one or more of the following therapies to help improve nerve health and the blood circulation in the feet: massage therapy, water therapy, acupuncture, magnetic insoles.
- Other natural treatment options for neuropathy may include: relaxation training, hypnosis, biofeedback training, acupuncture, transcutaneous electronic nerve stimulation (TENS) therapy.

2. Take a *food*-based nutritional supplement that provides two or more of the following nutrients to complement your super meal program, close any nutritional gaps and support your nerve/brain health.

- Evening primrose oil, black currant seed oil, or borage oil: contains gamma linolenic acid (GLA) that helps to maintain the myelin sheaths, support the communication between the brain and nerve cells, and increase absorption of Omega-3 EFAs.
- Fish/krill oil: contains DHA, an Omega-3 EFA that is important for the normal functions of the brain and nerves. DHA inhibits the production of amyloid precursor protein (APP), which prompts the production of amyloid fibrils in the brain.
- Glyconutrients: provide several essential monosaccharides that support cell-to-cell communications and the immune system.
- Phosphatidyl choline: supports the production of two vital components of the nervous system, acetylcholine (a neurotransmitter) and sphingomyelin (required for nerve cell protection), which are essential for the normal, healthy functioning of the nervous system and brain. The foods richest in phosphatidyl choline are beef liver, egg yolks and soya.
- Resveratrol: contains antioxidant properties that reduce oxidative stress in nerve cells. Food sources include dark grapes, red wine, blueberries, and cranberries.
- Turmeric: contains curcumin, an antioxidant that protects the nerves and reduces inflammation; and heals cuts and leg ulcers when applied topically. Studies with mice suggest curcumin can slow the progression of Alzheimer's. In addition, researchers found low incidences of neurological diseases such as

Alzheimer's in elderly Indian populations who consume curcumin as a regular part of their diet.

- Vitamin B-Complex: plays a crucial role in promoting and insuring nerve health as it provides nourishment for the nervous system, including the function of the brain and the production of its neurotransmitters, e.g. acetylcholine. Thiamine (B1) and biotin (B7) promote healthy nerves. Riboflavin (B2) aids in nerve insulation. Niacin (B3) assists nervous system function, while pyridoxine (B6) helps the body to use and absorb niacin and B12. A lack of B6 may cause carpal tunnel syndrome, painful neuropathy in your hands that may make it impossible to type or grip heavy objects. Also important is cyanocobalamin (B12), which helps nerves to function and avoid damage; and, is important to memory function as well as Alzheimer's prevention. Both B12 and folic acid (B9) deficiency can cause neuropathic leg and foot pain.
- Vitamin C: may help protect against deterioration of nerves and inhibit depletion of the neurotransmitter norepinephrine to prevent poor memory, loss of alertness, and clinical depression.
- Vitamin D: from sunlight, eggs, fish, cod liver oil may help the body defend against some cancers, diabetes, multiple sclerosis, and osteoporosis.
- Vitamin E: is important for the proper functioning of nerves and muscles, making it possible for them to function with less oxygen, thereby increasing endurance and stamina. A deficiency is often associated with symptoms of peripheral neuropathy. A recent study by Japanese researchers indicated Vitamin E might prevent and even reverse early neurodegenerative changes that would ultimately lead to Alzheimer's.

3. Take a *food*-based nutritional supplement that provides two or more of the following nutrients to complement your super meal program, close any nutritional gaps and support your brain health.
   - Betaine: is a polysaccharide in beets that lowers homocysteine and reduces inflammation that may affect the brain.
   - Cayenne pepper: stimulates the flow of blood to the brain, and accelerates the delivery of other key nutrients to the brain.

- Gingko biloba: contains the flavonoid compounds collectively known as "ginkgolides" that act specifically to dilate the smallest segment of the circulatory system, the micro-capillaries, which have a widespread affect on the body's organs, especially the brain. Researchers have also reported that ginkgo effectively increases blood circulation and oxygen levels in brain tissues. The flavonoids and organic acids in gingko biloba provide antioxidant properties to kill free radicals; increase the oxygen content to the brain by improving the blood flow in the small cerebral capillaries to enhance memory, increase mental focus and clarity; and, inhibit age related reduction in brain chemicals.
  Warning: Do not use gingko if you are taking a blood-thinning drug such as Coumadin or aspirin.
- L-carnosine: prevents the development of plaque that can contribute to senility and Alzheimer's disease. L-carnosine inhibits the activity of MAO B (monoamine oxidase B), which is an enzyme involved in breaking down some brain messengers (such as dopamine and serotonin), and, is known to increase the production of free radicals.
- Phosphatidyl serine (PS): is a natural nutrient found most notably in the cell membrane of neurons, comprising about 7 to 10 percent of its lipid content. PS assists in regulating membrane transfer of nutrients and neurotransmitters necessary for proper mental function. Therefore, PS is essential for nerve cell function and the production and release of neurotransmitters, supporting the integrity of nerve cell membranes and the formation of other important phospholipids to improve the health of the brain and nervous system. PS has been shown in numerous studies to help support memory and overall cognitive function, positive mood, and concentration. It also helps support the body's natural response to certain forms of stress. As a supplement, PS is primarily derived from soy.

Wellness Protocol for Cardiovascular Disease

Utilize the following specific steps as a guideline to help slow down, reverse or prevent cardiovascular (heart) disease.

1. Ensure that your doctor performs a series of stress tests to better evaluate the health of your heart and cardiovascular system. Request additional blood tests at least once a year for inflammation markers such as homocysteine, C-reactive protein, lipoprotein (a), fibrinogen.

2. Work with your dental hygienist to implement a thorough tooth and gum cleaning hygiene program to prevent periodontal disease and infections that can invade the arteries. Use an herbal-based powder and oral rinse to reduce bacteria growth and gum inflammation. Do not use the traditional toothpastes (which can be abrasive and toxic) or the oral rinses (which contain artificial sweeteners, preservatives, dyes, alcohol, and other unwanted chemicals).

3. To nourish and protect the cardiovascular system, eat carotenoid-rich foods such as red peppers, tomatoes, carrots, pumpkin, and cantaloupe to inhibit the formation of LDL cholesterol. Eat avocado, fish, and use extra virgin olive oil for the Omega-3s and to increase absorption of the fat-soluble carotenoids. Also, eat folate-rich foods such as spinach and lima beans to reduce homocysteine.

4. Review the following nutrients and their descriptions to identify the nutrients that are appropriate for your heart health and complement your super meal program by closing any nutritional gaps.

    *   Açai berries: are rich in oleic acid, which helps Omega-3 fish oils penetrate the cell membrane, making them more supple.
    *   Arginine: is an amino acid that increases the production of nitric oxide to relax artery walls. Foods rich in the arginine include fish, poultry, dairy, nuts, and chocolate.
    *   Astragalus: strengthens the beating and contraction of the heart, while increasing the level of energy production within heart cells.
    *   Betaine: is a natural polysaccharide found in beets that can lower homocysteine levels.
    *   Bilberry: is a bioflavonoid with active ingredients similar to those found in grapes and black currants including anti-inflammatory

factors, anti-clotting factors, and several properties which result in a collagen-stabilizing effect. This effect strengthens the veins by restoring the surrounding connective tissue sheath, decreasing their fragility and permeability. This helps to prevent blood pooling, clotting, and swelling that can lead to varicose veins and other venous conditions.

- Cayenne pepper (capsicum): contains the ingredient capsaicin, which gives peppers their heat. Capsaicin acts to reduce platelet stickiness and relieve pain. Cayenne acts as a circulatory stimulant that produces a speedy reaction in the circulatory system, removing the obstructions by natural evacuations and profuse perspiration; and, helps the arteries, veins and capillaries to regain their elasticity, causing blood pressure to adjust itself to normal. Cayenne regulates the flow of blood from the head to the feet so that the pressure is equalized. It influences the heart immediately, and then gradually extends its effects to the arteries, capillaries, and nerves (the frequency of the pulse is not increased, but is given more vigor). In equalizing the blood circulation, cayenne produces natural warmth; and in stimulating the peristaltic motion of the intestines, it aids in assimilation and elimination.

- CoQ10: is a powerful nutrient produced by the liver that acts as the "spark plug" for the mitochondria ("energy factories") within all cells, to produce energy -- CoQ10 works with acetyl-l-carnitine (ALC) and alpha lipoic acid (ALA) to produce adenosine triphosphate (ATP), the chemical form of energy in the body. CoQ10 provides antioxidant protection and nourishes the heart muscle and other hard-working organs including the liver, kidneys, brain, and pancreas. CoQ10 levels are reduced by statin drugs, (e.g. Lipitor), which, ironically, were designed to prevent heart disease, but may actually contribute to heart disease.

- D-Ribose: is a simple sugar molecule found in every cell of the body that supports the production of ATP (adenosine triphosphate) levels in the heart and skeletal muscles by fortifying the mitochondria and supporting the recycling of energy to provide continuous energy. Studies show that D-ribose provides an overall increase in physical energy levels, substantial increases in cardiovascular fitness and exercise, substantial reduction in recovery time following strenuous exercise or heavy labor, increased exercise performance and endurance, and substantial reduction in post-exercise stiffness and cramping. D-ribose works synergistically with CoQ10, l-carnitine, and magnesium.

- Fish/krill oil: contains DHA and EPA, preventing heart arrhythmia and sticky platelets, high blood pressure, high triglycerides, inflammation, and lowered immune function.
- Garlic: contains allicin, which enables red blood cells to release hydrogen sulphide to relax artery walls; inhibits red blood cells from sticking together; and, helps break down the buildup of plaque in the arterial walls. Similar to Vitamin E, onions, ginger, and Omega-3s, garlic helps to thin the blood. Garlic cloves provide the best health benefit when eaten raw or crushed to provide the allicin in its juice. Aged garlic provides similar or better health benefits. Garlic pills have no nutritional value.
- Ginger: is known as the "poor man's aspirin". Ginger thins the blood, lowers cholesterol and increases blood circulation to help prevent strokes and hardening of the arteries, based on research done at Cornell University Medical College. The active ingredient in ginger (gingerol) is proven effective in preventing recurrences of so-called "mini-strokes". It is believed that gingerol inhibits an enzyme that causes blood cells to clot. Ginger improves and stimulates circulation and relaxes the muscles surrounding blood vessels, facilitating the flow of blood throughout the body. As a circulatory stimulant (for the extremities), it works well with cayenne pepper, a circulatory stimulant (for the heart).
- Ginkgo biloba: contains flavonoids, including quercetin. Gingko acts as an antioxidant, anti-allergen, anti-inflammatory; and, as an oxygen-carrying agent, it increases the blood flow throughout the circulatory system as well as the brain. It may reduce plaque that builds up around artery walls. Ginkgo biloba has been used in the treatment of early-stage Alzheimer's disease, vascular dementia, and peripheral claudication.
Warning: Ginkgo can increase the risk of bleeding if used in combination with warfarin or antiplatelet agents.

- Glutathione (GSH): is called the "master antioxidant" because it is the regulator and regenerator of immune cells, it recharges other antioxidants (Vitamin C, E), it is the most valuable detoxifying agent in the human body, and it fights oxidation. Unlike other antioxidants, GSH is actually produced by the body. GSH is transported into the mitochondria, where it destroys free radicals, preventing damage to DNA, cell membranes, and protein. However, most GSH supplements do not work as advertised. Pre-cursors such as n-acetyl cysteine (NAC), artichoke, asparagus, broccoli, milk thistle, cruciferous vegetables and whey protein supplements with gamma-glutamylcysteine help the body produce GSH. GSH has more than 100 times the anti-oxidizing power of other antioxidants, dismantles fat molecules, is "turbocharged" by companion enzymes like GSH peroxides, and is regenerating. In addition, GSH plays a role in the detoxification of many xenobiotics (foreign compounds) both organic and inorganic; and, helps the immune response by optimizing macrophage functions, and by stabilizing the mitochondrial membrane to reduce cell death.
- Grapeseed extract: contains a concentration of the oligomeric proanthocyanidins (OPCs) found in grape seeds and skins that acts as a smooth muscle relaxant in blood vessels, to combat hypertension. It provides nutrient support to strengthen the walls of small capillaries to prevent capillary leakage in the legs, reducing fluid retention.
- Green tea: is rich in catechin polyphenols, particularly epigallocatechin gallate (EGCG), which is a powerful antioxidant that inhibits the abnormal formation of blood clots. Since green tea leaves are steamed instead of fermented like black tea leaves, they are more effective in preventing and fighting various diseases because the EGCG is not oxidized or converted into weaker compounds. Similarly, because white tea is even less processed than green tea, it provides more antioxidant and anti-cancerous benefits.

- Hawthorne berry: contains the flavonoids hypercide, rutin, and vitexin, which help the heart to pump more easily, and with more force. It also helps the beta cells conductivity from the nerve to muscle fibers, increases blood circulation in the heart, prevents stress-related heart attacks, and reduces angina pain and cardiac arrhythmia. Medical studies have established that when Hawthorne berry is present in the blood, the heart muscle can survive on less blood and oxygen. Also, if a heart attack occurs, the heart muscle can survive longer because the heart cells don't die as rapidly.
- L-carnitine: is synthesized in the body from two amino acids, l-lysine and l-methionine, and nourishes the heart by helping to transport fat to the mitochondria of each cell to burn the fat as fuel. More than 95% of the l-carnitine in the body resides in the heart muscle and the skeletal muscles.
  Note: L-carnitine and CoQ10 are two of the most powerful and important nutrients for the heart.
- Nattokinase: is a potent enzyme extracted from *fermented* soybeans that break down fibrin to dissolve blood clots. Fibrin is made up of sticky protein fibers that form a netlike plug to stop any bleeding. The body produces plasmin, an enzyme that dissolves fibrin, but plasmin levels tend to decrease with age.
- Onions: contain the flavonoid quercetin, which helps to prevent the oxidation of LDL cholesterol.
- Red clover: contains coumarins, which inhibit the liver/vitamin K factor to reduce blood clots. Red clover is a "blood cleanser" with high amounts of isoflavones, such as genistein.
- Resveratrol: is a flavonoid found in red wine and the skin of grapes and cranberries. It provides antioxidant protection from free radicals, which prevents hardening of the arteries and heart disease. It helps to thin the blood by inhibiting blood platelet aggregation; prevents narrowing of arteries by inhibiting the oxidation of LDL cholesterol; and, relaxes the artery walls by increasing the production of nitric oxide.
  Note: A concentrated source of resveratrol can be found in the plant polygonum cuspidatum, known as Japanese knotweed.

- Turmeric: contains the antioxidant curcumin and helps to thin the blood with aspirin-like effectiveness.
- Vitamin C (with bioflavonoids): provides antioxidant protection to prevent damage to the arterial walls and aids in the production of collagen to repair the arteries or other damaged tissues. Vitamin C helps to prevent the over-production of metabolic repair factors. Vitamin C is a water-soluble nutrient that "bathes" the outside of the cells to prevent the outer walls from becoming weak and breaking down. For example, have you ever noticed that older people tend to bruise more easily? Part of that is due to the lack of Vitamin C and the weakening of the cells closest to the outer skin layers. Wholefood Vitamin C, which includes bioflavonoids, rutin, Vitamin K, and enzymes, can actually help heal the heart by increasing the oxygen carrying capacity of the blood. Synthetic Vitamin C only contains ascorbic acid.
- Vitamin E (mixed tocopherols): is absorbed into the lipid portion of the cells to provide antioxidant protection inside of the cells; also, prevents fish oil from oxidizing too rapidly. It also prevents platelets from sticking to each other and to blood vessel walls.
  Note: CoQ10 and Vitamin E are fat-soluble and therefore are absorbed internal to the cells to protect the insides of the cells. Studies show that people who have had heart attacks tend to have low levels of these antioxidants in their bodies. Recent studies that indicated Vitamin E does not provide cardiovascular protection did not use the Vitamin E that consists of four tocopherols and four tocotrienols – the Vitamin E only contained the alpha tocopherol; and, some contained a synthetic form called dl-alpha tocopherol.
- Spiritual health: helps to control your emotions and reduce stress. Based on research from Johns Hopkins University, health of the heart can be affected by emotions, causing a surge in adrenaline and stress hormones that mimic a heart attack, possibly by constricting blood vessels. The MRI scans revealed no signs of actual heart attacks, but the subjects experienced measurable symptoms of cardiac distress.

Wellness Protocol for High Blood Pressure (HBP)

Your blood pressure is one of the most important tests that your doctor performs. It is the key indicator of your cardiovascular health, even more important than cholesterol. Utilize the following specific steps as a guideline to help reduce or prevent high blood pressure.

1. Eat foods rich in monounsaturated fats and Omega-3 EFAs, especially cold-water fish, flaxseed, nuts, extra virgin olive oil, organic flax oil, and avocado. If you don't like fish, take a pharmaceutical-grade fish oil capsule (1000 to 1500 mg daily), plus extra Vitamin E to protect the oil from peroxidation. Avocado contains folate, potassium, beta-sitosterol, Vitamin E, and fiber. Add ground flaxseed (1-2 tbsp.) to salads/beverages; drink filtered water; and, drink beverages such as hibiscus tea, which contains flavonoids that may help to lower blood pressure and does not contain caffeine.

2. Eat green leafy vegetables/grasses, which are rich sources of the common salts that can be converted to nitric oxide, which relaxes blood vessels. Eat *magnesium*-rich foods to equalize the levels of potassium and sodium and relax the artery muscles. Eat *potassium*-rich foods to lower the sodium level and maintain the balance of electrolytes to regulate blood pressure and muscle contraction. Potassium also aids in converting blood glucose into glycogen to be stored in the muscles and liver and released as needed. Also, eat some *calcium*-rich foods to support vascular muscle contraction.

    - Foods that are rich in *magnesium* include: green leafy vegetables (broccoli, spinach), tofu, tomato paste, sweet potato, black beans, nuts, seeds, baked beans, navy beans, peanut butter; beet greens, lima beans, black-eyed peas, pinto beans, whole grain cereals, squash, kidney beans, chickpeas, yogurt, lentils, okra.
    - Vegetables and fruits that are rich in *potassium* include: avocado, barley grass, wheat grass, bananas, beet greens, bell peppers, broccoli, cabbage, celery, collards, cucumbers, parsley, spinach, tomato, black-eyed peas, squash, black beans, lentils, navy beans, pinto beans; apricot, cantaloupe, grapefruit, honeydew, orange juice, papaya, peach.

- Vegetables, fruits and meat that have a moderate amount of *potassium* include: beets, carrots, ginger root, kale, mustard greens, okra, parsnips, pumpkin, sauerkraut, stringbeans, sweet potatoes; apple, cherries, banana, dates, grapes, lemons, oranges, mangos, pineapple, prune juice, raspberries, raisins, strawberries; halibut, flounder, rabbit, sardine, salmon, turkey.
- Foods that are rich in *calcium* include: low fat organic yogurt, sardines, salmon, mustard greens, oysters, broccoli, and tofu. The following foods offer the best form of calcium (that is soluble and easily assimilated): spinach, kale, broccoli, mustard greens, turnip greens, collard greens, sesame seeds, kelp, and seaweed.
- The following foods provide calcium but contain too much animal protein and fat: skim milk, Swiss cheese, cheddar cheese, cottage cheese. Too much animal protein causes the kidneys to overwork, removing calcium from your blood before it can be stored in the bones.
- *Caution:* Patients with renal disease, hyperkalemia, or taking potassium-sparing diuretics, usually need to restrict their potassium intake and should not try to follow a high potassium diet. Additionally, individuals who need to limit potassium intake should not use potassium chloride salt substitutes, which are often made from potassium chloride.

3. Avoid alcohol, tobacco, caffeine, soda, diet soda, and most drugs.
4. Obtain your own blood pressure monitor to record your blood pressure on a regular basis, especially if your blood pressure rises due to the "white coat syndrome". Check your blood pressure at the same times throughout the day. Also check your blood pressure when you are under stress or you don't feel well. Take your monitor with you when you visit your doctor to compare your readings.
5. If your blood pressure is only borderline high, discuss with your doctor to ensure that your blood pressure is being measured properly, especially since improper use of the blood pressure monitor may cause a false reading. Get additional diagnostic tests performed if the doctor is not certain or you are not making any progress.
6. Review the following nutrients and their descriptions to identify the nutrients that support your heart health and super meal program.

7. If you have been diagnosed with a **high volume of blood/fluids** (e.g. edema, water retention) due to high BUN, high sodium, low potassium serum levels, or cell dehydration, utilize one or more of the following nutrients.

    - Cayenne pepper: acts as a circulatory stimulant to expand the extremities of the circulatory system.
    - Celery (juice), cucumber, lemons, limes: act as natural diuretics.
    - Ginger: improves and stimulates circulation and relaxes the muscles surrounding the blood vessels.
    - Grapeseed extract: contains a concentration of the oligomeric proanthocyanidins (OPCs) found in grape seeds and skins that provides nutrient support to strengthen the walls of small capillaries to prevent capillary leakage in the legs, eyes and skin, reducing fluid retention.

8. If you have been diagnosed with **blood clots** or **thick, sticky blood** due to high triglycerides or high blood glucose, utilize one or two of the following to help "thin" the blood and reduce inflammation.

    - Bromelain: is an enzyme (found in the pineapple plant) that breaks down fibrin, a blood-clotting protein that can impede good circulation and prevent tissues from draining properly.
    - Garlic (raw/aged), onion: inhibit blood platelet aggregation.
    - Ginger: thins the blood, and has anti-inflammatory properties. Medical research conducted in both China and Russia has shown that ginger can help lower blood pressure.
    - L-carnitine: helps to metabolize fats in the blood.
    - Nattokinase: is a potent enzyme extracted from fermented soybeans that breaks down fibrin to dissolve blood clots.
    - Omega-3 EFAs: contain blood-thinning properties that help to lubricate the blood vessels, preventing clogging and hardening of the arteries. Food sources include fish oil, extra virgin olive oil, organic flaxseed oil, nuts and seeds.
    - Pine bark extract: contains bioflavonoids called oligomeric proanthocyanidins (OPCs) that reduce platelet aggregation preventing blood cells from sticking together and forming clumps in the blood.

- Red clover: is known as a "blood cleanser" with high amounts of isoflavones, such as genistein.
- Resveratrol: is a flavonoid in grape skins that inhibits blood platelet aggregation.
- Turmeric: contains curcumin, which helps to thin the blood with aspirin-like effectiveness.

9. If your doctor is able to determine that your **artery walls need to relax** to address narrowing (constriction), utilize one or more of the following.

- Arginine: increases production of nitric oxide to relax artery walls. Foods rich in arginine include fish, poultry, dairy, nuts, and chocolate.
- Celery stalk: contains a chemical oil called 3-n butyl phthalide that lowers blood pressure by relaxing the arteries and lowering the level of stress hormones called catacholamines.
  Note: Most people eat the stalk but actually it's the leaves that contain the most nutritional benefits.
- Exercise: on a consistent basis helps to increase the production of nitric oxide, which relaxes the artery walls.
- Grapeseed extract: contains a concentration of the oligomeric proanthocyanidins (OPCs) found in grape seeds and skins that acts as a smooth muscle relaxant in blood vessels to combat hypertension.
- Lysine, proline: are amino acids needed for collagen and elastin formation in the blood vessel walls, and to make lipoprotein (a) less sticky, preventing cholesterol from sticking to injured artery walls. Foods rich in lysine include: eggs, lima beans, raw milk, meat and Brewer's yeast. Foods rich in proline include meats.
- Magnesium: helps to relax the artery walls by maintaining an optimum mineral balance in the cells of the blood vessel walls. Foods rich in magnesium include green leafy vegetables and beans.
- Resveratrol: is a flavonoid in grape skins that increases production of nitric oxide to relax artery walls.
- Vitamin C: increases the production of prostacycline, which relaxes the artery walls and keeps blood viscosity from increasing.

10. If you have been diagnosed with **unbalanced hormone levels**, utilize some or all of the following:
    - Alkaline-forming foods: include raw vegetables and tart fruits that provide an array of vitamins, minerals, enzymes, fiber, and other nutrients to help provide antioxidant protection and biochemical/hormonal balance.
    - Exercise: helps to release endorphins and remove toxins to prevent hormonal imbalances.
    - Pine bark extract: reduces adrenaline stress reactions that trigger high blood pressure.
11. If you have been diagnosed with a **weak heart muscle**, utilize some of the following:
    - Astragalus: strengthens the beating and force of contraction of the heart muscle, while also increasing the level of energy production within heart cells.
    - CoQ10: provides the "spark" in the mitochondria to produce energy within the heart muscle.
    - D-Ribose: is a simple sugar molecule found in every cell of the body that supports the production of ATP (adenosine triphosphate) levels in the heart and skeletal muscles. It fortifies the mitochondria and supports the recycling of energy to provide continuous energy.
    - Exercise: on a consistent basis (with low-intensity) helps to gradually rebuild the strength and endurance of the muscle.
    - L-carnitine: provides nourishment to the heart muscle to break down fatty acids and produce energy by transporting fat to the mitochondria.
    - Magnesium: helps coordinate the activity of the heart muscle as well as the functioning of the nerves that initiate the heartbeat. It also helps to prevent spasms of the coronary arteries, an action that can cause the intense chest pain known as angina.
12. If you have been diagnosed with **inflammation** and **plaque buildup** (smaller diameter of artery walls), due to high homocysteine, high lipoprotein (a), or high C-reactive protein, refer to the next section for more detail.

Wellness Protocol for High Inflammation

If blood tests indicate a high level of homocysteine, C-reactive protein, fibrinogen, or cholesterol, utilize the following specific steps as a guideline to help reduce, reverse or prevent inflammation.

1. Eat foods that contain antioxidants and anti-inflammatory properties. Specifically, eat dark leafy greens and cruciferous vegetables such as broccoli, cabbage, Brussels sprouts, spinach, kale; red/yellow/orange vegetables such as peppers, carrots, squash, tomatoes; fruits such as avocado, blueberries, cherries, other berries, apples, apricots, oranges, grapefruit, red/black grapes, peaches; fish such as wild salmon and sardines; and, organic whole grains such as oat, quinoa and barley.

2. Review the following nutrients and their descriptions to identify the nutrients that are appropriate to reduce your internal inflammation and complement your super meal program by closing any nutritional gaps.

    To lower a high homocysteine:
    *   Betaine: is a natural polysaccharide found in beets that can lower homocysteine levels. Betaine can provide an additional benefit by increasing the production of S-adenosyl-methionine (SAMe), which is a metabolite of methionine that provides benefits to the joints, liver and one's mood (depression relief).
    *   Folic acid, Vitamin B6, Vitamin B12: are contained within green, leafy vegetables and legumes, e.g. spinach, broccoli, asparagus, avocado, beans, lentils, and organic whole grain cereals.
    *   Lecithin: contains choline, which may help to metabolize homocysteine.
    *   N-Acetyl Cysteine (NAC): is the stable form of the amino acid cysteine, which provides detoxifying and antioxidant protection by acting as a precursor to glutathione and contributing to its regeneration.

    To lower a high lipoprotein (a):
    *   Lysine, proline: are essential amino acids that make lipoprotein (a) less sticky by acting like teflon agents to prevent cholesterol from sticking to injured artery walls.

- N-Acetyl cysteine (NAC): breaks up the disulfide bonds between the LDL particle and the large glycoprotein apo(a) to lower lp(a).
- Niacin: reduces the production of lipoprotein (a), but until the artery wall damage is repaired, the liver will continue to produce the lipoprotein(a).
- Vitamin C (with bioflavonoids): helps to produce collagen to repair arterial walls and prevent the production of lipoprotein (a).

To lower a high C-reactive protein:
- Exercise: on a consistent basis (low to medium intensity) helps to prevent high inflammation.
- Omega-3 EFAs: reduce the production of pro-inflammatory cytokines and inhibit production of pro-inflammatory prostaglandins and leukotrienes.
- Quercetin: is one of the bioflavonoids with anti-inflammatory properties, found in rinds, barks, onions, and grape seeds.
- Turmeric: contains curcumin, which has powerful anti-inflammatory properties.
- No refined carbohydrates, other processed foods and high-fat animal products: which induce inflammation within the body.

To lower a high triglyceride level:
- L-carnitine: transports fat to the mitochondria to be burned as fuel, especially when exercising on a consistent basis.
- Fish/krill oil: contains EPA and DHA, which are needed for the transport and metabolism of both cholesterol and triglycerides. Fish/krill oil helps with inflammation, platelet stickiness, and triglycerides. Sources include wild salmon, sardines, albacore tuna, mackerel, herring, sablefish (black cod), and anchovies.
- Flaxseed: contains fiber and is one of the best vegetarian sources of Omega-3 essential fatty acids that has been shown to reduce serum triglyceride levels. Flax oil does not provide this benefit.
- Green tea: contains flavonoids (specifically, catechins) that may slow down the process that sends triglycerides into the bloodstream. So, drink a cup or two of green tea with your meals.
- Policosanol: is a phytochemical extract from sugar cane wax that may lower serum triglyceride levels.
- No refined sugar or refined flour foods, which raise triglycerides.

To lower a high LDL ("bad") cholesterol:

- Avocado: contains ten grams of fiber, and a plant chemical called beta-sitosterol – both help to lower cholesterol; also, contains monounsaturated fat, potassium, and antioxidants.
- Beta glucan: binds the cholesterol with bile acids for elimination in the feces. These soluble fibers also help to reduce the elevation in blood sugar levels by delaying gastric emptying so that dietary sugar is absorbed more gradually. Beta glucan is found in the cell walls of baker's yeast, grains (e.g. oat bran, barley bran, oat/rye sprouts) and mushrooms (e.g. maitake, reishi, shiitake).
- Fenugreek seeds: contain steroidal saponins (diosgenin, yamogenin, tigogenin, neotigogenin) that may inhibit cholesterol absorption and synthesis. They also contain a mucilaginous fiber that helps lower blood sugar levels by slowing the digestion of carbohydrates.
- Flaxseed: contains soluble and insoluble fiber and is one of the best vegetarian sources of Omega-3 essential fatty acids.
- Flaxseed oil: contains significant amounts of alpha linolenic acid (ALA) that may help lower cholesterol and blood pressure.
- Fiber: foods high in soluble and insoluble fiber include oat bran, pectin, dried beans, peas, flaxseed, apples (pectin), psyllium husk; and, green, leafy vegetables, especially broccoli, Brussel sprouts, spinach, kale.
  Note: If you are unable to consume at least 32 grams of fiber daily, then consider taking a daily fiber supplement.
  Studies show that the combination of 900 to 1800 mg of plant sterols and a daily minimum of 32 g of fiber work synergistically to block the absorption / reabsorption of cholesterol and remove it with the fecal waste.
- Garlic (raw/aged), Onions (raw/cooked): contain phytonutrients that help to decrease the amount of LDL cholesterol.
- Ginger root: contains nutrients that attenuate the development of atherosclerotic lesions, reducing the levels of LDL cholesterol and oxidized LDL cholesterol.

- Green tea: is rich in catechin polyphenols, particularly epigallocatechin gallate (EGCG), which is a powerful antioxidant that has been effective in lowering LDL cholesterol levels. In addition, green tea contains the flavonoid quercetin, which interrupts the oxidation of LDL cholesterol.
- Lecithin: inhibits intestinal absorption of cholesterol, increasing the excretion of cholesterol and bile acids.
- Monounsaturated fats: within olive oil, macadamia nuts, hazel nuts, pecans, and almonds may help to lower the LDL cholesterol and protect it from being oxidized. Omega-3 fats such as fish oil and flax oil are required for the transport and metabolism of both cholesterol and triglycerides.
- Niacin: lowers the LDL cholesterol, but can raise homocysteine levels. Consequently, have your doctor check your homocysteine level if you are taking niacin to lower your cholesterol.
- Phosphatidyl choline (PC): is the most abundant phospholipid in the body that is needed for cell membrane integrity and to facilitate the movement of fats in and out of cells. PC is required for the transport and metabolism of fats and cholesterol within the body, which is important for the healthy support of the endocrine, cardiovascular and hepatic systems.
- Plant sterols (phytosterols): are plant fats that block the absorption of dietary cholesterol filling up the absorption sites on the intestinal wall; and, block the reabsorption of cholesterol that is recirculated through the bile into the intestinal tract.

  Note: Clinical studies demonstrate that a daily minimum dosage of 900 to 1800 mg of plant sterols is very effective in reducing the LDL and total cholesterol. Specifically, plant sterol supplements in a very fine powder have proven to be more effective than tablets or liquids, especially when used in conjunction with a fiber supplement.

  Note: As of September 2000, the FDA authorized the use of labeling health claims about the role of plant sterol or plant stanol esters in lowering blood cholesterol levels to reduce the risk of coronary heart disease (CHD).

Note: A recent study from Canada discovered that plant sterols were effective in lowering cholesterol for everyone, but were dramatically more effective for Type 2 diabetics. Plant sterols reduced LDL cholesterol by about 26 percent for Type 2 diabetics and by about 15 percent for others after consuming a diet containing 1.8 g of plant sterols daily for three weeks.

- Policosanol: is a phytochemical extract from sugar cane wax that lowers cholesterol levels by slowing down cholesterol synthesis in the liver and increasing liver reabsorption of the LDL cholesterol. It also reduces the tendency of blood to clot by reducing the "stickiness" of blood platelets.
  Note: Based on the clinicals, ensure that the policosanol comes from sugar cane wax, not beeswax or rice extract.
- Polyunsaturated fats: such as sunflower, safflower, or soybean oil may help to lower the LDL cholesterol *but* they also lower the good HDL cholesterol. Do *not* cook with these oils because they break down and may form carcinogenic compounds.
- Soy protein: contains isoflavones that help to lower cholesterol. Specifically, the isoflavone genistein inhibits the oxidation of LDL cholesterol.
- Sunlight (at least 30 minutes/day): metabolizes cholesterol (in the skin) to produce Vitamin D and hormone precursors.
- Turmeric: contains curcumin, which reduces cholesterol by interfering with intestinal cholesterol uptake, increasing the conversion of cholesterol into bile acids, and increasing the excretion of bile acids.
- Vitamin C (with bioflavonoids): helps to protect and heal the artery walls.
- Vitamin D: produced naturally within the body due to exposure to sunlight; may prevent diabetes, some cancers (breast, prostate, colon), multiple sclerosis, and osteoporosis.
- Vitamin E (mixed tocopherols/tocotrienols): contains gamma tocotrienol, which suppresses the production of the HMG-CoA reductase enzyme involved in cholesterol production, resulting in less cholesterol being produced by the liver.

To reduce the oxidation of the LDL ("bad") cholesterol:
- Alpha lipoic acid: is a universal antioxidant that has the ability to conserve and prolong the life of Vitamin C and Vitamin E in the body, increasing their effectiveness.
- CoQ10, Vitamin E: are fat-soluble antioxidants that prevent the oxidation of LDL cholesterol and other lipids.
- Green tea, Onions: contain the flavonoid quercetin, which interrupts the oxidation of LDL cholesterol.
- Resveratrol: contains OPCs (within grape skins), which inhibit the oxidation of LDL cholesterol.
- Soy protein: contains the isoflavone genistein, which may inhibit the oxidation of LDL cholesterol.

To increase the size of small, dense LDL ("bad") cholesterol:
- Fish oil: contains docosahexaenoic acid (DHA), which helps to increase the LDL particle size.
- No processed foods: especially deep-fried foods and processed foods that contain hydrogenated oil (trans fats) such as margarine, potato chips, cookies, and other packaged foods.

To raise a low HDL ("good") cholesterol:
- Exercise: performed on a consistent basis with weight/resistance training may help to increase the HDL cholesterol.
- Monounsaturated fats: such as extra virgin olive oil, flaxseed, organic flax oil, walnuts, and avocados, contain Omega-3 EFAs and MUFAs that may help to increase HDL cholesterol.
- Red wine/grape skins: contain minute levels of resveratrol and other nutrients that may help to increase HDL cholesterol.

To lower a high fibrinogen level:
- Omega-3 EFAs: reduce the production of pro-inflammatory cytokines and inhibit the production of pro-inflammatory prostaglandins and leukotrienes.
- Other nutrients: bromelain, curcumin, garlic, green/white tea, nattokinase, serrapeptase.
- No saturated fat, tobacco: reduces exposure to the hormones and chemicals that increase the internal inflammation.

Chapter 16. Next Steps

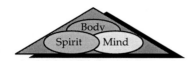

Now What?

According to Dr. Phil McGraw there are two factors that will prevent you moving from a condition that you claim you do <u>not</u> want (poor health), to a condition that you claim you <u>do</u> want (good health):

- The first is the advantages you get from the unwanted condition of poor health. Dr. Phil refers to this as "your payoff." For example, you may miss the doting you get from your family who feels sorry for you because of your illness. You may miss the convenience of taking a drug instead of making all these changes.

- The second is the disadvantages you avoid by not moving to the desired condition of good health. For example, you may not want to take on the responsibility for being accountable for your own health and the decisions you have to make because you can no longer blame the doctor or someone else for your poor health.

The underlying mechanism that drives these two factors is **behavior modification**. Trying to change your behavior after 20-30 years of eating and living a certain way is very difficult and challenging to say the least – but, not impossible. Consequently, if you do not face and address these two factors, then, the first time that you have to deal with a change that affects your daily life or the activities of your family members and friends, you will be tempted to revert to your old habits. In addition, when the journey starts to get a little rough, you will be tempted to fall back into your old habits. Instead of waiting for that to happen, develop a proactive plan that will address those problem areas *before* they occur.

Note: If you need help in developing a proactive plan that is customized to your lifestyle and your health needs, contact our wellness center (800-813-1927, 800-954-0366) or visit our website <u>www.deathtodiabetes.com</u>.

The Excuses

During my presentations and many of the diabetic support group meetings that I either attended or facilitated, I heard almost every excuse imaginable, many of them disguised to rationalize eating foods that most people know are bad for them. Bottomline, most people really don't want to change their lifestyle or eating habits -- even if it's killing them. The following is a summary of the key types of excuses and specific countermeasures to successfully overcome these excuses.

Time:
- Some people feel that, due to their busy schedules and family commitments, they do not have the time to prepare meals and eat properly.
- There is no time to acquire knowledge, no time to eat, no time to prepare meals properly, no time to shop for groceries, no time to get a physical exam; no time to exercise; no time due to long work hours. Potatoes, rice, macaroni, pasta, pizza, and frozen dinners are easy foods to prepare, requiring very little time.
- Very little time is required to obtain food from fast food restaurants.

Countermeasures:
- Prepare meals on the weekends, and store them in freezer bags.
- Purchase frozen vegetables and fruits to save preparation time when cooking.
- Use healthy snack foods such as nuts, seeds, pulse food, and fruits.
- Use nutritional supplements that can easily be added to your beverages to turn them into quick super meals, e.g. ground flaxseed, super greens powder, whey protein powder, soy protein powder.
- Exercise while on the phone or watching TV. Get up 15 minutes earlier in the morning to exercise or exercise as soon as you get home before life gets in the way. Walk after lunch. Try mall-walking.
- Purchase an exercise machine that will motivate you to exercise and make it easier to exercise while on the phone or watching TV.
- *Benefit:* You will save the time that you would have spent with doctors, drugstores, hospitals, sick days, etc.

Lifestyle:
- Many people enjoy their lifestyle and lack the motivation to give up any of their freedoms.
- Many people just don't like to exercise. Reasons include time, boredom, pain, sweat, cost, and community involvement.
- Many families do not sit down and eat together anymore.

Countermeasures:
- If you have any disease, then, your current *life*style is really your *death*style – give it up before it gives you up.
- Become a community advocate for change, e.g. support getting bicycle and walking lanes added in your neighborhood.
- Learn ways to enjoy exercise. If you make exercise fun, the time will fly by. Exercise with a friend or the family. Make it a social event. Keep track of your exercise progress to provide motivation. Make exercise a fun activity, e.g. go hiking, participate in a walk-a-thon.
- Set aside at least two days each week to eat together as a family.
- *Benefit:* You will enjoy a higher quality of life and slow down the biological clock.

Food Addiction, Enjoyment:
- Some people are addicted to the chemicals in the "dead" foods, which cause the toxic overloads and the biochemical and hormonal imbalances. Unfortunately, some people don't realize that they have a chemical addiction to the "dead" food.
- Some people are "addicted" to the freedom and lifestyle that the convenience of prepared/fast foods brings to their lives.
- The foods that are unhealthy include many of the good-tasting foods, which are easy to acquire and easy to prepare.

Countermeasures:
- Change your definition of food. Many of your favorite foods are poison to your body. Would you consume arsenic if it taste good? Start eating more of the healthy foods and gradually convert each unhealthy (favorite) food to a healthier version.
- Reduce the number of times that you eat out. Also, reduce your time spent watching TV, especially the food commercials and the news.
- *Benefit:* You will enjoy food without sacrificing your health.

Finances:
- Potatoes, rice, macaroni, pasta are inexpensive foods, and easy to prepare, especially for a large family.
- Some people feel that it costs more to eat healthy.
- Many people can't afford to buy exercise equipment or join a gym.

Countermeasures:
- Spend the same amount of money on meat, but buy a smaller amount of a higher quality meat, e.g. lean, no antibiotics. Buy foods that will heal your body so that you can reduce the money you're spending on doctors, drugs and hospitals.
- Reduce eating out at fast food restaurants.
- *Benefit:* You will eventually begin to save money because eating healthy requires less food (fuel), less drugs, less doctor visits, less medical bills, etc.

Denial/Spirit:
- Some people rationalize: "Well, you gotta die of something some time!" (*Author's Note:* I hear this excuse all the time).
- Some people feel fine while others don't believe that they are seriously sick (Illusion of Health, State of Denial).
- Some people are unaware of the extra weight they're carrying.
- Most people don't realize that they are as addicted to food as drug addicts are addicted to drugs.
- Some people have a negative outlook on life.
- Some people are stubborn, and refuse to make the necessary changes to their nutrition, exercise, and lifestyle.
- There is a defense mechanism that tries to "protect" us when, after years of being told one thing ("there's no cure for diabetes") that the opposite might be true. Some people will actually spend energy trying to convince themselves and others that "It can't be true – it can't be that simple."; or "That's impossible – I've been living with this disease a long time, I should know."

Countermeasures:
- Improve your spiritual health, emotional health, and family health.
- Believe that God will help you, but don't sit around waiting for God – take action, listen to your surroundings.

- Increase your knowledge about nutrition and disease.
- Accept the fact that you will make mistakes. We all make mistakes, but how you respond will determine your level of success.
- Don't waste energy trying to convince yourself and others that you can't get your disease under control. It would be more fruitful using that energy to attempt to improve your health.
- *Benefit:* Spiritual health allows you to focus on your faith and ability to help others, with a de-emphasis on drugs. This supports Apostle Paul's requirement to glorify God in our body, as well as our spirit: "Know ye not that your body is the temple of the Holy Ghost . . . therefore glorify God in your body, and in your spirit, which are God's." (1 Corinthians 6:19-20)
- *Benefit:* Emotional health allows you to be happier, with no anxiety or frustration; and, your energy is no longer spent on being unhealthy, overweight, tired, or living in pain.
- *Benefit:* Family health becomes your legacy. Your children will not follow today's trend of more obese children and more children becoming Type 2 diabetics. Keep in mind that obesity in childhood carries into adulthood more than 75% of the time.

Knowledge:
- Many people are brainwashed by the food industry and TV advertising about processed foods, fast foods, snack foods, and soda beverages – most are chemicals disguised as "food".
- Some people don't really believe that eating properly can make that much of a difference; and, even if it did, it takes too long to reap the benefits. It's easier to just take a drug.
- Some people are not aware that some of their family members or friends may not want them to succeed.
- Because drugs are so effective at lowering blood glucose, blood pressure, and cholesterol, many people believe that the drugs are really working to improve their health.
- Most people have developed an acceptance of over-the-counter and prescription drugs as a way-of-life and a belief that they actually work to heal the body.

- Some people are not aware of the effects that food chemicals can have on their health.
- People are not aware of how to easily convert their favorite foods to healthier versions with very little effort.
- Some people aren't certain what to do with the glucose readings.
- Some diabetics believe they're okay because they're on pills instead of insulin.
- Some diabetics successfully control their glucose level for a while, but they give up when they don't understand why they eventually lose control.
- Some people waste their hard-earned money on worthless vitamin "rocks".

Countermeasures:
- Educate yourself and your family members about nutrition, drugs, disease, vitamins, and other supplements.
- Join a support group and become an active participant.
- Learn who your friends are. As Earvin (Magic) Johnson said: "When you face a crisis, you know who your true friends are."
- Take a class in nutrition, diabetes or exercise.
- Attend a health fair, a wellness meeting, or a medical conference.
- Become an advocate in your church or other community group.
- *Benefit:* You will feel a lot more comfortable with the decisions you make about your health once you've armed yourself with the knowledge. This knowledge will give you an inner strength that you didn't know that you had. And, as this inner strength builds over time, you will become more empowered – because, *strength over time is power*. This newly discovered power will help you become an advocate within your family and, if you choose to do so, your community. And, more importantly, your family's health will be greatly improved.

Did any of those excuses sound familiar to you? You can defeat these excuses by planning ahead with some of these countermeasures.

Author's Personal Note: Thanks to my mother and daughter, who supplied many of the countermeasures.

The 10 Steps to Reverse Type 2 Diabetes

The following is a summary of the 10 key steps to control and possibly reverse your diabetes.

1. Increase your **knowledge** about diabetes and its complications, nutrition, exercise, and drugs. Visit your local library, go to medical-related websites, take classes, and talk to other (healthy) diabetics.

2. Eat the **5 "live" super foods**, especially bright-colored vegetables, fruits, raw juices, sea vegetables, grasses, plant protein, plant oils, whole grains, legumes, filtered water, and cold-water fish. Eat **4-5 super meals/snacks** each day. Buy a steamer for your vegetables.

3. Reduce/stop eating the **5 "dead" processed foods**, especially white flour, sugar, 'enriched' foods, starches, animal meat, trans fats, drugs.

4. Increase your **blood glucose testing** to at least 4 times a day, including a post-meal test to customize your nutritional profile. Use a **journal/logbook** to record, track, analyze and make changes.

5. Take a **wholefood** or **food-based supplement** to complement your nutritional program and accelerate the healing process.

6. Perform **cleansing/detoxification** to remove the toxins and waste.

7. **Exercise** consistently by stretching/walking 30 to 45 minutes four to six times a week. And, add 10 to 15 minutes of weight/resistance (anaerobics) exercise on alternate days.

8. Utilize exercise, prayer, yoga, or other meditation techniques to relax, help relieve the stress, and connect with your **inner spirit**. Find some quiet time for yourself each day, even if it's only 5 minutes. Join a local support group to get information and share your problems with other diabetics. Your insight may help someone in the group and will motivate you to continue making progress.

9. Work with your **doctor** and other healthcare professionals to communicate your health goals and build your relationships. Ensure your treatment is focused on repairing your body and reducing your drug usage/dependency and not just suppressing the symptoms.

10. Develop an overall (proactive) **wellness plan**. Address any excuses or barriers you may have before proceeding with your recovery plan.

Epilogue

Initially after my recovery, my daughter would call at least once a week and ask me how I was doing; plus, she would ask a couple of questions about diabetes, weight loss and nutrition. Then, she would ask me to send her an e-mail to summarize our discussion. After a couple months of this, Cynthia called and told me that she had been sharing what we talked about with her friends and other people at work. She said: "Dad, this is the last time I'll bug you about this . . . this stuff really makes sense and it works! It's not just for diabetics. Dad, you should write a book! Several people asked for copies of the e-mail information you sent me. They liked what they read, but they have more questions."

About a year ago a co-worker went to the hospital with a case of diabetes, high blood pressure and hypertriglyceridemia. He tried the super meal program and within four months, he had significantly reduced his blood pressure, triglycerides and glucose level and was able to reduce the amount of medication he was taking. He had so much energy, he started building a barn.

Another person from one of the local churches called to thank me and said although she'd been a diabetic for several years with little glucose control, she was able to get her glucose under control within two weeks by following the super meal program.

A person at work tried the super meal program and said he had more energy and felt better than he had felt for the past several years. Similar to what my daughter had said, he stated: "Your super meal program will work for anybody! So, when are you going to write a book?"

Another co-worker had a son who had just been diagnosed as diabetic, and he was really concerned with what to do to help him. About a month or so later, he called and said: "Thank you! My son is doing so much better! His glucose level is almost back to normal! Can you send me some more information?"

During a presentation to the staff of a correctional facility, someone asked where they could get more extensive information about my super meal program. A similar question came up during one of my talks to a group of health and wellness consultants. When I showed a biomedical engineering professor a copy of my notes and my biochemical flow charts, he remarked, "It looks like you've written a thesis, is it available?" I began to realize that maybe my mother, daughter, and others were right -- maybe I should write a book.

There are so many stories, many of them about people that I haven't even met yet. For example, someone called me from Virginia concerning her husband who is diabetic. In a matter of a few months, he lost over 20 pounds and lowered his average glucose level within the normal range. And there are other stories that I don't even know about. I realize that this is all anecdotal, but the information in this book would have been enough for me when I was initially struggling with my diabetes and things looked pretty grim.

At one of the church presentations, someone said to me: "I'm waiting for God to get me through my diabetes; and, no disrespect, but you ain't God." Everyone laughed and I smiled nodding in agreement trying to decide what to say when someone said, "Yeah, he ain't God, but maybe God sent this man to help us. By all accounts, he should be dead, but instead he's here giving us hope about a disease where there was little hope." That's probably one of the better reasons that I've heard that may explain why I didn't die when I was in the diabetic coma.

Several years ago, my mother felt that I needed to spend more time in church, but I felt that I was too busy, but would eventually get around to it. My mother said, "If you don't figure out a way, God will figure it out for you." Well, as usual, my mother was right. During the first year after my recovery I spent at least a couple days each week in a church or other forum talking about diabetes, heart disease, nutrition, and spiritual health. During one of my phone conversations with my mother, she said: "Hmm-mm . . . a few years ago you were too busy to go to church just once a week; now, you're visiting churches a couple times a week, and sometimes spending a weekend at a church conference . . . doesn't God have a sense of humor?"

I am not certain what the future holds, but, I plan to continue participating in health fairs and providing presentations to the local churches and other community groups. These venues have provided me with invaluable information into the struggles that people have with diabetes and its complications.

In my enthusiasm to share my experiences and insights as a diabetic, I hope this information will prove to be as invaluable to you as it has been for me and others that I have met during these past three years. There is a saying that "Knowledge is power." If that's true, then this book can provide you with power. But, I believe that the *real* power resides within those of you who *use* this knowledge and take the action to become healthier. So hopefully, something in this book hits a chord with you such that you are going to take some action, any action to improve your health or that of a loved one.

Back in the 1990s I was a volunteer math tutor for several years. During that time I learned two important facts about students: one, they made the same basic mistakes with math; and, two, the successful students took the responsibility for their mistakes and corrected them to improve their grades. I've discovered something similar working with diabetics: one, they make the same basic mistakes (with food, exercise, testing); and, two, the successful diabetics took the responsibility for their mistakes and corrected them to improve their health. Hopefully, you will become one of those successful diabetics.

In the meantime, there is so much more I could not fit into this book about nutrition, supplements, exercise, spirit, health planning, and systemic diseases such as heart disease, cancer, osteoporosis, arthritis, allergies, acid reflux, and leaky gut syndrome. And, some people have expressed an interest in smaller versions of my oversized flow charts and diagrams that I use during my presentations, including my "health & wellness" pyramid that goes beyond the traditional food pyramid. Other related activities include developing a training course about this program, developing an audio CD for the visually-impaired, teaching nutritionists how to develop a nutritional profile, and designing a biomedical engineering course about operational models and their applications to new technologies and diagnostic failure analysis methodologies. God willing, maybe, these activities will be the foundation for a new book.

A couple of months after I had left the hospital, I told my mother what the doctors said: "According to medical science, I should be dead. According to medical science, I should have lost one or both feet to amputation. According to medical science, I should . . ." My mother interrupted me and said: "Boy, you tell them doctors that there is a science (listen to me now) . . . there is a science that is bigger, much bigger than *medical* science – that science, it's called *God's* science, and God's science can fix any disease. Besides, God has other plans for you now."

Well, Mother, I guess one of those plans was for me to write this book.

Update by the Author
I am currently working with a health services company (Parwel) to provide diabetes education and health services to organizations and corporations that are health-conscious and aware of the importance of their employees' health. I am also conducting diabetes wellness classes and workshops; and providing health coaching to wellness groups, individuals and families.

Because of the overwhelming response to my workshops and because some people don't have time to read my book, I developed a DVD, and, with my daughter's help, I am currently developing a cookbook, meal planner, workbook, audio book CD set, and a wellness journal.

Go to www.deathtodiabetes.com for an up-to-date list of new products and services; or, go to www.YouTube.com to see me in action.

Contact Information
Websites: www.DeathToDiabetes.com, www.parwel.com
Email: engineer@deathtodiabetes.com
Phone numbers: 800-813-1927, 800-954-0366 (W), 585-671-0577
Business address: 940 Holt Road #190   Webster, NY 14580

CHAPTER 16

Chapter 17. Recipes of Super Meals

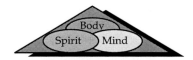

Preparation

The following are some general meal planning tips – some that I obtained from my mother and others that I obtained from nutrition-minded people:

- Obtain the following kitchen appliances/tools (mandatory):
  - A steamer to properly steam vegetables and prevent overcooking
  - A water filter to provide filtered water
  - A blender to prepare blended juices and replace bottled juices/beverages, especially soda and diet soda
  - A juicer to produce fresh raw vegetable, grass and fruit juices
  - Enameled cast iron cookware, stoneware, glassware, or some nonstick cookware to reduce the use of cooking oils
  - A Foreman grill to drain the fat from the meat
- Obtain the following kitchen appliances/tools (optional):
  - A large pot to prepare vegetable soups
  - Glassware-like containers to protect fresh vegetables and fruits; and, to store and freeze future meals, including soups
  - A freezer to allow you to stock up on foods that are on sale
  - A pressure cooker or portable convection oven (to save time when cooking)
  - A coffee grinder (to grind up fresh flaxseeds)
- Depending on your health needs and finances, purchase organic, fresh, or frozen vegetables and fruits instead of canned. It is not necessary that all your food be organic unless you have a concern with pesticides and other harmful chemicals. The key is that you replace the "dead" processed foods with the "live" vegetables, fruits, nuts, seeds. Use the Alternative Foods table (Figure 16, page 354) and the Resources list (page 374) as a guide when you start shopping.

- Prepare vegetable soups and casseroles that are less time-consuming, healthy, and inexpensive, especially if you have a large family.
- If you choose to adopt the mentality that there is a war going on inside your body, then, grocery shopping is your way of selecting the right foods to obtain the "weapons and ammunition" to fight the "enemy" known as diabetes. In general, avoid the middle aisles of the large grocery stores because that's where they usually stock the processed foods. Try to stay on the outside perimeter of the store.

Cooking Tips

Beans, Grains, Nuts & Seeds
- Add canned beans to soups, salads, and casseroles to provide fiber, but, rinse the beans to remove the excess sodium.
- Soak beans (and discard the water) to break down the gas-producing sugars, stachyose and raffinose.
- Use barley in almost any recipe that calls for rice, e.g. stuffed peppers, rice pilaf -- to provide more whole grain fiber.
- Use barley flour when making fresh bread or pasta.
- Use whole grains such as amaranth and quinoa because of their higher content of fiber, selenium, Vitamin E, and protein. Replace refined white flour and all-purpose flour with oat flour, soy flour, etc.
- Avoid roasted nuts because roasting oxidizes the fat. Always soak nuts/seeds to break down the enzyme inhibitors which interfere with digestion (The enzyme inhibitors are nature's defense mechanism of not being eaten before they can sprout and grow). Soak the nuts/seeds in a bowl of distilled water for 5-8 hours. Remove and discard the grains that float as they are likely rancid. Drain and rinse. Refrigerate nuts to protect the fat from turning rancid.

Desserts
- When making brownies, replace the semisweet chocolate with unsweetened cocoa and the butter with a cup of pureed prunes, which keep the brownies moist.
- When making a chocolate cake, replace the chocolate with cocoa, use fewer egg yolks, and reduce the amount of butter by substituting some nonfat yogurt.

- Add a handful of walnuts and a half-cup of blueberries to your bowl of ice cream to provide some fiber and protein and slow down the absorption of the sugar.
- Make your own homemade ice cream with low fat cream and fresh fruit. If you purchase your ice cream, do not buy the low fat versions because they contain more sugar and are less filling. Instead buy the rich ice cream, but eat less of it with some nuts and fruit.
- Sherbet, sorbet, ice milk, and low fat frozen yogurt are alternatives to the rich ice cream, but, be careful not to overeat them because they tend to be less filling and contain more sugar.

Fats, Oils
- Use rice bran oil, olive oil or cold-pressed macadamia nut oil for low heat stir-frying and sautéing foods. Use "light" olive oil for baking because it has little or no olive taste. Use a nonstick cooking spray made with olive oil but do not use it in a high heat environment. Use extra virgin olive oil to flavor salads and foods after cooking. Rice bran oil is rich in Vitamin E tocopherols and tocotrienols, a unique antioxidant known as gamma oryzanol, high quantities of phytosterols, polyphenols and squalene; and has a high smoke point.
- Use extra virgin coconut oil for cooking because this saturated fat is very healthy and can handle the heat.
- Instead of butter, spread a pat of extra virgin coconut oil onto a slice of sprouted grain bread and lightly toast. (Thanks, Cynthia)
- Mix 1-2 tablespoons of extra virgin olive oil into your tub of (soft) margarine spread.
- Avoid the clear vegetable oils such as corn, sunflower. Extra virgin olive oil (or rice bran oil) is the preferred oil for salads. and steamed vegetables, as it provides antioxidants and helps the body absorb the vegetable's fat-soluble nutrients (e.g. carotenoids).
- Extra virgin olive oil does not stay liquid when it is refrigerated. Mix extra virgin olive oil (60%) with flax oil (40%) or with macadamia nut oil to create your own new "super" oil that will remain more liquid when stored in the refrigerator. (Thanks, Larry P.)
- Reduce cooking with oil, which breaks down when overheated and forms harmful chemicals. If you decide to cook with oil, add the oil

to the food before cooking, and use stoneware to not overcook or "burn" the oil. Do not reheat or reuse oil. Avoid deep-frying, which creates carcinogens such as acrylamide.

- Freshly ground flaxseed is much healthier than flax oil, but it should be consumed almost immediately because the ALA oil in it goes rancid very quickly when exposed to air. Because polyunsaturated oils such as flaxseed or walnut oil become rancid when exposed to heat, light, and oxygen for too long, they should be stored in dark glass, tightly closed containers in the refrigerator. Only purchase organic flax oil that is being refrigerated in an opaque container (to keep out light) and has an expiration date. Refrigerate the flax oil after opening the bottle and try to use it up within 3 months because flax oil does not retain its vital nutrients even under proper care.

- But, if you decide to deep-fry, when high heat is used, use a healthy saturated fat such as organic or extra virgin coconut oil. And, use a flash-fryer to sear the outside of the food and prevent the oil from seeping into the food. Do not deep-fry with a polyunsaturated oil or shortening, which is a form of polyunsaturated fat that has been hydrogenised and transformed into a trans fat.

Meats, Fish, Dairy

- Cook wild salmon slowly (250° for 12-18 minutes, depending on size and thickness) to seal in the juices. Salmon is done when it turns translucent to opaque, and flakes separate easily with a fork. Use a light brushing of olive oil to help avoid salmon sticking to a grill or baking sheet. When grilling start with the skin side up and flip only once. The skin side has the rich oils, which will be drawn into the salmon by the heat below. Also, to prevent sticking, cut a potato in half and run it lengthwise down the hot grill – the starch will act as a natural lubricant. For seasoning, use a simple brushing with olive oil, sea salt, pepper, or a mix of olive oil, chopped fresh mint and cilantro.

- Fish can be broiled, baked, grilled, or steamed, but, be careful not to overcook and dry out the fish. Shrimp, lobster, and scallops are good choices for stir-frying with vegetables.

- If you miss fried fish, coat the fish in egg whites and bread crumbs, then bake until crispy. Squeeze some lemon or orange juice and sprinkle some dill over the fish. Top the fish with some fresh parsley, basil or thyme for added flavor.
- If possible avoid grilling, broiling or frying animal meat, especially red meat. Toxic compounds are created that have been linked to several cancers. To reduce these levels of carcinogens, use lean cuts only, marinate them, and flip them frequently on the grill to reduce the cooking time. Avoid smoked and processed meats such as bacon, sausage, ham, hot dogs, bologna, and lunch meats, which have been linked to cancer, multiple sclerosis, and Type 2 diabetes.
- If you eat beef, eat only the lean beef. The leanest cuts usually carry the label "USDA Select". Select beef contains 40% less fat than "prime" and 20% less fat than "choice". If financially possible, eat only organic USDA certified meat. Avoid the meat if it has a lot of marbling – this indicates a lot of fat. Cut away any visible fat before cooking the meat to reduce the fat and toxin intake. While broiling meat, let the fat drip off, but don't let it drain on hot charcoal or a hot burner because this will produce undesirable fumes.
- Use ground turkey or chicken in place of ground beef for lasagna, soups, stuffed peppers, burgers, etc. to reduce your saturated fat intake. If you really prefer the beef, then, use organic, free-range beef and use 20-25% less meat. Other meat options include wild game such as venison and bear because they provide Omega-3 EFAs and conjugated linoleic acid (CLA).
- Marinade meat overnight in something flavorful, e.g. olive oil, garlic, ginger, and light soy sauce. Use olive oil as part of the marinade to "break down" the harmful saturated fats and to increase the flavor.
- Sauté your meats with red and green peppers, onions, garlic, mushrooms, tomatoes, and other vegetables that you like to give the meat a better flavor and reduce the amount of meat that you would normally eat because of the extra vegetables.
- To reduce the amount of arachidonic acid in steaks and roasts: trim all the visible fat from the steak, then place it in a large resealable plastic bag along with a mixture of 1 cup of red wine and 1 cup of olive oil or light sesame oil. Allow the meat to marinate in this

mixture in the refrigerator for a full 24 hours, flipping the bag and contents over a couple of times. Take the steak out, drain it for an hour or so, discard the marinade, rub the beef with some pepper or other spices to taste, then grill it.

Note: The wine acts as a solvent to leach out a fair amount of the fat in the steak, which is replaced in part by the fat in the olive or sesame oil. The oil permeates the steak, giving it a juicy succulent taste and makes it healthier. You can use this technique with roasts as well.

- If you miss fried chicken, coat the skinless chicken with skim milk, egg whites, a small amount of organic flour, cornflake crumbs, herbs and spices; and, and bake at 375°. Another option is to coat the chicken, then flash-fry the chicken for 30 seconds in a nonstick pan coated with a teaspoon of olive or rice bran oil to crisp the outside; then, bake the chicken at 400° for approximately 40 minutes.
- If you really like fried foods, then, use a flash fryer that will sear the food on the outside and prevent the absorption of the oil into the meat. But, you should eventually transition away from fried foods.
- Eat organic eggs raw for optimum nutrition. Do not scramble the eggs as the heat damages the protein and other nutrients.

Seasoning, Spices, Garlic, Sugar

- Use herbs, organic spices, mushrooms, pure extracts and condiments such as cayenne, cilantro, thyme, garlic, onions, rosemary, sage, black pepper, organic mustard, organic salad oil, organic apple cider vinegar, and organic ketchup. This will eliminate the use of table salt, refined sugars, high fructose corn syrup, hydrogenated oils and other chemicals hidden within traditional spices and condiments.
- Since cooking kills garlic's anti-tumor properties, eat aged garlic or add the raw garlic to your food when it is almost finished cooking. Or, chop up your garlic and let it set for 10 minutes before adding it to anything about to be cooked. This enables naturally present enzymes in the garlic to start a chemical reaction producing the compounds that fight tumors.

Note: Try aged garlic if you are sensitive to the allicin in raw garlic.
- Use a couple sprays of liquid "buttery" spreads on top of steamed vegetables to enhance the taste. Also, use mushrooms, onions, peppers, garlic, and other spices to reduce the need for table salt.

- Season food, especially meat, the night before to allow the seasoning to be absorbed and reduce the need for salt.
- In place of refined sugar, use xylitol or stevia. Other options include agave nectar or an organic cane juice. These products do not cause the "sugar rush". Also, use pure extracts or organic spices such as cinnamon and ginger. In place of brown sugar use an organic sugar cane such as muscovado sugar.
- For those recipes that call for more than a cup of flour, replace a half a cup of the flour with a half a cup of carrot pulp or applesauce to add more fiber and nutrients.
- Chop and crush garlic, and sauté it in olive oil to add to soups, stews, and other dishes. Also, add fresh ground garlic to salad dressings and marinades. Do not use garlic salt because it's loaded with sodium and does not provide the same health benefits as fresh, crushed garlic.

Vegetables
- Eat most of your vegetables raw to obtain their enzymes to facilitate proper digestion. Since cooking kills most of the enzymes, take a plant-based enzyme supplement with each meal if you don't like raw.
- Slice and add red, yellow, and orange peppers and mushrooms to your vegetables before steaming for additional flavor and antioxidant protection. Be careful not to over steam -- if the vegetables are limp or discolored, then, you overcooked them.
- When stir frying, place the vegetables into the pan last so that they are not overcooked.
- For variety, roast the vegetables (e.g. turnips, butternut squash, sweet potatoes). Cube the vegetables, coat them with a small amount of olive/coconut oil and season them with thyme and other spices. Place them on a nonstick baking sheet (glassware) and slow-roast them for an hour and a half.
- Select mushrooms with smooth, unblemished caps. Don't add mushrooms in the early stages of preparing a cooked dish as they will become tough and flavorless. Instead add the mushrooms toward the end of cooking to improve the flavor and tenderness.

Eating out at Restaurants
- Avoid entrées that are fried, sautéed drenched in oil, cheese, or other fat. Order entrées that are baked, broiled, grilled or poached because they are normally lower in fat. Ask for the butter or other oil to be provided in a side dish so that you can control the amount.

- Be careful of salads that may be drenched with a high fat salad dressing, or contain lots of breadcrumbs or croutons. Ask for a low-calorie, low-fat dressing or use the higher fat version sparingly.
- Order one steamed green vegetable and another bright-colored vegetable instead of rice, pasta, mashed potatoes, or French fries.
- Because portion sizes served in most restaurants are very large, automatically cut your plate in half and place half the meal in a doggie-bag to take home and enjoy with a later meal; or, share it with a friend. Keep your portion of lean meat, pork, skinless chicken or fish to the size of a deck of cards (3 oz).

Recipes

The following recipes of super meals, smoothies and snacks are very simple recipes, some of which I developed and some of which I obtained from health-oriented websites and modified to suit my taste and health needs during my recovery. Some of the recipes/tips are also provided by my mother, daughter, Larry, Sylvia, and Alfreda. The primary purpose of these recipes is to give you examples of a super meal or snack so that you can use your own creativity to design your own super meals and snacks to suit your taste, health needs and lifestyle. You can modify your current meals; or, buy one of the many creative recipe books that provide great ideas about preparing healthy and tasty meals. And, don't forget that you can convert many of your own favorite meal recipes to super meal recipes by using the planning tips from the previous section and the Alternative Healthier Foods table (Figure 16) in the Appendix.

The recipes include: Breakfast (with Spinach); Breakfast (Omelette); Breakfast "Quickie" (Juice Drink); Broccoli & Chicken; Cabbage & Fish; Chicken & Vegetables (Stir-Fry); Chicken, Broccoli & Rice; Chili; Oatmeal; Omelette; Raw Juice; Salad #1 (Carrots & Raisins); Salad #2 (Spinach, Salmon & Walnuts); Shrimp Gumbo; Smoothie #1 (Fruit, Nuts & Yogurt); Smoothie #2 (Berries & Flaxseed); Snack #1 (Nuts & Fruit); Snack #2 (Turkey Sandwich); Snack #3 (Juice Drink); Snack #4 (Mix 'n Match); Stuffed Green Peppers; and, Super Dessert.

Note: Refer to my soon-to-be-released cookbook and 90-day meal planner book for a more comprehensive set of super meal recipes and meal planning guidelines.

Breakfast (with Spinach)

Ingredients:

1 oz. of baked wild salmon	½ onion (sliced)
(leftover from dinner the night before)	½ green (or red) pepper
1 slice of soy cheese	1 tbsp. virgin olive oil
2 cups of fresh or frozen spinach	1 tsp. organic butter
(or 1 cup Brussel sprouts)	16 ounces filtered water

Directions:

Preheat oven to 350°.

Place the spinach (or other vegetable) in a steamer with water, place on the stove and turn on medium for 5-7 minutes. Add part of an onion and/or red/yellow pepper.

Sprinkle a pinch of cayenne powder or other seasonings on top of the salmon for additional flavor, e.g. garlic, peppers. Sprinkle a couple drops of extra virgin olive oil on top of the salmon (to keep it moist) and place in the pre-heated oven for no more than 2 minutes. Add 1 slice of soy cheese on top of the salmon approximately 1 minute before removing from the oven.

When ready, remove the spinach from the steamer and place in a small bowl. Add 1 tbsp. of extra virgin olive (or organic flaxseed oil) on top of the spinach (or other vegetable). If you like a "buttery" taste for your vegetables, add a teaspoon of organic butter, a teaspoon of macadamia nut oil, or spray a couple ounces of liquid "buttery" spread on top of the spinach. When you start to eat the spinach, the butter will trigger a signal that helps to satisfy your taste buds.

If you prefer more of a bitter taste, sprinkle 1 tablespoon of organic apple cider vinegar on top of the spinach; or, squeeze a whole lemon on top of the spinach (to break down any oxalic acid).

Remove the salmon from the oven and place on a small plate.

Prepare a glass of filtered water with a slice of lemon.

Options:

Use other vegetable such as broccoli, cauliflower, and Brussel sprouts. For a variety, mix these vegetables with snow peas, stringbeans, red/yellow/orange peppers or carrots.

Add a clove of garlic or shiitake mushrooms for additional flavor.

A protein option replacement for the salmon is 2 lightly scrambled (organic) eggs but this will require more time to prepare. Other protein options include 1 ounce of organic skinless chicken breast, or other fish: canned tuna, canned wild salmon, or sardines.

A carbohydrate option for the spinach is 16 ounces of raw carrot juice. Add a tbsp. of flaxseed or wheat grass powder and a scoop of protein/fiber powder to the juice.

Note: Aged garlic is produced when it is sliced, macerated and kept in water or alcohol for up to two years before being turned into a dietary supplement. The resulting aged garlic extract does not contain allicin but is high in water soluble phytochemicals such as diallyl sulphides that provide numerous health benefits. [Reference: The Garlic Cure].

Breakfast (Omelette)

Ingredients:

5 egg whites
1 cup mushrooms
1 onion (diced)
1 red pepper (diced)

2 organic eggs
1 tbsp. virgin olive oil
1 ½ cups broccoli
(Option: 2 cups spinach)

Directions:
Sauté the vegetables in a medium frying pan or wok until tender (but still firm).
Mix 5 egg whites and 2 organic eggs, and add on top of the vegetables.
Stir and cook for about 2-3 minutes, add organic spices. Prepare a glass of filtered
water.

Breakfast "Quickie" (Juice Drink)

Many of us just don't have time to fix breakfast in the morning. Here is a "quickie" that
takes less than a minute to prepare and it still contains all 4 macronutrients!

Ingredients:

2 cups organic (bottled) berry juice
or 2 cups yogurt
½ cup filtered water (optional)

2 tbsp. ground flaxseed
or 2 tbsp. fiber/protein powder
(with 1 tbsp. organic flax oil)

Directions:
Place the juice (or yogurt) into a container with a lid.
Add the protein powder and flax oil or the ground flax seed to the juice/yogurt.
Screw on the lid and shake up the drink (or stir the yogurt) until the powder has
dissolved.
Add 1 to 2 pieces of ice if you like your drink cold, shake for several seconds.

Broccoli & Chicken

Ingredients:

1 cup broccoli florets
1 cup snow peas
½ cup grapes

½ cup onion, chopped
1 tsp. ginger
¼ cup filtered water

3 ounces of boneless, skinless chicken breast (cut lengthwise into thin strips)

Directions:
In a wok or large nonstick pan, heat the olive oil over a medium-high heat. Add the
chicken and sauté, turning frequently until lightly browned, about 5 minutes.
Add broccoli, snow peas, onion, ginger, and water. Continue cooking, stirring often,
until the chicken is done, water is reduced to a glaze, and vegetables are tender, about 20
minutes. If the pan dries out, add water in tablespoon increments to keep moist.
Prepare a glass of filtered water. Eat the grapes for dessert.

Cabbage & Fish

Ingredients:

1 cabbage	2-3 hot peppers
1 onion	1 green pepper
3-4 carrots	1-2 garlic cloves
2 tbsp. olive oil	2 pieces of fish (tilapia)

Directions:

Grate the cabbage and place in a large pot. Mix in the other ingredients.
Cook for 30 minutes or until done. If it starts to dry out during cooking, add water in tablespoon increments to keep moist. Bake the two pieces of fish. Prepare a glass of filtered water.

Chicken & Vegetables (Stir-Fry)

Ingredients:

1½ tsp. olive oil	¾ cup snow peas
3 tsp. gingerroot, minced	1/3 cup water chestnuts
2 tsp. garlic, minced	1½ cup scallions
2 cups mushrooms, sliced	2 cups cauliflower
2 cups cabbage, shredded	1 tbsp. soy sauce
4 ounces chicken tenderloin in ½-inch cubes	½ cup chicken broth

Directions:

Heat ¾ tsp. oil in a medium-size nonstick sauté pan. Add chicken, 1 tsp. ginger, and 1 tsp. garlic. Stir-fry until chicken is cooked and garlic is lightly brown.
In a separate nonstick pan, heat the remaining oil and stir in the mushrooms. Cook for 2 minutes. Add cabbage, snow peas, water chestnuts, scallions, cauliflower, soy sauce, broth, and remaining ginger and garlic. Stir-fry until cabbage and cauliflower are tender. But, be careful not to overcook.
Place vegetables on a serving dish and top with the chicken.
Prepare a glass of filtered water.

Chicken, Broccoli & Rice

Ingredients:

1 lb. chicken breast (skinless, boneless)
1 can cream of broccoli soup
½ tsp. cayenne pepper (or black pepper)
¾ cup carrots (thinly sliced)

1 cup nonfat milk
2 tbsp. margarine
2 cups broccoli
1 ½ cups whole grain rice

Directions:

Place the margarine, chicken breast, and carrots in a skillet and cook until tender and crisp. Add the broccoli. Cook the (whole grain) rice separately.
Stir in the soup, milk, and pepper.
Reduce heat to low, cover and simmer 10 minutes until vegetables are tender.
Stir in the rice, cover and remove from the heat.
Let stand for 5 minutes. Fluff with fork before serving.
Prepare a glass of filtered water.
Note: This is one of my mother's recipes.

Chili

Ingredients:

1 ½ tsp. olive oil
½ medium onion, chopped
½ green bell pepper, seeded & chopped
¾ cup soybean hamburger
1 tsp. chili powder
½ cup canned kidney beans

¼ tsp. sea salt
1 garlic clove, chopped
½ cup filtered water
2 oz. soy cheese (grated)
½ tsp. ground cumin
1 cup canned crushed tomatoes

Directions:

Heat oil in a large nonstick sauté pan over a medium heat.
Sauté the onion and green pepper in the oil for 5 minutes or until the onion turns translucent.
Mix in the chili powder, cumin, salt, and garlic and cook for 2 minutes.
Add the hamburger and water. Stir in the tomatoes and kidney beans. Cover and simmer 15 to 30 minutes to blend flavors.
Serve in a bowl, sprinkled with grated cheese.
Prepare a glass of filtered water.
Tip: Place onions in the freezer for 30 minutes to avoid tearing up when slicing onions.

Oatmeal

Ingredients:

1 cup cooked organic oatmeal
1 cup (21 grams) of protein powder
3 cups water (or 3 cups organic apple juice)

3 tsp. slivered almonds
1 tsp. sea salt

Directions:

Mix 3 cups of water (or apple juice) with the oatmeal and bring to a boil. Let simmer for approximately 30 minutes. Add the almonds.
Mix in the protein powder before serving. Prepare a glass of filtered water.

Omelette

Ingredients:

1 cup red & green bell peppers, chopped
2 cups mushrooms, sliced
¼ tsp. garlic, minced
¼ tsp. Worcestershire sauce
¼ tsp. dill
1 dash of lemon herb seasoning
1 cup egg substitute
½ cup mandarin orange sections

1 ½ tsp. olive oil
¾ cup onion, chopped
¼ tsp. dried parsley
¼ tsp. dried oregano
¼ tsp. cilantro
¼ tsp. chili powder
2 cups alfalfa sprouts
½ cup organic salsa

Directions:

In a nonstick sauté pan, heat the oil over a medium-high heat.
In a medium-size bowl, combine the onion, peppers, and mushrooms. Add the garlic, oregano, dill, chili powder, parsley, Worcestershire sauce, cilantro, and lemon herb seasoning. Spoon mixture into the sauté pan and sauté for 3 minutes but do not overcook the vegetables.
Pour the egg substitute into the sauté pan, stir to distribute the vegetables, and cook until almost set. Sprinkle sprouts onto half of the omelette and fold over.
Remove to serve plate. Decorate with orange sections, and top the omelette with the salsa.

Raw Juice

If you have never juiced before, start with carrots and spinach; then, move to other vegetables like cucumber, celery and cabbage; and grasses such as wheat and barley. Keep in mind that since carrots, beets, apples and other fruits contain a lot of fructose (sugar), always ensure that you are consuming them with water, and some nuts/seeds that contain protein and fat to slow down the absorption of the carbohydrates. If you do not have the patience to prepare your own juice, then, you can try bottled organic juices sold in health food stores. Although these processed juices contain sugar, they contain no high fructose corn syrup and preservatives.

Ingredients:

7 to 8 medium-size carrots	1 medium-size apple
2 tbsp. ground flaxseed	½ tsp. cinnamon

Directions:
Clean the carrots and apple. Cut off the tops of the carrots.
Place the carrots in the juicer, then the apple.
Pour the juice into a container with a lid.
Add the ground flaxseed and shake up the container until the flaxseed dissolves.

Options:
- If you don't like to juice or don't have the time, mix 16 ounces of low-sodium V-8 juice with a tbsp. of flax oil and 2 scoops of super green powder. (Thanks, Larry P.)
- Add 1-2 scoops of wheat/barley grass powder to provide maximum nutrients for nourishment, cleansing, detox, and repair.
- **P**lace the green super food powder under your tongue to accelerate (sublingual) absorption into your bloodstream. (Thanks, Sylvia P.)

Salad #1 (Carrots & Raisins)

Ingredients:

2 ½ cups shredded carrots (3-4 large carrots)	½ cup raisins
¾ cup organic mayonnaise	¾ cup chopped celery
½ cup chopped walnuts/almonds	¼ tsp. sea salt

Directions:
Combine and mix the ingredients in a medium bowl.
Prepare a glass of filtered water.

Salad #2 (Spinach, Salmon & Walnuts)

Ingredients:

1 can (15 oz.) wild salmon (backbone and skin removed)
4 cups baby spinach leaves   ¼ cup finely chopped walnuts
2 Tbsp. walnut oil   ½ cup finely chopped celery
2 small cloves garlic, minced   ¼ cup light canola mayonnaise
1 Tbsp. freshly squeezed lemon juice   1 tsp. freshly ground black pepper
8 cherry tomatoes, cut in half
2 Tbsp. organic vinegar
¼ tsp. sea salt

Directions:

Place the oil, vinegar, garlic, celery, salt, pepper in a medium/large bowl and mix together. Then, mix in the spinach and top with the salmon.
Place the cherry tomato halves around the sides and sprinkle the top with the walnuts.

Shrimp Gumbo

Ingredients:

1 ½ tsp. extra virgin olive oil   ½ tsp. garlic, minced
1 cup celery, sliced   ¼ tsp. chili powder
1 cup onions, chopped   1/8 tsp. celery seed

6 oz. small shrimp, shelled & deveined   ¼ tsp. paprika
1 cup tomatoes, chopped   ½ cup frozen okra, sliced
¼ cup frozen corn kernels   ½ tsp. lemon herb seasoning
½ to 1 tsp. hot pepper sauce   ½ cup lemon/lime-flavored water

Directions:

Heat oil in a medium-size nonstick sauté pan. Add the celery, onion, tomatoes, okra, corn, hot pepper sauce, garlic, chili powder, and celery seed. Cook until the vegetables are tender. Mix in the shrimp, paprika, lemon herb seasoning, and flavored water. Simmer 3 to 5 minutes until the shrimp are cooked. Spoon into a medium-size bowl and serve. Prepare a glass of filtered water (16 ounces).

Smoothie #1 (Fruit, Nuts & Yogurt)

Ingredients:

1 cup 1% milk
4 tsp. slivered almonds
1 cup strawberries (or other fruit)

½ cup plain low-fat yogurt
½ cup tangerine segments
14 grams protein powder

Directions:
Place all ingredients except the protein powder into a blender. Blend until smooth. Add the protein powder and blend until smooth.

Smoothie #2 (Berries & Flaxseed)

This type of smoothie will reduce the cravings for sugar and other sweet foods while providing key nutrients such as EFAs, fiber, enzymes, water, and antioxidants.

Ingredients:

½ cup of blueberries or "black" grapes
½ cup of cherries, strawberries
½ cup organic berry juice (optional)

1 apple, sliced
2 cups of filtered water
2 tbsp. ground flaxseed

Directions:
Place the fruit, flaxseed, water and juice into a blender and blend on high until smooth.
Note: If the fruit is frozen, place them into the blender one at a time and blend to prevent the blender from binding.
Add 2 to 3 pieces of ice if you like your drink cold, blend until smooth.

Options:
- Add 1 to 2 scoops of a high-quality whey (or soy) protein powder or fiber/protein wholefood supplement to turn this smoothie into a "replacement meal".
- If you plan to exercise during the day, add 1-2 tbsp. of pure liquid carnitine to facilitate fat burning.

Snack #1 (Nuts & Fruit)

Ingredients:

1 apple (12 to 15 grapes or other fruit)
1 glass filtered water

½ cup walnuts/almonds

Directions:
(No cooking preparation required).

Snack #2 (Turkey Sandwich)

Ingredients:

2 slices of sprouted grain bread
1 slice soy cheese
1 tbsp. organic mayonnaise or mustard
1 tomato (sliced)

1 cup lettuce
3 ounces turkey breast
½ cup walnuts

Directions:

Cut the turkey breast into several thin slices. Add the mayonnaise (or mustard) and lettuce to each slice of bread. Add the slice of cheese and tomato onto each piece of bread. Place the turkey slices onto each slice of bread. Prepare a glass of filtered water. Eat the walnuts separately.
Option: Toast the bread and/or warm up the turkey breast with olive oil.

Snack #3 (Juice Drink)

Ingredients:

16 ounces organic fruit juice
2 tbsp. soy protein/glyconutrient powder

1 tbsp. ground flaxseed
1 glass of filtered water (8 ounces)

Directions:

Place the juice into a container with a lid. Add the ground flaxseed and protein powder to the juice and shake up until the flaxseed and protein powder have dissolved. Drink the water separately or add a few ounces to the drink to dilute the sugar content of the juice.

Snack #4 (Mix 'n Match)

Carbohydrate:

25 grapes
20 cherries
1 cup berries
½ oz. organic dark chocolate
8 saltine crackers
6 baked tortilla chips
3 graham cracker squares

Protein/Fat

½ oz. organic cheddar cheese
1 oz. organic feta cheese
2 oz. organic soy cheese
1 tbsp. organic peanut butter
Handful of walnuts/almonds
3 oz. guacamole
(mashed seasoned avocado)

Directions:

Mix and match: take one item from the Carbohydrate column and one item from the Protein/Fat column. Prepare a glass of filtered water.
Note: There are high quality pulse foods that can be used as snack foods. These pulse foods contain dates, oats, sesame seeds, amaranth, quinoa, almonds, cashews, hazelnuts, figs, walnut oil, grapeseed oil, and other nutrients. Refer to the Resource List on page 374 for specific websites that provide these super foods.

Stuffed Green Peppers

Ingredients:

1 pound lean ground beef
¼ tsp. black pepper
2 garlic cloves (chopped/crushed)
3 medium green peppers
3 8-ounce cans organic tomato sauce
3 tbsp. Parmesan cheese, grated (optional)

1 tsp. sea salt
¼ tsp. cayenne pepper
½ cup onion, finely chopped
½ cup Minute Rice
¼ cup filtered water

Directions:

Preheat oven to 425°F. In medium glass bowl, crumble ground beef; stir in onion. Heat 5 to 6 minutes until beef is browned, stirring once; drain. Stir in 1 ½ cans tomato sauce, water, 1 tbsp. cheese, salt, pepper, and garlic. Heat, covered, 3 ½ to 5 minutes, stir in rice; let stand, covered, 7 minutes.

Meanwhile, cut peppers in half lengthwise; remove seeds and rinse. Spoon beef rice filling into each half; place in oblong baking dish. Top with remaining sauce and cheese, and add chopped/crushed garlic.

Heat, covered 15 to 18 minutes until peppers are tender.

Prepare a pot of green tea.

Note: This is one of my mother's recipes.

Super Dessert

Ingredients:

½ cup of blueberries or strawberries
1 (frozen) banana
⅓ cup ground almonds

1 cup organic yogurt or organic egg
1 cup almond milk/raw milk
1 tbsp. raw honey

Directions:

Place the ingredients into a blender and blend on high until smooth.

Add more yogurt to thicken; or add water or almond milk if the mixture is too thick.

Note: This recipe is for people (like the author) who love ice cream desserts.

Option: Add 1-2 tbsp. of pure liquid carnitine to facilitate fat burning.

Thanks to Sylvia P. for this recipe.

APPENDIX

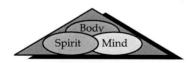

Super Meal Model

The following diagram is a more detailed breakout of the Super Meal Model described in Chapter 7. Examples of "live" super foods are listed under the bolded, underlined text headings.

Super Meal Model	
[At least 4 daily meals/snacks]	
### Carbohydrates	### Proteins
•**Vegetables** [5 to 7 cups/day] e.g. broccoli, spinach, Brussel sprouts, kale, stringbeans, peppers, cauliflower, cabbage •**Fruits** [2 to 3 cups/day] e.g. blackberries, blueberries, cherries, apples, grapes, lemons, pears, strawberries •**Some Whole Grains** [0.5 to 1 cup/day] e.g. barley, alfalfa, oat, rice germ/bran •Processed Foods [<1 serving/day] e.g. refined white flour products, white rice, potatoes, bread, pasta, macaroni, crackers, donuts, pastries, biscuits, cakes, snacks; wheat; refined white sugar products, sucrose, high fructose corn syrup, soda, potato chips, cookies, honey, candy, some cereals, ketchup.	•**Plant Protein (Legumes, Soy)** [1 to 2 cups/day] e.g. beans, lentils, nuts, seeds; tofu, tempeh, miso, soy milk, soy protein powder; spirulina, chlorella •**Fish/Seafood** [3 to 4 5-ounce servings/week] e.g. wild salmon, trout, tuna, sardines, mackerel; organic shrimp, crab, lobster •**Meat/Dairy (Lean/Organic)** [1-2 servings/day] e.g. organic, lean (no skin) chicken, beef, turkey, lamb; free-range eggs; goat's milk, cheese •Meat/Dairy [<1 serving/day] e.g. chicken, beef, turkey, lamb; eggs; cow's milk, cheese
### Fats	### Liquids
•**Monounsaturated Fats** [2 to 3 tbsp./day] e.g. extra virgin olive oil, macadamia nut oil, hazelnuts, almonds, Brazil nuts, cashews, avocado, sesame seeds, pumpkin seeds •**Polyunsaturated Fats** [1 to 2 tbsp./day] e.g. Omega-3s: flaxseed, flax oil, hemp oil, pumpkin seeds, walnuts, oily fish; Omega-6s: borage oil, evening primrose oil •Saturated Fats [<1 serving/day] e.g. animal fats, butter, lard, red meat, poultry skin, cheese, cream, milk; palm oil •Trans Fats [0 servings/day] e.g. partially hydrogenated oil in margarine, French fries, potato chips, pretzels, cookies, fried foods, processed foods	•**Pure Water** [6 to 9 cups/day] e.g. pure water, filtered water, distilled water •**Water in raw juices** [2 to 6 cups/day] e.g. raw vegetable juice, raw fruit juice, blended juice •Tap Water; Water in bottled, canned beverages, juices, coffee [<1 cup/day] Notes: 1.Eat foods from each of these 4 groups for every meal or snack. 2. Eat more of the foods with the bolded text headings. 3. Use nutritional **food**-based supplements.
7 Nutrient Factors: Vitamins, Minerals, Fiber, Antioxidants, Enzymes, Oils, Water	

Figure 15. Super Meal Model

Alternatives for Favorite Foods

The following are some of the alternative healthier foods for some of your favorite, but less-nutritious, foods.

Favorite Foods	Alternative (Healthier) Foods
Beverages	
Soda, Diet soda, cola, most bottled juices	Blended juice, raw juice, organic juice; fresh/frozen apples, grapes, low-sodium V-8 juice; wheat grass juice
Tap water	Filtered water (carbon, reverse osmosis); raw juice
Coffee	Green/white tea, herbal tea (decaffeinated); roasted chicory; soy coffee
Seasonings, Sweeteners	
Sugar, artificial sweeteners	Xylitol, stevia, agave nectar; raw honey Spices: cinnamon, cloves, ginger, nutmeg, fennel, allspice.
Milk chocolate	Carob, unsweetened, dark chocolate, cocoa
Salt	Sea salt, peppers, onions, garlic, other organic spices; mushrooms
Breads	
Bagel	Whole grain bagel; bagel with cream
White bread, wheat bread; refined white flour	Sprouted grain bread; manna bread; organic whole grain bread, sourdough bread; oat flour, soy flour
Cereals	
Corn flakes, breakfast cereals	High fiber organic grain cereals, rice germ/bran
Grits, cream of wheat, instant oats	Organic whole grain oatmeal, oat bran
Dairy	
Cow's cheese	Soy cheese, lite cheese, mozzarella, organic cheese, goat cheese, cottage cheese, organic yogurt
Chicken's eggs	Organic eggs from free-range chickens; Egg substitute, egg whites; raw, soft-boiled
Cow's milk (homogenized, pasteurized)	Goat's milk, raw milk; raw almond milk; organic soy milk, organic milk

Favorite Foods	Alternative (Healthier) Foods
Fats & Oils	
Butter	Extra virgin coconut oil, raw almond butter; organic butter; macadamia nut oil
Margarine (stick)	Soft margarine (in a tub), e.g. Smart/Earth Balance spread, Spectrum soy spread
Vegetable oils (e.g. corn, soybean); salad dressing	Extra virgin olive oil, macadamia nut oil, organic rice bran oil, flaxseed oil
Vinegar	Organic apple cider vinegar
Meats & Seafood	
Beef, ground beef	Ground turkey; very lean beef, organic beef, veal; wild game: venison, bear Beef with visible fat trimmed and soaked in olive oil/red wine
Bacon, sausage, ham, pork, hot dogs, lunch meats	Turkey bacon; soy bacon/sausage; organic bacon/sausage
Chicken, turkey	Organic (skinless) chicken, turkey
Fried meats	Baked, broiled meats, wild salmon, fish; Flash-fried foods (with virgin coconut oil); organic seafood
Grains, Vegetables	
Potatoes, French fries; white rice, white pasta, fried rice	Cauliflower; sweet potatoes, jicama; organic brown rice, whole grain pasta, potato skins; beans Land vegetables/fruits; sea vegetables; pulse food (parched vegetables)
Iceberg Lettuce	Romaine lettuce, spinach, barley grass, sprouts; wheat grass
Snacks, Desserts, Vitamins	
Potato Chips, Candy, Cookies	Nuts & seeds, organic potato chips, organic cookies, vegetable chips, pulse food; Tortilla chips with guacamole
Ice Cream	Homemade ice cream; organic ice cream (Add walnuts or raw egg and fresh fruit to provide protein, Omega-3s and fiber); Sherbet, frozen yogurt, soy dessert; homemade smoothies with whole fruits
Vitamin Pills	Wholefood or natural 100% additive-free pharmaceutical-grade supplements only

Figure 16. Alternative Healthier Foods

References: Websites & Books

The following is a list of the references and resources that I used to help write this book:

Traditional websites and institutions:
World Health Organization www.who.int/topics/diabetes_mellitus/en/
American Association of Naturopathic Physicians   www.naturopathic.org
American Naturopathic Medical Association www.anma.com
American Diabetes Association www.diabetes.org/home.jsp
American Heart Association www.americanheart.org
Canadian Association of Naturopathic Doctors www.naturopathicassoc.ca
Canadian Diabetes Association www.diabetes.ca/section_main/welcome.asp
Center for Disease Control www.cdc.gov/ www.cdc.gov/diabetes
Center for Drug Evaluation and Research www.fda.gov/cder
John Hopkins Hospital & Health System www.hopkinshospital.org/health_info
Juvenile Diabetes Research Foundation www.jdf.org
National Inst. of Diabetes & Digestive & Kidney Diseases www.niddk.nih.gov/
National Library of Medicine www.ncbi.nlm.nih.gov
National Medical Association www.nmanet.org/
Naturopathic Medicine Network www.pandamedicine.com/medicine.html
USDA National Nutrient Database www.nal.usda.gov/fnic/foodcomp
U.S. Food & Drug Administration www.fda.gov

General medical/health/wellness websites:
www.webmd.com www.healthfinder.gov/library
www.diabetesmonitor.com
www.alternativemedicine.com
www.bodymindspiritjourneys.com

Organic food, Other websites:
www.allorganiclinks.com   www.organicvalley.coop
www.mayoclinic.org www.homeopathy-ecch.org www.dlife.com
www.wholefoodsmarket.com   www.wholefoodscoop.org

Books and Newsletters:

- The Bible
- Biochemistry, Berg, Jeremy M.; Tymoczko, John L. & Stryer, Lubert
- Diabetes Meals on the Run, Betty Wedman-St. Louis, PhD., R.D.
- Endocrinology: An Integrated Approach, Nussey, S.S. and Whitehead, S.A.
- Hallelujah: A Lifetime of Memories with Recipes, Maya Angelou
- Healthy Heart Longer Life, Joseph Goldstrich, M.D.
- Holy Lockdown, Jeremiah Camara
- The Insulin Control Diet, Calvin Ezrin, M.D., Robert Kowalski
- The Mind-Body Prescription, John E. Sarno, M.D.
- Natural Hormonal Enhancement, Rob Faigin
- The Power of Intention, Dr. Wayne Dyer
- Sugars That Heal: Science of Glyconutrients, Emil Mondoa, Mindy Kitei
- Quick Cooking for Diabetes, Louise Blair, Norma McGough, Diabetes UK
- You: The Owner's Manual, Mehmet Oz, M.D., Michael Roizen, M.D.
- The Zone Diet, Barry Sears, M.D.
- The Garlic Cure, James Scheer, Lynn Allison, Charlie Fox

Clinical References

The following is a list of the clinical references and resources that I used to help write this book and substantiate many of the claims and nutritional recommendations.

Acetyl-L-carnitine, L-carnitine

1. Double-blind parallel design pilot study of acetyl levocarnitine in patients with Alzheimer's disease. Arch Neurol 1992; 49: 1137 -41. Sano M, Bell K, Cote L, et al..
2. Clinical pharmacodynamics of acetyl-L-carnitine in patients with Parkinson's disease. Int J Clin Pharmacol Res 1990; 10.139-43. Puca FM, Genco S, Specchio LM, et al.
3. Acetyl-L-carnitine for symptomatic diabetic neuropathy [letter]. Diabetologia 1995; 38: 123. Quatraro A, Roca P, Donzella C, Acampora R, Marfella R, Giugliano D
4. Effect of acetyl-L-carnitine in the treatment of painful peripheral neuropathies in HIV+ patients. J Peripher Nerv Syst 1997; 2:250-2. Scarpini E, Sacilotto G, Baron P, Cusini M, Scarlato G.
5. L-carnitine improves glucose disposal in type 2 diabetic patients. J. Am. Coll. Nutr. 1999; 18(1): 77-82. Mingrone, G. et al.

Alpha lipoic acid:

6. Alpha lipoic acid treatment decreases serum lactate and pyruvate concentrations and improves glucose effectiveness in lean and obese patients with type 2 diabetes. *Diabetes Care* 1999;22:280–7. Konrad T, Vicini P, Kusterer K, et al.
7. Alpha-lipoic acid in the treatment of diabetic peripheral and cardiac autonomic neuropathy. Diabetes 46 Suppl 2: S62-6. Ziegler, D. and F. A. Gries (1997).
8. Effects of treatment with the antioxidant alpha-lipoic acid on cardiac autonomic neuropathy in NIDDM patients. A 4-month randomized controlled multicenter trial (DEKAN Study). *Diabetes Care* 1997;20:369-73. Ziegler D, Schatz H, Conrad F, et al.
9. Effects of alpha-lipoic acid on microcirculation in patients with peripheral diabetic neuropathy. These results demonstrate that in patients with diabetic polyneuropathy ALA improves microcirculation. Haak E,. University Hospital, Frankfurt, Germany.

10. The radical scavenger a-lipoic acid enhances insulin sensitivity in patients with NIDDM; a placebo-controlled trial. Presented at Oxidants and Antioxidants in Biology, Santa Barbara, California, February 27-March 1, 1997. Jacob, S. et al.
11. Lipoic acid decreases lipid peroxidation and protein glycosylation and increases (Na+ + K+)- and Ca++-ATPase activities in high glucose-treated red blood cells (RBC). Free Radical Biol. Med. 1998; 25: S94 (Abstr. 268); see also Free Radical Biol. Med. 2000; 29(11): 1122-8. Jain, S.K., Lim, G.
12. Antioxidant properties of lipoic acid and its therapeutic effects in prevention of diabetes complications and cataracts. Ann. N.Y. Acad. Sci. 1994; 738: 257-64. Packer, L.

Cardiovascular health, High blood pressure:
13. Action of plant sterols on inhibition of cholesterol absorption. 1991; *Eur J Clin Pharmacol* 40(1): S59-63. Heinemann, T., G. Kullak-Ublick, et al.
14. Effects of garlic on fibrinolysis and platelet aggregation. 1993; *Arzneimittelforschung* 43(2): 119-22. Legnani, C., M. Frascaro, et al.
15. Flax facts. A grain for good health. Diabetes Self Manag. 2003 Nov-Dec;20(6):18, 20-2. PMID: 14971334. Campbell AP.
16. Inhibition of whole blood platelet aggregation by compounds in garlic clove extracts. 1992; *Thromb Res* 65(2): 141-56. Lawson, L., D. Ransom, et al.
17. Rice bran oil lowers serum total and LDL cholesterol. 1991; Atherosclerosis 88(2-3): 133-142. Nicolosi, R., L. Ausman, et al.
18. The effect of a salmon diet on blood clotting, platelet aggregation and fatty acids. 1991; *Lipids* 26(2): 87-96. Nelson, G., P. Schmidt, et al.
19. Carnitine May Attenuate Free Fatty Acid-Induced Endothelial Dysfunction. Ann N Y Acad Sci. 2004 Nov;1033:189-97. PMID: 15591016. Shankar SS, Mirzamohammadi B, Walsh JP, Steinberg HO.
20. The effect of fish oil on blood pressure. 1993; *Am J Clin Nutr* 57(1): 57-64. Morris, M., J. Taylor, et al.
21. Cardiovascular wellness can be achieved with nutrients such as CoQ10, grapeseed extract, hawthorn, garlic, green tea, selenium, Vitamin C, Vitamin E. 2003 article by Heather Granato at www.naturalproductsinsider.com/articles/311feat1.html.
22. The natural treatment of hypertension. J Clin Hypertens (Greenwich). Agents with some evidence of benefit include coenzyme Q10, fish oil, garlic, vitamin C, and L-arginine. 2004 May;6(5):242-8. Wilburn AJ, King DS, Glisson J, Rockhold RW, Wofford MR., University of Mississippi School of Pharmacy, University, MS.
23. AGEs and their interaction with AGE-receptors in vascular disease and diabetes mellitus. I. The AGE concept. Cardiovascular Research. 1998; 37(3):586-600. Bierhaus A, Hofmann MA, Ziegler R, et al.
24. Carnosine is a novel peptide modulator of intracellular calcium and contractility in cardiac cells. Am J Physiol 1997; 272(1 Pt 2):H462-8. Zaloga GP, Roberts PR, Black KW.
25. Diabetic cardiomyopathy and carnitine deficiency. J. Diabetes Complications 1999; 13: 86-90. Malone, J.I. et al.
26. C-reactive protein, dietary n-3 fatty acids, and the extent of coronary artery disease. Am. J. Cardiol. 2001 Nov 15: 88(10): 1139-42. Madsen, T. et al.
27. Prophylactic aspirin and risk of peptic ulcer bleeding. Conclusion: No conventionally used prophylactic aspirin regimen seems free of the risk of peptic ulcer complications. BMJ, Apr 1995; 310: 827 - 830. John Weil, Duncan Colin-Jones, Michael Langman, David Lawson, Richard Logan, Michael Murphy, Michael Rawlins, Martin Vessey, and Paul Wainwright.

Cholesterol (Plant sterols, Policosanol, Resveratrol), Homocysteine:
28. High cholesterol may protect against infections and atherosclerosis. *Quart J Med* 2003;96:927-934.Ravnskov U.

29. Inhibition of human LDL oxidation by resveratrol. *Lancet.* 1993;341:1103–1104. Frankel EN, Waterhouse AL, Kinsella JE.

30. Cholesterol-lowering effect of stanol ester in a US population of mildly hypercholesterolemic men and women: a randomized controlled trial. Mayo Clinic Proceedings. 1999;74(12):1198-1206. Nguyen TT, Dale LC, von Bergmann K, Croghan IT.

31. Comparison of the efficacy and tolerability of policosanol with that of fluvastatin in older hypercholesterolemic women. Policosanol significantly lowered low density lipoprotein cholesterol (29.2%), total cholesterol (19.3%), triglycerides (7%), and significantly increased high density lipoprotein cholesterol (19.8%). *Clin Drug Invest 21(2):103-113, 2001.* J.C. Fernández, R. Más, National Center for Scientific Research, Havana City, Cuba; G. Castaño, Medical Surgical Research Center, Havana City, Cuba; R. Menéndez, A.M. Amor, R.M. González, E. Alvarez, National Center for Scientific Research, Havana City, Cuba

32. U.S. Department of Health and Human Services. FDA authorizes new coronary heart disease health claim for plant sterol and plant stanol esters. Posted September 5, 2000. Available at: www.fda.gov/bbs/topics/answers/ans01033.html. U.S. Food & Drug Administration.

33. Incremental reduction of serum total cholesterol and low-density lipoprotein cholesterol with the addition of plant stanol ester-containing spread to statin therapy. American Journal of Cardiology. 2000;86(1):46-52. Blair SN, Capuzzi DM, Gottlieb SO, Nguyen TT, Morgan JM, Cater NB.

34. Plant stanol ester: review of cholesterol-lowering efficacy and implications for coronary heart disease risk reduction. Preventive Cardiology. 2000;3(3):121-130. Cater NB.

35. Effect of carnitine on blood lipid pattern in diabetic patients. L-carnitine (1 mg per 2.2 pounds of body weight), both cholesterol and triglycerides dropped 25-39% in just ten days. *Nutr Rep Int* 1984;29:1071-9. Abdel-Aziz MT, Abdou MS, Soliman K, et al.

Cholesterol (Statin drugs):

36. The myotoxicity of statins. Adverse reactions involving skeletal muscle are the most common (reported incidence 1-7%). The recent withdrawal of cerivastatin because of deaths from rhabdomyolysis, of which 25% were related to gemfibrozil-cerivastatin combination therapy, has focused attention on myotoxicity associated with statins and in particular with statin-fibrate combinations. Cerivastatin was associated with a 10-fold higher incidence of myotoxicity than any other statin, suggesting that there may be differences in myotoxic potential between agents. Potential differences in myotoxicity between agents may relate to the physicochemical, pharmacokinetic and pharmacodynamic properties of individual drugs. Evans M, Rees A., Dept. of Diabetes and Endocrinology, University Hospital of Wales, UK.

37. Myotoxicity and rhabdomyolysis due to statins. Rhabdomyolysis is a rare but potentially fatal complication associated with the use of cholesterol synthesis inhibitors (statins). Myopathy is present when plasma activity levels of creatinine kinase are raised to in excess of 10 times the upper limit of the normal value. Muscular complaints which may be indicative of myotoxicity and subsequent myopathy are present in 1-7% of statin users. Rhabdomyolysis was clearly more prevalent under cerivastatin users than the users of other statins and was therefore recently withdrawn from the market. Statins should be withdrawn immediately if myopathy is suspected. Ned Tijdschr Geneeskd. 2001 Dec 8;145(49):2371-6. Banga JD., Universitair Medisch Centrum Utrecht,

38. Rhabdomyolysis associated with cerivastatin and cyclosporine combination therapy. Med Clin (Barc). 2002 May 18;118(18):716-7. Spanish. Nicolas De Prado I, Miras Lopez M, Moran Sanchez S, Mercader Martinez J.

39. Statins have many benefits. Like all medications, statins have potential side effects. The most common side effects are: Nausea, Diarrhea, Constipation, Muscle aching. In addition, two potentially serious side effects are elevated liver enzymes and statin myopathy. Mayo Clinic. www.mayoclinic.com/invoke.cfm?id=AN00587

40. Biochemical and clinical consequences of inhibiting coenzyme Q10 biosynthesis by lipid-lowering HMG-CoA reductase inhibitors (Statins): a critical overview. *Adv Ther.* Jul/Aug 1998;15(4):218-228. Bliznakov EG, Wilkins DJ.

Chromium, Brewer's yeast:

41. The case for supplemental chromium and a survey of clinical studies with chromium picolinate. J Appl Nutr 1991;43:59-66. McCarty MF.
42. The effects of chromium supplementation on serum glucose and lipids in non-insulin-dependent diabetics. 1992; *Metabolism* 41(7): 768-71. Abram, A., B. Brooks, et al.
43. Chromium picolinate increases membrane fluidity and rate of insulin internalization. 1992; *J Inorg Biochem* 46(4): 243-50. Evans, G. and T. Bowman.
44. Role of chromium in barley in modulating the symptoms of diabetes. 1991; *Ann Nutr Metab* 35(2): 65-70. Mahdi, G. and D. Naismith.
45. Effect of chromium chloride supplementation on glucose tolerance and serum lipids including high-density lipoprotein of adult men. Am J Clin Nutr 1981;34:2670–8. Riales R, Albrink MJ.
46. Chromium, glucose intolerance and diabetes. *J Amer Coll Nutr.* 1998;17:548-555, Anderson RA.
47. Chromium in the prevention and control of diabetes. *Diabetes Metab.* 2000; 26:22-27, Anderson RA.
48. Elevated intake of supplemental chromium improved glucose and insulin variables in individuals with type 2 diabetes. *Diabetes.* 1997;46:1786-1791, Anderson RA.
49. Beneficial effect of chromium-rich yeast on glucose tolerance and blood lipids in elderly subjects. *Diabetes* 1980;29:919-25. Offenbacher EG, Pi-Sunyer FX.
50. Beneficial effect of chromium supplementation on serum triglyceride levels in NIDDM. *Diabetes Care* 1994;17:1449-52. Lee NA, Reasner CA.
51. Elevated intakes of supplemental chromium improve glucose and insulin variables in individuals with type 2 diabetes. Diabetes 1997; 46: 1786-91. Anderson, R.A. et al.

CoQ10:

52. Antioxidative effect of dietary coenzyme Q10 in human blood plasma. Int J Vitam Nutr Res 1994;64:311–5. Weber C, Jakobsen TS, Mortensen SA, et al.
53. Inhibition of LDL oxidation by ubiquinol-10. A protective mechanism for coenzyme Q in atherogenesis? Mol Aspects Med 1997;18:S85–103. Thomas SR, Neuzil J, Stocker R.
54. Evidence of plasma CoQ10-lowering effects of HMG-CoA reductase inhibitors. 1993; J Clin Pharmacol 33(3): 226-9. Ghirlanda, G., A. Oradei, et al.
55. Effect of coenzyme Q7 treatment on blood sugar and ketone bodies of diabetics. Blood sugar levels fell substantially in 31% of diabetics after supplementing with 120 mg per day of CoQ7, a substance similar to CoQ10. *J Vitaminol (Kyoto)* 1966;12:293-8. Shigeta Y, Izumi K, Abe H.
56. Impact of ubiquinone (coenzyme Q10) treatment on glycemic control, insulin requirement and well-being in patients with Type 1 diabetes mellitus. Supplementation of 100 mg CoQ10 per day for three months did not improve glucose control or reduce the need for insulin. *Diabet Med* 1999;16:312-8.Henriksen JE, Bruun Andersen C, Hother-Nielsen O, et al.
57. Can correction of sub-optimal coenzyme Q status improve beta-cell function in type II diabetics- Med. Hypotheses 1999 May; 52(5): 397-400. McCarty, M.F.
58. Toward Practical Prevention of Type 2 Diabetes. Other nutrients that might prove to aid diabetic glycemic control, and thus have potential for prevention, include coenzyme Q and conjugated linoleic acids (CLA). Supplementation with these nutrients may prove to be a practical strategy for diabetes prevention. Med Hypotheses 2000 (May); 54 (5): 786–793. McCarty MF, Pantox Laboratories, San Diego, USA.
59. Coenzyme Q10 Administration and its Potential for Treatment of Neurodegenerative Diseases. Oral administration of CoQ10 significantly decreased elevated lactate levels in

patients with Huntington's disease. These studies therefore raise the prospect that administration of CoQ10 may be useful for the treatment of neurodegenerative diseases. Biofactors 1999; 9 (2–4): 261–266. Beal MF, Neurochemistry Laboratory, Massachusetts General Hospital, Boston, MA.

60. A Possible Role of Coenzyme Q10 in the Etiology and Treatment of Parkinson's Disease. Data suggests that CoQ10 may play a role in cellular dysfunction found in PD and may be a potential protective agent for parkinsonian patients. Biofactors 1999; 9 (2–4): 267–272. Shults CW, Haas RH, Beal MF, Dept. of Neurosciences, University of California, San Diego, CA.

Diabetes (Type 1):

61. Possible regeneration of the Islets of Langerhans in Streptozotocin-diabetic rats given Gymnema sylvestre leaf extract, *J. Ethnopharmacology* 30:265-279 (1990). Shanmugasundaram, E.R.B. et al (Dr Ambedkar Institute of Diabetes, Kilpauk Medical College Hospital, Madras, India).

62. Effect of nicotinamide therapy upon B-cell function in newly diagnosed type 1 (insulin-dependent) diabetics. *Diabetologia* 1989;32:160–2. Mendola G, Casamitjana R, Gomis R.

63. Relationship between cows' milk consumption and incidence of IDDM in childhood. *Diabetes Care* 1991;14:1081–3. Dahl-Jorgensen K, Joner G, Hanssen KF.

64. Type I (insulin-dependent) diabetes mellitus and cow milk: casein variant consumption. *Diabetologia* 1999;42:292-6. Elliott RB, Harris DP, Hill JP, et al.

65. A bovine albumin peptide as a possible trigger of insulin-dependent diabetes mellitus. Children antibodies cross-react with and damage the insulin-producing cells of the pancreas. *N Engl J Med* 1992;327:302-7. Karajalainen J, Martin JM, Knip M, et al.

66. Cow's milk exposure and type I diabetes mellitus. Preliminary studies have found that early introduction of cows' milk formula feeding increases the risk of developing type 1 diabetes. *Diabetes Care* 1994;17:13-9. Gerstein H.

67. Biotin status and plasma glucose in diabetics. Type 1 diabetics were given 16 mg of biotin per day for one week, their fasting glucose levels dropped by 50%. *Ann NY Acad Sci* 1985;447:389-92. Coggeshall JC, Heggers JP, Robson MC, Baker H.

68. A population based strategy to prevent insulin-dependent diabetes using nicotinamide. Healthy children at high risk for type 1 diabetes (such as the healthy siblings of children with type 1 diabetes) may be protected from the disease by supplementing with niacinamide, but only under doctor supervision. *J Pediatr Endocrinol Metab* 1996;9:501-9, Elliott RB, Picher CC, Fergusson DM, Stewart AW.

69. The Deutsche Nicotinamide Intervention Study. An attempt to prevent type 1 diabetes. Supplementing with niacinamide may not help prevent type 1 diabetes. *Diabetes* 1998;47:980-4. Lampeter EF, Klinghammer A, Scherbaum WA, et al.

70. Insulin Cells Persist in Long-standing Diabetes. Study showed that the majority (88 percent) with type 1 diabetes for up to 60 years still had detectable insulin-producing beta cells in their pancreas. According to Dr. P. C. Butler: Type 1 could, theoretically, be cured by stopping the beta cells from being destroyed. Therefore, type 1 diabetes may be reversible by targeted inhibition of beta cell destruction. Additional studies being funded by the Juvenile Diabetes Research Foundation. Reuters Health, June 2005; Diabetes Today; Dr. P. C. Butler, University of California, Los Angeles, CA.

Diabetes (Type 2), Metabolic Syndrome X:

71. Maturity-onset diabetes mellitus--toward a physiological appropriate management. Therapy includes: GTF, to directly enhance the efficacy of insulin; weight loss, exercise, and fasting, to help reduce tissue resistance to insulin; mitochondrial "metavitamins", to optimize the oxidative disposal of excess substrate; a high-fiber, low-fat diet, which appears superior to traditional diabetic diets as a promoter of glucose tolerance. Following a prolonged fast, obese diabetics show substantial improvement in most parameters of insulin function--an effect which is to some degree independent of weight loss; long-term remission of diabetes may be possible if the benefits of therapeutic fasting are conserved by appropriate metabolic measures. Med Hypotheses. 1981 Oct;7(10):1265-85. Review. McCarty MF.

72. Dietary factors determining diabetes and impaired glucose tolerance. A 20-year follow-up of the Finnish and Dutch cohorts of the Seven Countries Study. Eating carbohydrate-rich foods such as beans, peas, oats with low glycemic indices is associated with a *low* risk of type 2 diabetes. *Diabetes Care* 1995;18:1104-12. Feskens EJ, Virtanen SM, Rasanen L, et al.

73. Beneficial effects of high dietary fiber intake in patients with type 2 diabetes mellitus. Six-weeks study, 50 grams/day of fiber from high fiber foods (e.g. leafy green vegetables, granola, fruit, etc.): average glucose level 10% lower; insulin levels 12% lower; significant reductions in total cholesterol, triglycerides, and LDL ("bad") cholesterol; slight decreases in glycosylated hemoglobin -- compared to participants eating the ADA diet (24 grams/day). *New Engl J Med* 2000;342:1392-8. Chandalia M, Garg A, Lutjohann D, et al.

74. Diabetes mellitus -- a free radical-associated disease. 1993; *Z Gesamte Inn Med* 48(5): 223-32. Kahler, W., B. Kuklinski, et al.

75. Comparison of effects of high and low carbohydrate diets on plasma lipoproteins and insulin sensitivity in patients with mild NIDDM. 1992; *Diabetes* 41(10): 1278-85. Garg, A., S. Grundy, et al.

76. A high-monounsaturated fat/low-carbohydrate diet improves peripheral insulin sensitivity in non-insulin-dependent diabetic patients. 1992; *Metabolism* 41(12): 1373-8. Parillo, M., A. Rivellese, et al.

77. Effect of high intakes of fruit and vegetables on redox status in type 2 onset diabetes: a pilot study. Int J Vitam Nutr Res. 2004 Sep;74(5):313-20. PMID: 15628668. Giammarioli S, Filesi C, Vitale B, Cantagallo A, Dragoni F, Sanzini E.

78. Effect of Vitamin C Supplementation on Blood Sugar and Antioxidative Status in Types II Diabetes Mellitus Patients. Taehan Kanho Hakhoe Chi. 2003 Apr;33(2):170-8. Korean. PMID: 15314445. Park HS, Lee YM.

79. Dietary antioxidant intake and risk of type 2 diabetes. This study supports the hypothesis that development of type 2 diabetes may be reduced by the intake of antioxidants in the diet. Montonen J, Knekt P, Jarvinen R, Reunanen A., National Public Health Institute, Dept. of Health & Functional Capacity, Helsinki, Finland.

80. Experiences with a diet-training program in patients with obesity associated diseases including follow-up. Z Gesamte Inn Med. 1989 Sep 1;44(17):509-12. Hantzschel U, Kraus E, Dempe A.

81. European stroke prevention study: effectiveness of antiplatelet therapy in diabetic patients. 1992; *Stroke* 23(6): 851-4. Sivenius, J., M. Laakso, et al.

82. Weight gain during insulin therapy in patients with type 2 diabetes mellitus. Diabetes Res Clin Pract. 2004 Sep;65 Suppl 1:S23-7. PMID: 15315867. Heller S., UK.

83. AGEs and their interaction with AGE-receptors in vascular disease and diabetes mellitus. I. The AGE concept. Cardiovascular Research. 1998; 37(3):586-600. Bierhaus A, Hofmann MA, Ziegler R, et al.

84. Cystic fibrosis-related diabetes. Diabet Med. 2003 Jun;20(6):425-36. Mackie AD, Thornton SJ, Edenborough FP., Diabetes and Endocrine Centre and Adult Cystic Fibrosis Unit, Northern General Hospital, Sheffield, UK.

85. Does a vegetarian diet reduce the occurrence of diabetes? Vegetarians have a low risk of type 2 diabetes. *Am J Publ Health* 1985;75:507-12. Snowdon DA, Phillips RL.

86. Insulin sensitivity and abdominal obesity in African-American, Hispanic, and non-Hispanic white men and women. Excess abdominal weight makes the body less sensitive to insulin. *Diabetes* 1996;45:1547-55. Karter AJ, Mayer-Davis EJ, Selby JV, et al.

87. Intra-abdominal fat is associated with decreased insulin sensitivity in healthy young men. *Metabolism* 1991;40:600-3. Park KS, Hree BD, Lee K-U, et al.

88. Weight loss in obese subjects prevents the progression of impaired glucose tolerance to type II diabetes. *Diabetes Care* 1994;17:372. Long SD, Swanson MS, O'Brien K, et al.

89. Caloric restriction per se is a significant factor in improvements in glycemic control and insulin sensitivity during weight loss in obese NIDDM patients. *Diabetes Care* 1994;17:30. Wing RR, Marcuse MD, Blair EH, et al.

90. Tobacco and end stage diabetic nephropathy. People with diabetes who smoke are at higher risk for kidney damage. *BMJ* 1987;295:581-2. Stegmayr B, Lithner F.

91. Insulin-dependent diabetes mellitus mortality-the risk of cigarette smoking. People with diabetes who smoke are at higher risk for heart disease. *Circulation* 1990;82:37-43. Scala C, LaPorte RE, Dorman JS, et al.

92. Therapeutic evaluation of the effect of biotin on hyperglycemia in patients with non-insulin dependent diabetes mellitus. Fasting glucose levels dropped using 9 mg per day for two months in type 2 diabetics. *J Clin Biochem Nutr* 1993;14:211-8. Maebashi M, Makino Y, Furukawa Y, et al.

93. Body composition, visceral fat, leptin, and insulin resistance in Asian Indian men. *J Clin Endocrinol Metab*84 :137 –144,1999. Banerji MA, Faridi N, Atluri R, Chaiken RL Lebovitz HE.

94. Leptin secretion from subcutaneous and visceral adipose tissue in women. *Diabetes*47 :913 – 917,1998. Van Harmelen V, Raynisdottir S, Eriksson P, Thörne A, Hoffstedt J, Lönnqvist F, Arner P.

95. C-reactive protein, interleukin 6, and risk of developing type 2 diabetes mellitus. JAMA 2001 Jul 18; 286(3): 327-34. Pradhan, A. et al.

96. Advanced glycation end products: a nephrologist's perspective. Am. J. Kidney Dis. 2000 Mar; 35(3): 365-80. Raj, D.S. et al.

97. Zinc and insulin sensitivity. Biol. Trace Elem. Res. 1992; 32: 305-10. Faure, P. et al.

98. Caffeine: a cause of insulin resistance- Diabetes Care 2002; 25: 399-400. Biaggioni, I., Davis, S.N.

99. Caffeine can decrease insulin sensitivity in humans. Diabetes Care 2002; 25: 364-9. Keijzers, G. et al.

100. Sleep Deprivation Promotes Insulin Resistance 2001. Ford-Martin, P.

101. Effects of varying carbohydrate content of diet in patients with non-insulin-dependent diabetes mellitus. JAMA 1994; 271: 1421-8. Garg, A., Bantle, J., Henry, R. et al.

102. Treatment of periodontal disease in diabetics reduces glycated hemoglobin. J. Periodontol. 1997 Aug; 68(8): 713-9. Grossi, S.G. et al.

103. Decrease Your Sleep and Increase Your Risk of Diabetes 2001, The Lancet October 23, 1999;354:1435-1439. Mercola, J.

104. Effect of eicosapentaenoic acid ethyl ester v. oleic acid-risk safflower oil on insulin resistance in type 2 diabetic model rats with hypertricylglycerolaemia. Br. J. Nutr. 2002 Feb; 87(2): 157-62. Minami, A. et al.

105. Polyol pathway hyperactivity is closely related to carnitine deficiency in the pathogenesis of diabetic neuropathy of streptozotocin-diabetic rats. J. Pharmacol. Exp. Ther. 1998; 287: 897-902. Nakamura, J. et al.

106. Type 2 diabetes can be prevented with lifestyle change. Presented at the American Diabetes' Association's 60th Annual Scientific Session, San Antonio, Texas, June 9-13, 2000. Tuomilehto, J.

107. Prevention of type 2 diabetes mellitus by changes in lifestyle among subjects with impaired glucose tolerance. N. Engl. J. Med. 2001 May 3; 344(18): 1343-50. Tuomilehto, J. et al.

108. The effect of sugar cereal with and without a mixed meal on glycemic response in children with diabetes. J. Pediatr. Gastroenterol. Nutr. 1991 Aug; 13(2): 155-60. Wang, S.R. et al.

109. Prevalence of hyperinsulinemia in patients with high blood pressure. J. Intern. Med. 1992; 231: 235-40. Zavaroni, I., Mazza, S., Dall'aglio, E. et al.

110. Use of Gymnema sylvestre leaf extract in the control of blood glucose in insulin-dependent diabetes mellitus, J. *Ethnopharmacology* 30:281-294 (1990). Shanmugasundaram, E.R.B. et al.

111. Cinnamon improves glucose and lipids of people with type 2 diabetes. *Diabetes Care* 2003 Dec;26(12):3215-8. Khan A, Safdar M, Khan MMA, Khattak KN, Anderson RA.

Exercise:

112. Exercise and the nitric oxide vasodilator system. Sports Med. 2003;33(14):1013-35. Review. PMID: 14599231. Maiorana A, O'Driscoll G, Taylor R, Green D., Australia

113. Role of exercise training on cardiovascular disease in persons who have type 2 diabetes and hypertension. Cardiol Clin. 2004 Nov;22(4):569-86. PMID: 15501624. Stewart KJ.

114. Influence of resistance exercise training on glucose control in women with type 2 diabetes. Metabolism. 2004 Mar;53(3):284-9. PMID: 15015138. Fenicchia LM, Kanaley JA, Azevedo JL Jr, Miller CS, Weinstock RS, Carhart RL, Ploutz-Snyder LL.

115. Insulin resistance and associated metabolic abnormalities in muscle: effects of exercise. Obes Rev. 2001 Feb;2(1):47-59. Review. PMID: 12119637. Perez-Martin A, Raynaud E, Mercier J., France

116. High-intensity resistance training improves glycemic control in older patients with type 2 diabetes. Diabetes Care. 2002 Oct;25(10):1729-36. PMID: 12351469. Dunstan DW, Daly RM, Owen N, Jolley D, De Courten M, Shaw J, Zimmet P., Australia

117. Effects of L-carnitine supplementation on physical performance and energy metabolism of endurance-trained athletes: a double blind crossover field study. *Eur J Appl Physiol* 1996;73:434–9. Colombani P, Wenk C, Kunz I, et al.

118. Effects of postprandial exercise on glycemic response in IDDM subjects, improves insulin sensitivity. *Diabetes Care* 1994;17:1203. Rasmussen OW, Lauszus FF, Hermansen K.

119. Physical activity and reduced occurrence of non-insulin-dependent diabetes mellitus. *N Engl J Med* 1991;325:147-52. Helmrich SP, Ragland DR, Leung RW, Paffenbarger RS.

120. Effects of exercise on glycemic control and body mass in type II diabetes mellitus. JAMA 2001; 286(10): 1218-27. Boule, N.G. et al.

121. Physical activity and reduced occurrence of non-insulin-dependent diabetes mellitus. N. Engl. J. Med. 1991 Jul 18; 325(3): 147-52. Helmrich, S.P. et al.

Eye health:

122. Scientific basis for medical therapy of cataracts by antioxidants. 1992; *Am J Clin Nutr* 53(1 Suppl). Weisburger, J.

123. Antioxidant nutrition and cataract in women: a study. 1993; *Nutr Rev* 51(3): 84-6. Bunce, G.

124. Diabetic cataracts and flavonoids. *Science*. 1977;195:205–206. Varma SD, Mizuno A, Kinoshita JH.

125. Role of nutrients in delaying cataracts. 1992; *Ann N Y Acad Sci* 669(1): 11-23. Taylor, A.

126. A possible role for vitamins C and E in cataract prevention. 1991; *Am J Clin Nutr* 53(1 Suppl): 346S-351S. Robertson, J., A. Donner, et al.

127. The role of the carotenoids, lutein and zeaxanthin, in protecting against age-related macular degeneration: A review based on controversial evidence. Nutr J. 2003 Dec 11;2(1):20. PMID: 14670087. Mozaffarieh M, Sacu S, Wedrich A., Vienna, Austria.

128. Zinc and the eye. J Am Coll Nutr. 2001 Apr;20(2 Suppl):106-18. Review. PMID: 11349933. Grahn BH, Paterson PG, Gottschall-Pass KT, Zhang Z., Saskatoon, Canada.

129. Health benefits of omega-3 fatty acids. Nurs Stand. 2004 Aug 11-17;18(48):38-42. Review. PMID: 15366399. Ruxton C.

130. Efficacy of N-acetyl carnosine in the treatment of cataracts. Drugs R D. 2002;3(2):87-103. Babizhayev MA, Deyev AI, Yermakova VN, Semiletov YA, Davydova NG, Doroshenko VS,

Zhukotskii AV, Goldman IM., Innovative Vision Products, Inc., County of Newcastle, Delaware.

131. Bilberry may lower the risk of some diabetic complications, such as diabetic cataracts and retinopathy. One preliminary trial found that supplementation with a standardized extract of bilberry improved signs of retinal damage in some people with diabetic retinopathy. *Klin Monatsblatt Augenheilk* 1981;178:386-9. Scharrer A, Ober M. Anthocyanoside in der Behandlung von Retinopathien.

132. Epidemiologic evidence of a role for the antioxidant vitamins and carotenoids in cataract prevention. Am J Clin Nutr. 1991;53:352S-355S. Jacques PF, Chylack LT.

Fiber

133. Diets containing soluble oat extracts improve glucose and insulin responses of moderately hypercholesterolemic men and women. *Am J Clin Nutr* 1995;61:379-84. Hallfrisch J, Scholfield DJ, Behall KM.

134. Beneficial effects of viscous dietary fiber from Konjac-mannan in subjects with the insulin resistance syndrome: results of a controlled metabolic trial. *Diabetes Care* 2000;23:9-14. Vuksan V, Sievenpiper JL, Owen R, et al.

135. Hypoglycemic effect of 1-3 ounces of powdered fenugreek seeds in non-insulin dependent diabetic subjects. *Nutr Res* 1990;10:731-9. Sharma RD, Raghuram TC.

136. Effect of konjac fiber (glucomannan) on glucose and lipids. Reduces the elevation of blood sugar levels that is typical after a meal. *Eur J Clin Nutr* 1995;49(Suppl. 3):S190-7. Doi K.

137. Effect of Konjac food on blood glucose level in patients with diabetes. Overall diabetic control is improved with glucomannan-enriched diets. *Biomed Environ Sci* 1990;3:123-31. Huang CY, Zhang MY, Peng SS, et al.

138. Konjac-mannan (glucomannan) improves glycemia and other associated risk factors for coronary heart disease in type 2 diabetes in controlled study. A randomized controlled metabolic trial. *Diabetes Care* 1999;22:913-9. Vuksan V, Jenkins DJ, Spadafora P, et al.

139. Effects of psyllium on glucose and serum lipid responses in men with type 2 diabetes and hypercholesterolemia. In a double-blind trial, supplementing of 5.1 grams of psyllium per day for eight weeks lowered blood glucose levels by 11% to 19.2%, total cholesterol by 8.9%, and LDL (bad) cholesterol by 13%, compared to a placebo. *Am J Clin Nutr* 1999;70:466-73. Anderson JW, Allgood LD, Turner J, et al.

140. Supplementation with dietary fiber improves fecal incontinence. Nurs Res 2001 Jul-Aug; 50(4): 203-13. Bliss DZ, Jung HJ, Savik K, Lowry A, LeMoine M, Jensen L, Werner C, Schaffer K. 2001.

141. Dietary protein and soluble fiber reduce ambulatory blood pressure in treated hypertensives. Hypertension 2001 Oct; 38(4): 821-6. Burke V, Hodgson JM, Beilin LJ, Giangiulioi N, Rogers P, Puddey IB. 2001.

Fish oil:

142. The long-term outcome of patients with IgA nephropathy treated with fish oil in a controlled trial. Mayo Nephrology Collaborative Group. *J Am Soc Nephrol* 1999;10:1772-7. Donadio JV Jr, Grande JP, Bergstralh EJ, et al.

143. Biological effects of omega-3 fatty acids in diabetes mellitus. *Diabetes Care* 1991;14:1160-79. Malasanos TH, Stacpoole PW.

144. Effect of fish oil concentrate on lipoprotein composition in NIDDM. *Diabetes* 1988; 37:1567-73. Schectman G, Kaul S, Kassebah AH.

145. Effects of n-3 polyunsaturated fatty acids on glucose homeostasis and blood pressure in hypertension. *Ann Intern Med* 1995;123:911-8. Toft I, Bonaa KH, Ingebretsen OC, et al.

146. The independent and combined effects of aerobic exercise and dietary fish intake on serum lipids and glycemic control in NIDDM. *Diabetes Care* 1997; 20:913-21. Dunstan DW, Burke V, Mori TA, et al.

147. Effect of high fiber intake in fish oil-treated patients with non-insulin-dependent diabetes mellitus *Am J Clin Nutr* 1997; 66:1183-7. Sheehan JP, Wei IW, Ulchaker M, Tserng KY.

148. Effect of garlic and fish-oil supplementation on serum lipid and lipoprotein concentrations in hypercholesterolemic men. *Am J Clin Nutr* 1997; 65:445-50. Adler AJ, Holub BJ.

149. Intake of mercury from fish, lipid peroxidation, and the risk of myocardial infarction and coronary, cardiovascular, and any death in eastern Finnish men. Circulation 1995;91:645-55. Salonen JT, Seppanen K, Nyyssonen K, et al.

150. Fish diet, fish oil and docosahexaenoic acid rich oil lower fasting and postprandial plasma lipid levels. Eur J Clin Nutr 1996;50:765-71. Agren JJ, Hanninen O, Julkunen A, et al.

151. Effects of fish oil supplementation in rheumatoid arthritis. Ann Rheum Dis 1990;49:76-80. van der Tempel H, Tulleken JE, Limburg PC, et al.

152. Effect of eicosapentaenoic acid ethyl on albuminuria of non-insulin dependent diabetic patients. Diabetes Res Clin Pract 1995;28:35-40. Shimizu H, Ohtani K, Tanaka Y, et al.

153. Fish oil improves arterial compliance in non-insulin-dependent diabetes mellitus. Arterioscler Thromb 1994;14:1425-9. McVeigh GE, Brennan GM, Cohn JN, et al.

154. Short report: the effect of fish oil on blood pressure and high-density lipoprotein-cholesterol levels in phase I of the trials of hypertension prevention. J Hypertens 1994;12:209-13. Sacks FM, Hebert P, Appel LJ, et al.

155. Effect of eicosapentaenoic acid and docosahexaenoic acid on oxidative stress and inflammatory markers in treated-hypertensive type 2 diabetic subjects. This study is the first report demonstrating that either EPA or DHA reduce in vivo oxidant stress without changing markers of inflammation, in treated hypertensive, type 2 diabetic subjects. Mori TA, Woodman RJ, Burke V, Puddey IB, Croft KD, Beilin LJ., Dept. of Medicine, The University of Western Australia.

156. Neuroprotective effect of docosahexaenoic acid-enriched phospholipids in experimental diabetic neuropathy. These results demonstrate a protective effect of daily doses of DHA on experimental diabetic neuropathy. Coste TC, Gerbi A, Vague P, Pieroni G, Raccah D., Faculte de Medecine Timone, Marseille, France.

Glyconutrients; Ginkgo biloba, Ginseng, Fenugreek:

157. Effects of nutraceutical and glyconutrients in diabetes mellitus: decreased glucose levels, improved healing of foot ulcers, weight loss, reduced medications. Proc Fisher Inst Med Res. 1997; 1: 19-23, McDaniel CF;Dykman KD;McDaniel R;Ford C;Tone C

158. Nutraceuticals and glyconutrients decrease blood glucose and pain in an individual with non-insulin dependent diabetes and myofascial pain syndrome. Proc Fisher Inst Med Res. 1997; 1: 30-31, McDaniel CF;Stevens EW

159. Effect of glyconutritionals on oxidative stress. GlycoScience & Nutrition. 2001:2(12):1-10. Goux WJ, Boyd S, Tone CM, et al.

160. American ginseng (*Panax quinquefolius* L.) reduces postprandial glycemia in non-diabetic subjects and subjects with type 2 diabetes mellitus. *Arch Intern Med* 2000;160:1009-13. Vuksan V, Sivenpiper JL, Koo VY, et al.

161. The effect of 3-month ingestion of Ginkgo biloba extract on pancreatic ß-cell function in response to glucose loading in normal glucose-tolerant individuals. J Clin Pharmacol 2000;40:647-4. Kudolo GB.

162. Effect of fenugreek seeds on blood glucose and serum lipids in type 1 diabetes. Eur J Clin Nutr 1990;44:301-6. Sharma RD, Raghuram TC, Sudhakar Rao N.

163. Use of fenugreek seed powder in the management of non-insulin dependent diabetes mellitus. Nutr Res 1996;16:1131-9. Sharma RD, Sakar A, Hazra DK, et al.

164. American ginseng (3 grams/day) reduces postprandial glycemia in non-diabetic subjects and subjects with type 2 diabetes mellitus. *Arch Intern Med* 2000;160:1009-13. Vuksan V, Sivenpiper JL, Koo VY, et al.

165. Ginkgo biloba extract and folic acid in the therapy of changes caused by autonomic neuropathy. Ginkgo biloba extract may prove useful for prevention and treatment of early-

stage diabetic neuropathy. Other herbs:fenugreek seeds and eleuthero (Siberian ginseng). Acta Med Austriaca 1989;16:35-7 [in German]. Koltringer P, Langsteger W, Lind P, et al.

Grape seed extract, Resveratrol:
166. Grape seed extract induces apoptotic death of human prostate carcinoma DU145 cells via caspases activation accompanied by dissipation of mitochondrial membrane potential and cytochrome c release. Carcinogenesis. 2002 Nov;23(11):1869-76. Agarwal C, Singh RP, Agarwal R., Dept. of Pharmaceutical Sciences, University of Colorado, Denver, CO.
167. Inhibition of human LDL oxidation by resveratrol. *Lancet.* 1993;341:1103–1104. Frankel EN, Waterhouse AL, Kinsella JE.
168. Biological effects of resveratrol. Resveratrol is a common phytoalexin found in grape skins, peanuts, and red wine. Acts as an antioxidant, promotes nitric oxide production, inhibits platelet aggregation, increases high-density lipoprotein cholesterol; can function as a cancer chemo-preventive agent; has been reported to have some estrogenic properties; exhibits anti-inflammatory, neuroprotective, and antiviral properties. Antioxid Redox Signal. 2001 Dec;3(6):1041-64, Bhat KPL, Kosmeder JW 2nd, Pezzuto JM., Dept. of Medicinal Chemistry and Pharmacognosy, University of Illinois Cancer Center, University of Illinois at Chicago.
169. Benefits of resveratrol in women's health. Supplementation may be a potential alternative to conventional HRT for cardio-protection and osteoporosis prevention and may confer other potential health benefits in women. Drugs Exp Clin Res. 2001;27(5-6):233-48. Bagchi D, Das DK, Tosaki A, Bagchi M, Kothari SC., Dept. of Pharmacy Sciences, Creighton University School of Pharmacy and Allied Health Professions.
170. Neuroprotective effects of resveratrol against beta-amyloid-induced neurotoxicity in rat hippocampal neurons: involvement of protein kinase C. Resveratrol, an active ingredient of red wine extracts, has been shown to exhibit neuroprotective effects in several experimental models. Br J Pharmacol. 2004 Mar;141(6):997-1005.

Gymnema sylvestre, Bitter melon:
171. Anti-diabetic effect of Gymnema montanum leaves: effect on lipid peroxidation induced oxidative stress in experimental diabetes. Pharmacol Res. 2003 Dec;48(6):551-6. PMID: 14527818. Ananthan R, Baskar C, NarmathaBai V, Pari L, Latha M, Ramkumar KM.
172. Anti-diabetic effect of a leaf extract from Gymnema sylvestre in non-insulin-dependent diabetes mellitus patients. J Ethnopharmacol 1990;30:295–305. Baskaran K, Ahmath BK, Shanmugasundaram KR, Shanmugasundaram ERB.
173. Effect of extended release gymnema sylvestre leaf extract (Beta Fast GXR) alone or in combination with oral hypoglycemics or insulin regimens for type 1 and type 2 diabetes. Diabetes In Control Newsletter 2001;76. Joffe DJ, Freed SH.
174. New hypoglycemic constituents in "gymnemic acid" from Gymnema sylvestre. Chem Pharm Bull (Tokyo) 1996;44:469–71. Murakami N, Murakami T, Kadoya M, et al.
175. Insulinotropic activity of G. sylvestre, R.Br. and Indian medicinal herb used in controlling diabetes mellitus. Pharmacol Res Commun 1981;13:475–86. Shanmugasundaram KR, Panneerselvam C, Sumudram P, Shanmugasundaram ERB.
176. Bitter melon (Momordica charantia): a review of efficacy and safety. Am J Health Syst Pharm. 2003 Feb 15;60(4):356-9. Review. PMID: 12625217. Basch E, Gabardi S, Ulbricht C.
177. Effect of bitter melon (Momordica charantia Linn) on level and function of natural killer cells in cervical cancer patients with radiotherapy. J Med Assoc Thai 2003;Jan, 86(1):61-68. Pongnikorn S, Fongmoon D, Kasinrerk W, Limtrakul PN.
178. Improvement of glucose tolerance due to Momordica charantia (bitter melon slices). *BMJ* 1981;282:1823-4. Leatherdale BA, Panesar RK, Singh G, et al.
179. Anti-diabetic and adaptogenic properties of Momordica charantia extract (bitter melon): An experimental and clinical evaluation. *Phytother Res* 1993;7:285-9. Srivastava Y, Venkatakrishna-bhatt H, Verma Y, et al.

180. Effect of Extended Release Gymnema Sylvestre Leaf Extract (Beta Fast GXR) Alone or In Combination With Oral Hypoglycemics or Insulin Regimens for Type 1 and Type 2 Diabetes. The use of Gymnema Sylvestre (Beta Fast GXR®) supplementation in all patients with diabetes has a positive result. Reducing postprandial blood glucose significantly caused a decrease of HbA1c, therefore reducing the complications from diabetes. Diabetes In Control Newsletter, Issue 76 (1) : 30 Oct 2001. Joffe, DJ; Freed, SH.

181. Possible regeneration of the islets of Langerhans in streptozotocin diabetic rats given Gymnema sylvestre leaf extracts. J Ethnopharmacol 1990;30:265-79. Shanmugasundaram ERB, Leela Gopinath K, Radha Shanmugasundaram K, Rajendran VM.

Neuropathy, Nephropathy

182. The effect of gamma-linolenic acid on human diabetic peripheral neuropathy: a double-blind placebo-controlled trial. 4 grams of evening primrose oil per day for six months improved nerve function and relieved pain symptoms of diabetic neuropathy. *Diabet Med* 1990;7:319-23. Jamal GA, Carmichael H.

183. Regression of diabetic neuropathy with total vegetarian (vegan) diet. *J Nutr Med* 1994;4:431-9. Crane MG, Sample C.

184. Biotin for diabetic peripheral neuropathy. Biotin may also reduce pain. *Biomed Pharmacother* 1990;44:511-4. Koutsikos D, Agroyannis B, Tzanatos-Exarchou H.

185. The effect of gamma-linolenic acid on human diabetic peripheral neuropathy: a double-blind placebo-controlled trial. Supplementing with 4 grams of evening primrose oil per day for six months improved nerve function and relieved pain symptoms of diabetic neuropathy. *Diabet Med* 1990;7:319-23. Jamal GA, Carmichael H.

186. L-acetyl-carnitine as a new therapeutic approach for peripheral neuropathies with pain. 1 gram per day by injection reduced pain from diabetic nerve damage. *Int J Clin Pharmacol Res* 1995;15:9-15. Onofrj M, Fulgente T, Mechionda D, et al.

187. Treatment of painful diabetic neuropathy with topical capsaicin. A multicenter, double-blind, vehicle-controlled study. The Capsaicin Study Group. Double-blind trials have shown that topical application of creams containing 0.025-0.075% capsaicin (from cayenne can relieve symptoms of diabetic neuropathy (numbness and tingling in the extremities). Four or more applications per day may be required to relieve severe pain, but this should be done only under a doctor's supervision. *Arch Intern Med* 1991;151:2225-9.

Nutrition, Vitamins, Other Supplements:

188. Antioxidant nutrient intake and diabetic retinopathy. The San Luis Valley Diabetes Study. *Ophthalmology* 1998;105:2264–70. Mayer-Davis E, Bell RA, Reboussin BA, et al.

189. Inhibition of whole blood platelet aggregation by compounds in garlic clove extracts. 1992; *Thromb Res* 65(2): 141-56. Lawson, L., D. Ransom, et al.

190. The effect of a salmon diet on blood clotting, platelet aggregation and fatty acids. 1991; *Lipids* 26(2): 87-96. Nelson, G., P. Schmidt, et al.

191. Comparison of effects of high and low carb diets on plasma lipoproteins and insulin sensitivity in patients with NIDDM. 1992; *Diabetes* 41(10): 1278-85. Garg, A., S. Grundy.

192. A high-monounsaturated fat/low-carbohydrate diet improves peripheral insulin sensitivity in non-insulin-dependent diabetic patients. 1992; *Metabolism* 41(12): 1373-8. Parillo, M., A. Rivellese, et al.

193. Effects of dietary carbohydrate and fat intake on glucose and lipoprotein metabolism in individuals with diabetes mellitus. 1991; *Diabetes Care* 14(9): 774-85. Hollenbeck, C. and A. Coulston.

194. Carnosine: an endogenous neuroprotector in the ischemic brain. Cell Mol Neurobiol. 1999; 19(1):45-56. Stvolinsky SL, Kukley ML, Dobrota D, et al.

195. Action of carnosine and beta-alanine on wound healing. Surgery. 1986; 100(5):815-21. Nagai K, Suda T, Kawasaki K, et al.

196. Breakfast Foods and the Health Benefits of Inulin and Oligofructose. K. Niness. Orafti Active Food Ingredients, Malvern PA. Copyright 1999 American Association of Cereal Chemists, Inc.

197. Comparison of the effects of psyllium and wheat bran on gastrointestinal transit time and stool characteristics. J Am Diet Assoc 1988;88:323-6. Stevens J. VanSoest PJ, Robertson JB, Levitsky DA.

198. Improved insulin response and action by chronic magnesium administration in aged NIDDM subjects. Double-blind research indicates that supplementing with magnesium improves insulin production in elderly people with type 2 diabetes. *Diabetes Care* 1989;12:265-9. Paolisso G, Sgambato S, Pizza G, et al.

199. Magnesium supplementation in the treatment of diabetes. Connection between magnesium deficiency and insulin resistance. Doctors recommend a daily 200-600 mg magnesium supplement for diabetics with normal kidney function. *Diabetes Care* 1992;15:1065-7. American Diabetes Association.

200. Vitamin D and pancreatic islet function. Vitamin D is needed to maintain adequate blood levels of insulin. *J Endocrine Invest* 1988;11:577-84. Labriji-Mestaghanmi H, Billaudel B, Garnier PE, Sutter BCJ.

201. Inadequate vitamin D status: does it contribute to the disorders comprising syndrome 'X'? Vitamin D receptors have been found in the pancreas where insulin is made and preliminary evidence suggests that supplementation can increase insulin levels in some people with type 2 diabetes; prolonged supplementation might also help reduce blood sugar levels. *Br J Nutr* 1998;79:315-27 [review]. Boucher BJ.

202. Preventing complications of diabetes. Doctors have suggested that quercetin might help people with diabetes because of its ability to reduce levels of sorbitol. *Townsend Letter* 1985;32:307 [editorial]. Gaby A.

203. Oral vanadyl sulfate improves insulin sensitivity in NIDDM but not in obese non-diabetic subjects. *Diabetes* 1996;45:659-66. Halberstam M, Cohen N, Schlimovich P, et al.

204. Biotin for diabetic peripheral neuropathy. Biomed. Pharmacother. 1990; 44: 511-4. Koutsikos, D. et al.

205. Therapeutic evaluation of the effect of biotin on hyperglycemia in patients with non-insulin dependent diabetes mellitus. J. Clin. Biochem. Nutr. 1993; 14: 211-18. Maebashi, M. et al.

206. Cinnamon improves glucose and lipids of people with type 2 diabetes. *Diabetes Care* 2003 Dec;26(12):3215-8. Khan A, Safdar M, Khan MMA, Khattak KN, Anderson RA.

207. Effect of Drinking Soda Sweetened with Aspartame or High Fructose Corn Syrup on Food Intake and Body Weight. American Journal of Clinical Nutrition, 1990 51, 963-96. Tordoff, M. and Alleva, A.M.

208. Effects of sweetness perception and caloric value of a preload on short term intake, Physiol Behav 1983 Jan;30(1):1-9. Brala PM, Hagen RL.

Obesity:

209. Leptin levels in type 2 diabetes: associations with measures of insulin resistance and insulin secretion. The main determinants for leptin levels in type 2 diabetic subjects as in healthy subjects - insulin secretion and the degree of insulin resistance also seem to contribute significantly to leptin levels. Horm Metab Res. 2003 Feb;35(2):92-6. Wauters M, Considine RV, Yudkin JS, Peiffer F, De Leeuw I, Van Gaal LF., Dept. of Diabetology, Metabolism and Clinical Nutrition, University Hospital Antwerp, Belgium.

210. Dietary fish as a major component of a weight-loss diet: effect on serum lipids, glucose, and insulin metabolism in overweight hypertensive subjects. *Am J Clin Nutr* 1999;70:817-25. Mori TA, Bao DQ, Burke V.

211. Long-term exercise training with constant energy intake. 1: Effect on body composition and selected metabolic variables. Int. J. Obesity 14:57-73, 1990. Bouchard C., A. Tremblay, A. Nadeau, J. Dussault, J.-P. Despres, G. Theriault, P.J. Lupien, O. Serresse, M.R. Boulay, and G. Fournier.

212. Body composition, visceral fat, leptin, and insulin resistance in Asian Indian men. *J Clin Endocrinol Metab*84 :137 –144,1999. Banerji MA, Faridi N, Atluri R, Chaiken RL Lebovitz HE.
213. Obesity as a disease. Br. Med. Bull. 1997; 53: 307-21. Jung, R.
214. Fat metabolism during exercise. Sports Science Exchange, 8(6), article 59. Coyle, E.F. 1995.
215. Sex differences in endurance capacity and metabolic response to prolonged, heavy exercise. European Journal of Applied Physiology, 52, 446-450; 1984. Frogerg, K., & Pedersen, P.K.
216. Energy expenditure in different modes of exercise. American College of Sports Medicine Current Comment, June, 2002. Kravitz, L. & Vella, C.A.
217. Long-term exercise training with constant energy intake. 1: Effect on body composition and selected metabolic variables. Int. J. Obesity 14:57-73, 1990. Bouchard C., A. Tremblay, A. Nadeau, J. Dussault, J.-P. Despres, G. Theriault, P.J. Lupien, O. Serresse, M.R. Boulay, and G. Fournier.

Omega-3, Omega-6 EFAs, Monounsaturated Fats:
218. The effect of dietary omega-3 fatty acids on coronary atherosclerosis. A randomized, double-blind, placebo-controlled trial. Ann Intern Med 1999;130:554-62. von Schacky C, Angerer P, Kothny W, et al.
219. Biological effects of omega-3 fatty acids in diabetes mellitus. Diabetes Care 1991;14:1160-79. Malasanos TH, Stacpoole PW.
220. Effects of n-3 polyunsaturated fatty acids on glucose homeostasis and blood pressure in essential hypertension. *Ann Intern Med* 1995;123:911-8. Toft I, Bonaa KH, Ingebretsen OC.
221. Arterial compliance in obese subjects is improved with dietary plant n-3 fatty acid from flaxseed oil despite increased LDL oxidizability. *Arterioscler Thromb Vasc Biol.* July 1997;17(6):1163-1170. Nestel PJ, Pomeroy SE, Sasahara T, et al.
222. Dietary supplementation of omega-3 polyunsaturated fatty acids improves insulin sensitivity in non-insulin-dependent diabetes. *Diabetes Res* 1987;4:141–7. Popp-Snijders C, Schouten JA, Heine RJ, et al.
223. Dietary fish as a major component of a weight-loss diet: effect on serum lipids, glucose, and insulin metabolism in overweight hypertensive subjects. *Am J Clin Nutr.* 1999;70:817-825. Mori TA, Bao, DQ, Burke V, et al.
224. Dietary fat and risk for advanced age-related macular degeneration. *Arch Opthalmol.* 2001;119(8):1191-1199. Seddon JM, Rosner B, Sperduto RD, Yannuzzi L, Haller JA, Blair NP, Willett W.
225. Fish oil supplementation in type 2 diabetes: a quantitative systematic review. *Diabetes Care.* 2000;23:1407-1415. Montori V, Farmer A, Wollan PC, Dinneen SF.
226. The effect of fish oil on hypertension, plasma lipids and hemostasis in hypertensive, obese, dyslipidemic patients with and without diabetes mellitus. *Prostaglandins Leukot Essent Fatty Acids.* 1999;61(2):83-87. Yosefy C, Viskoper JR, Laszt A, Priluk R, Guita E, Varon D, et al.
227. Olive oil supplementation decreases LDL oxidation. 1993; *Harefuah* 124(1): 1-4. Aviram, M. and E. Kassem.
228. The effects of monounsaturated-fat enriched diet and polyunsaturated-fat enriched diet on lipid and glucose metabolism in subjects with impaired glucose tolerance. *Eur J Clin Nutr* 1996;50:592–8. Sarkkinen E, Schwab U, Niskanen L, et al.
229. Comparison of a high-carbohydrate diet with a high-monounsaturated-fat diet in patients with non-insulin dependent diabetes mellitus. *N Engl J Med* 1988;319:829–34. Garg A, Bananome A, Grundy SM, et al.
230. Beneficial effects of increasing monounsaturated fat intake in adolescents with type 1 diabetes. *Diabetes Res Clin Pract* 2000;48:193–9. Donaghue KC, Pena MM, Chan AK, et al.
231. Docosahexaenoic and eicosapentaenoic acids in plasma phospholipids are divergently associated with high density lipoprotein. Arterioscler Thromb. 1992;12(6):675-681. Bonaa KH, Bjerve KS, Nordoy A.
232. Effects of docosahexanoic acid on serum lipoproteins in patients with combined hyperlipidemia. A randomized, double-blind, placebo-controlled trial. *J Am Coll Nutr.*

1997;16:3:236-243. Davidson MH, Maki KC, Kalkowski J, Schaefer EJ, Torri SA, Drennan KB.

233. Similar effects of rapeseed oil (canola oil) and olive oil in a lipid-lowering diet for patients with hyperlipoproteinemia. The results indicate lipid-lowering diets containing either rapeseed oil or olive oil have similar effects on serum lipoprotein concentration and glucose tolerance in hyperlipidemic subjects. J Am Coll Nutr. 1995 Dec;14(6):643-51. Nydahl M, Gustafsson IB, Ohrvall M, Vessby B., Univ. of Uppsala, Sweden.

234. Food safety and health effects of canola oil. Canola oil contains 55% of the monounsaturated fatty acid; oleic acid, 25% linoleic acid and 10% alpha-linolenate [polyunsaturated fatty acid (PUFA)], and only 4% of the saturated fatty acids (SFAs) that have been implicated as factors in hypercholesterolemia. It is very low in erucic acid--a fatty acid suspected to have pathogenic potential in diets high in the original rapeseed oil in experimental animals. J Am Coll Nutr. 1989 Oct;8(5):360-75. Review. Dupont J, White PJ, Johnston KM, Heggtveit HA, McDonald BE, Grundy SM, Bonanome A., Dept. of Food and Nutrition, Iowa State University, Ames.

Saturated Fats/Coconut Oil

235. Effects of sunflower oil and coconut oil on protein and fat retention, fatty acid pattern of back fat and blood parameters in piglets. Fat content in the coconut oil fed animals, after only 34 days, was 15.9%, in the control group, 18.6%. Arch. Tieremahr (East Germany) 34(l), 19-33, 1984. [and in the sunflower oil fed animals. 21:1%.]. F. Berschauer et al.

236. Effect of fish oil and coconut oil on antioxidant defense system and lipid peroxidation in rat liver. The rate of lipid peroxidation in isolated microsomes was three-fold higher in rats fed fish oil as compared to rats with coconut oil diet. These results suggest that fish oil feeding at an amount compatible with human diet, although decreasing plasma lipids, actually challenges the antioxidant defense system, thus increasing the susceptibility of tissues to free radical oxidative damage. Free Radical Res. Commun. (Switzerland) 12-13 (1), 147-152, 1991. M. D'Aquino et al.

Vegetables & Fruits

237. Effect of high intakes of fruit and vegetables on redox status in type 2 onset diabetes: a pilot study. Int J Vitam Nutr Res. 2004 Sep;74(5):313-20. PMID: 15628668. Giammarioli S, Filesi C, Vitale B, Cantagallo A, Dragoni F, Sanzini E.

238. Five to nine daily servings of vegetables and fruit lower stroke risk. Journal of the American Medical Association, 4/12/1995, pp. 1113-1117. Harvard Heart Letter, September 195.

239. Effect of high intakes of fruit and vegetables on redox status in type 2 onset diabetes: a pilot study. Int J Vitam Nutr Res. 2004 Sep;74(5):313-20. A high consumption of fruit and vegetables by diabetic patients not receiving pharmacological treatment, reduces oxidative stress and seems to produce an improvement in some redox status parameters. Giammarioli S, Filesi C, Vitale B, Cantagallo A, Dragoni F, Sanzini E., Istituto Superiore di Sanita, National Centre for Food Quality and Risk Assessment, Rome, Italy.

240. Brassicia vegetable & breast cancer risk. *JAMA*, 2001. Terry P, Wolk A, Magnusson C.

241. Broccoli sprouts: An exceptionally rich source of inducers of enzymes that protect against chemical carcinogens. *Proc. Natl. Acad. Sci.* 1997;94:10367-10372. Fahey JW, Zhang Y. Talalya P.

242. The Health Benefits of Fruits and Vegetables: A Scientific Overview for Health Professionals. Better Health Foundation, 2002, p16. Hyson D.

243. The effect of fruit and vegetable intake on risk for coronary heart disease in women. Arch Intern Med. 2001;134:1106-1114. Joshipura KJ, Hu FB, Manson JE, et al.

244. The role of folate, antioxidant vitamins and other constituents in fruits and vegetables in the prevention of cardiovascular disease: The epidemiological evidence. Int J Vitam Nutr Res. 2001;71(1):5-17. Eichholzer M, Luthy J, Gutzwiller F, Stahelin HB.

245. Dietary folate from vegetables and citrus fruits decreases plasma homocysteine concentrations in humans in a dietary controlled trial. J Nutr. 1999:129:1135-1139.
246. Effect of high fiber vegetable, fruit, nut dish on serum lipids, and colonic function. Metabolism, 2001;50(4):494-503. Jenkins DA, Kendall CWC, Popovich DG et al.
247. Influence of increased fruit and vegetable intake on plasma and lipoprotein carotenoids and LDL oxidation in smokers and non-smokers. Clin Chem. 2000;46(11):1818-1829.
248. Fruit and vegetable consumption and diabetes mellitus incidence among U.S. adults. Prev Med. 2001;32:33-39. Ford ES, Mokdad AH.
249. Fruit and vegetable intake and population glycosylated hemoglobin levels: the EPIC-Norfolk study. Eur J Clin Nutrition. 2001;55:342-348.
250. Potassium, magnesium, and fruit and vegetable intakes are associated with greater bone density in elderly men and women. Am J Clin Nutr. 1999;69:727-736. Tucker KL, Hannan MT, Honglei C, Cupples LA, Wilson P, Kiel DP.

Vitamin Bs:
251. B vitamins and nerve health. Japanese researchers studied how B vitamins helped nerves repair themselves and transmit their vital information. Gen Pharmacol 1996;27(6)995-1000.
252. B vitamins and nerve health. A German study found B vitamins enhanced nerve health. Ex Clin Endocrinol Diabetes 1996;104(4):311-6.
253. Study discovered that taking B-6 can relieve nerve pain. Adv Perit Dial 2000;16:308-12.
254. Biotin and peripheral neuropathy. French scientists administering high doses of biotin to people suffering from severe peripheral neuropathy noted marked pain relief within a couple of months. (The researchers kept giving the people in the study supplements for two years.) These scientists concluded that biotin is crucial for keeping nerves functioning properly, and they suggested that biotin be used routinely for the prevention and management of neuropathy. Biomed Pharmacother 1990;44(10):511-4.
255. Riboflavin and nerve pain. In the 1990s Cubans suffered an epidemic of nerve pain. When medical experts gave them riboflavin and antioxidant nutrients, their problems decreased. Am J Clin Nutr 2000;71:1676-81S.

Vitamin C:
256. Effect of vitamin C on glycosylation of proteins, may reduce glycosylation. *Diabetes* 1992;41:167-73. Davie SJ, Gould BJ, Yudkin JS.
257. Does diabetes mellitus increase the requirement for vitamin C? Vitamin C lowers sorbitol, a sugar that can accumulate and damage the eyes, nerves, and kidneys. *Nutr Rev* 1996;54:193-202 [review]. Will JC, Tyers T.
258. Magnesium and ascorbic acid supplementation in diabetes mellitus, may improve glucose tolerance. *Ann Nutr Metab* 1995;39:217-23. Eriksson J, Kohvakka A.
259. High-dose vitamin C supplementation increases plasma glucose. Many doctors suggest diabetics supplement with 1-3 grams per day of vitamin C. However, higher amounts could be problematic: in one person, 4.5 grams per day increased blood sugar levels. *Diabetes Care* 1999;22:1218 [letter]. Branch DR.
260. Antioxidant nutrient intake, including both vitamins E and C, and diabetic retinopathy. The San Luis Valley Diabetes Study. Note: Outcome of trial might reflect that sicker people are more likely to take supplements in hopes of getting better. *Ophthalmology* 1998;105:2264-70. Mayer-Davis E, Bell RA, Reboussin BA, et al.
261. Vitamin C and hyperglycemia in the European Prospective Investigation in Cancer-Norfolk (EPIC-Norfolk) study; a population-based study. Diabetes Care 2000 Jun; 23(6): 726-32. Sargeant, L.A. et al.
262. Effect of Vitamin C Supplementation on Blood Sugar and Antioxidative Status in Types II Diabetes Mellitus Patients. Taehan Kanho Hakhoe Chi. 2003 Apr;33(2):170-8. Korean. PMID: 15314445. Park HS, Lee YM.

Vitamin E:

263. Low vitamin E status is a potential risk factor for insulin-dependent diabetes mellitus. *J Intern Med* 1999;245:99–102. Knekt P, Reunanen A, Marniumi J, et al.

264. Increased risk of non-insulin dependent diabetes mellitus at low plasma vitamin E concentrations: a four year follow up study in men. *BMJ* 1995;311:1124–7. Salonen JT, Nyssonen K, Tuomainen T-P, et al.

265. Vitamin E: more than an antioxidant. 1993; *Clin Cardiol* 16(4 Suppl): 116-8. Steiner, M.

266. Effect of Vitamin E on diabetes mellitus. 1992; *Taiwan I Hsueh Hui Tsa Chih* 91(3): 270-5. Wu, H., T. Tai, et al.

267. Vitamin E reduction of protein glycosylation in diabetes. New prospect for prevention of diabetic complications. 1991; Diabetes Care 14(1): 68-72. Ceriello, A., D. Giugliano, et al.

268. Vitamin E improves insulin action in non-insulin-dependent diabetics. 1993; Am J Clin Nutr 57(5): 650-6. Paolisso, G., A. D'Amore, et al.

269. The effect of supplemental vitamin E on serum parameters in diabetics, post coronary and normal subjects. *Nutr Rep Int* 1985;31:1171–80. Bierenbaum ML, Noonan FJ, Machlin LJ, et al.

270. Pharmacologic doses of vitamin E improve insulin action in healthy subjects and non-insulin dependent diabetic patients. *Am J Clin Nutr* 1993;57:650–6. Paolisso G, D'Amore A, Giugliano D, et al.

271. Reversal of defective nerve condition with vitamin E supplementation in type 2 diabetes. *Diabetes Care* 1998;21:1915–8. Tütüncü NB, Bayraktar M, Varli K.

272. Low vitamin E status is a potential risk factor for type 1 insulin-dependent diabetes mellitus. *J Intern Med* 1999;245:99-102. Knekt P, Reunanen A, Marniumi J, et al.

273. Increased risk of non-insulin dependent diabetes mellitus at low plasma vitamin E concentrations: a four year follow up study in men. *BMJ* 1995;311:1124-7. Salonen JT, Nyssonen K, Tuomainen T-P, et al.

274. The effect of supplemental vitamin E on serum parameters in diabetics, post coronary and normal subjects, improved glucose tolerance. *Nutr Rep Int* 1985;31:1171-80. Bierenbaum ML, Noonan FJ, Machlin LJ, et al.

275. Pharmacologic doses of vitamin E improve insulin action in healthy subjects and non-insulin dependent diabetic patients. *Am J Clin Nutr* 1993;57:650-6. Paolisso G, D'Amore A, Giugliano D, et al.

276. Reversal of defective nerve condition with vitamin E supplementation in type 2 diabetes. *Diabetes Care* 1998;21:1915-8. Tütüncü NB, Bayraktar M, Varli K.

277. Reversal of defective nerve condition with vitamin E supplementation (for 6 mos.) in type 2 diabetes. *Diabetes Care* 1998;21:1915-8. Tütüncü NB, Bayraktar M, Varli K.

278. Vitamin E reduction of protein glycosylation in diabetes. *Diabetes Care* 1991;14:68-72. Ceriello A, Giugliano D, Quatraro A, et al.

279. Vitamin E Shows Promise in Treating Diabetes 2001 Jun 5. Washington,D.C.: Hearst Newspapers. Devaraj,S.

280. Vitamin E Helps Protect the Breasts, *Prevention*, April, 1977. London, Robert.

Resources

During my return trips to churches and other community groups, I discovered that many people were happy to know that there were foods and nutritional supplements that provided health benefits without the need for drugs. However, some people were frustrated trying to find these foods and nutritional supplements in their local grocery and health food stores. Here are some resources that you can use as a starting point.

Author's website
www.DeathToDiabetes.com 1-800-813-1927, 1-585-671-0577
Exercise equipment, kitchen utensils, juicers, etc.
www.hsn.com 1-800-284-3100
www.qvc.com 1-888-345-1515
www.shopnbc.com 1-800-676-5523
Glyconutrient food, wholefood supplements, pulse food
www.mannapages.com/dmcculley 1-800-281-4469
www.enivamembers.com/207858 1-866-999-9191
www.myforevergreen.org/519407/ 1-801-655-1000
www.healthalert.com 1-800-231-8063
Omega-3 oils, flaxseed, fish oil supplements
www.pizzeys.com 1-877-804-6444
www.omegaflo.com 1-800-661-FLAX (3529)
www.yourvitamins.com 1-800-800-1200
Organic food resources (meat, dairy, recipes)
www.allorganiclinks.com/General_Organic_Information
Skincare products (additive-free, latest technologies)
Isomers Laboratories, Toronto, Canada 1-416-787-2465
Vitamins, herbs, nutritional supplements (additive-free)
www.yourvitamins.com 1-800-800-1200
www.800herbdoc.com 1-800-HERBDOC (1-800-437-2362)
www.mountainroseherbs.com 1-800-879-3337
Wild salmon, tuna
www.vitalchoice.com 1-800-608-4825
www.seabear.com 1-800-645-FISH (3474)

Author's Update & the Book Cover Design

Update: DeWayne McCulley grew up in Western Pennsylvania (Farrell, Pa) with two strong, caring and hardworking parents and seven brothers and sisters. He was blessed with great teachers and professors, who taught him the wonders of mathematics and science. DeWayne believes he was fortunate to have worked as an engineer for Xerox, where he learned about diagnostics and how/why electronics and software fail and how to design systems that can be diagnosed and repaired.

Today the author is working with Parwel, a health services company to provide diabetes education and health coaching to corporations, organizations, families, and individuals.

Email: engineer@deathtodiabetes.com
Phone numbers: 800-813-1927, 800-954-0366, 585-671-0577

Book Cover Design: DeWayne wanted a book title and a cover design that was clear and powerful, but conveyed a positive, uplifting message of hope and sincerity -- while conveying the purpose of his book. First, DeWayne came up with the phrase "death to diabetes" to indicate hope and the end (or death) of this serious disease. Then, he needed a cover design that "connected" with the phrase. DeWayne remembered that he had a dream about graveyards when he was in the hospital, but it didn't make any sense at that time. Although, some people thought that a photograph of a graveyard was "too dark", DeWayne felt that people would "get it" and see the graveyard and the word "Diabetes" on a headstone as a positive, powerful message. Finally, trying to find a book cover designer that "understood" DeWayne's vision was not easy. Fortunately, he found one (Katiuscia Lanza) accidentally when he was looking in the yellow pages for someone that could make him a large sign for an upcoming health fair. Coincidentally, because of the recent loss of her grandfather, Kat understood exactly what DeWayne was looking for and was able to find a local cemetery for the book's unique cover design.

Death to Diabetes

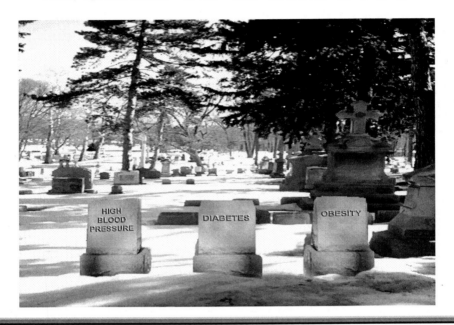

Health & Wellness Services

Contact the wellness center if you need help with your health planning. Services include: personal health coaching (telephone, online, in person), healthy lifestyle risk assessment, customized nutrition programs/meal planning, diabetes education classes/workshops, reviews of medical blood test results, discounts for multiple products/services; certified instruction for healthcare professionals, family wellness planning/coaching; and corporate wellness training.

Contact the author to register for a free telephone seminar or obtain one of his free popular CDs with your next purchase.

Websites: www.DeathToDiabetes.com, www.parwel.com

Email: engineer@deathtodiabetes.com

Phone numbers: 800-813-1927, 800-954-0366, 585-671-0577

376

INDEX

A

B

INDEX

Death to Diabetes

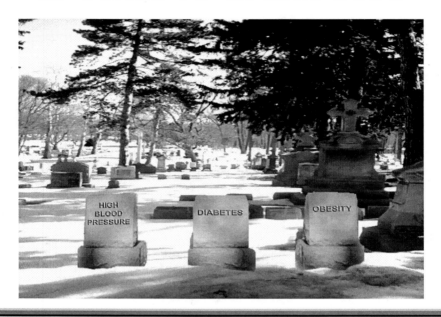

Health & Wellness Services

Contact the wellness center if you need help with your health planning. Services include: personal health coaching (telephone, online, in person), healthy lifestyle risk assessment, customized nutrition programs/meal planning, diabetes education classes/workshops, reviews of medical blood test results, discounts for multiple products/services; certified instruction for healthcare professionals, family wellness planning/coaching; and corporate wellness training.

Contact the author to register for a free telephone seminar or obtain one of his free popular CDs with your next purchase.

Websites: www.DeathToDiabetes.com, www.parwel.com

Email: engineer@deathtodiabetes.com

Phone numbers: 800-813-1927, 800-954-0366, 585-671-0577

Videos: www.YouTube.com

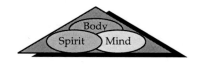

God's Food for Thought

When a car manufacturer makes an automobile, they put it through hundreds of tests. Then, they define a set of maintenance and repair procedures that explain how the car should be serviced and maintained to run at peak performance. These procedures are published in a book called the Automobile Owners Manual. This manual will tell you what oil and gasoline to use, and give you all the information needed to make your car run at peak performance.

God has given us an Owners Manual called the **Bible**. The Bible explains how to keep the body healthy and operating at peak performance. But God's Manual has been neglected, and our hospitals are full. Today we have more disease than ever because we choose to eat man's processed foods and chemicals instead of God's nutrient-rich foods.

First Corinthians 10:31: "Whether therefore ye eat, or drink, or whatsoever ye do, do all to the glory of God." Give glory by eating and drinking right. **First Corinthians 6:19-20** says why: "What? know ye not that your body is the temple of the Holy Ghost which is in you, which ye have of God, and ye are not your own? For ye are bought with a price: therefore glorify God in your body, and in your spirit, which are God's."

God wants to dwell in you, but He cannot dwell in a defiled body – it's not our body, it's God's to use for His glory. God then gets very explicit in this area. **First Corinthians 3:16-17:** "Know ye not that ye are the temple of God, and that the Spirit of God dwelleth in you? If any man defile the temple of God, him shall God destroy; for the temple of God is holy, which temple ye are." God says if we willfully defile the body, He will destroy us!

There are a lot of people today who will not follow God's laws of health, and then when they get sick and diseased, they blame God. A person says, "Oh, why is God allowing me to die of emphysema?" Yet that person smoked cigarettes for 30 years! That's not God's fault. God is reasonable. He says, "If you obey, you will prosper and have no disease."

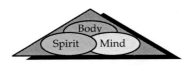

We should desire to honor God by the way we treat our bodies. Why? Because God says that we're that important. And because our health matters to the one who made us and loves us. As a result, we should eat healthy because we're worth it and because we're called to something noble and great! If family or finances is not a strong-enough motivation, then, what God requires should be a strong-enough motivation that should stick with us in the long run.

What you believe is the very foundation of who you are. If you believe that you will be poor because you were born into poverty, then you are – not you will be; you are. We only have today; actually, we only have right now, the very moment we're in. This moment determines the next moment, determines the next moment and so on. What do you believe, right now? If you believe in the ways of the world and live your life according to those conditions, you are a victim. If you believe the Word of God you are His heir, a victor, and have dominion over all the earth. You walk by faith, not by sight. A victor never thinks of defeat, but lives each moment with a Kingdom mentality of faith.

Therefore, become a *victor* of wellness, not a *victim* of disease and drugs.

Bible Quotes about Nutrition

"He causeth the grass to grow for cattle, and herbs for the use of man." Psalms 104:14

"For one believeth he may eat all things, anyone who is weak eateth herbs." Romans 14:2

"And the fruit thereof shall be for meat, and the leaf thereof for medicine." Ezekiel 47:12

"My people perish through lack of knowledge." Hosea 4:6

Contact Information

Contact the wellness center if you need help with your health planning.

Websites: www.DeathToDiabetes.com, www.parwel.com

Email: engineer@deathtodiabetes.com

Phone numbers: 800-813-1927, 800-954-0366, 585-671-0577
